Human Reproduction

Human Reproduction:
Growth and Development

Edited by

Donald R. Coustan, M.D.

Chairman, Department of Obstetrics and Gynecology, Brown University School of Medicine; Obstetrician and Gynecologist-in-Chief, Women and Infants' Hospital of Rhode Island, Providence, Rhode Island

Associate Editors

Ray V. Haning, Jr., M.D.

Associate Professor of Obstetrics and Gynecology, Brown University School of Medicine; Director, Division of Reproductive Endocrinology, Women and Infants' Hospital of Rhode Island, Providence, Rhode Island

Don B. Singer, M.D.

Professor of Pathology, Brown University School of Medicine; Pathologist-in-Chief, Women and Infants' Hospital of Rhode Island and Rhode Island Hospital, Providence, Rhode Island

Little, Brown and Company
Boston   New York   Toronto   London

First Edition

Library of Congress Cataloging-in-Publication Data
Human reproduction : growth and development / edited by Donald R.
    Coustan, associate editors, Ray V. Haning, Jr., Don B. Singer.
        p.   cm.
    Includes bibliographical references and index.
    ISBN 0-316-15827-5
    1. Obstetrics.   I. Coustan, Donald R.
    [DNLM: 1. Fetal Development–physiology.   2. Prenatal Care.
3. Pregnancy Complications.   WQ 210 H918 1994]
RG524.H85   1994
618.2–dc20
DNLM/DLC
for Library of Congress   94-22477
                                                                      CIP

Printed in the United States of America
ICP

Editorial: Nancy E. Chorpenning, Rebecca Marnhout
Production Editor: Cathleen Cote
Copyeditor: Sharon Hogan
Indexer: Barbara Farabaugh
Production Services: Michael Bass & Associates

This book is lovingly dedicated to the memory of Dr. John Evrard, one of the founders of the Brown University School of Medicine course entitled Human Reproduction: Growth and Development. He taught us all a great deal about science, clinical medicine, and human relations. He treated medical students with love and respect, and they adored him.

Contents

Contributing Authors

Cydney I. Afriat, C.N.M., M.S.N., R.D.M.S.
Clinical Teaching Associate, Obstetrics and Gynecology, Brown University School of Medicine; Nurse Midwife, Department of Obstetrics and Gynecology, Women and Infants' Hospital of Rhode Island, Providence, Rhode Island
13. Antepartum Care; 18. Birth

Diane J. Angelini, Ed.D., C.N.M.
Clinical Assistant Professor of Obstetrics and Gynecology, Brown University School of Medicine; Director, Nurse-Midwifery, Department of Obstetrics and Gynecology, Women and Infants' Hospital of Rhode Island, Providence, Rhode Island
20. The Puerperium

William Cashore, M.D.
Professor of Pediatrics, Brown University School of Medicine; Associate Chief, Department of Pediatrics, Women and Infants' Hospital of Rhode Island, Providence, Rhode Island
6. Neonatal Adaptations; 22. Care of the Newborn

Donald R. Coustan, M.D.
Chairman, Department of Obstetrics and Gynecology, Brown University School of Medicine; Obstetrician and Gynecologist-in-Chief, Women and Infants' Hospital of Rhode Island, Providence, Rhode Island
9. Fetal Physiology; 10. Maternal Physiology; 14. Prescribing During Pregnancy; 16. Fetal Assessment; 18. Birth; 19. Obstetric Analgesia and Anesthesia; 20. The Puerperium; 24. Obstetric Complications

Gary Frishman, M.D.
Assistant Professor of Obstetrics and Gynecology, Brown University School of Medicine; Gynecologic Endocrinology Specialist, Division of Reproductive Endocrinology, Women and Infants' Hospital of Rhode Island, Providence, Rhode Island
2. Gametogenesis, Fertilization, and Implantation; 12. Abortions, Miscarriages, and Ectopic Pregnancies

Ray V. Haning, Jr., M.D.
Associate Professor of Obstetrics and Gynecology, Brown University School of Medicine; Director, Division of Reproductive Endocrinology, Women and Infants' Hospital of Rhode Island, Providence, Rhode Island
1. The Menstrual Cycle; 11. Diagnosis of Pregnancy

David L. Meryash, M.D.
Associate Professor of Clinical Pediatrics, Cornell University Medical College, New York; Chief, Division of Child Development and Human Genetics, North Shore University Hospital, Manhasset, New York
7. Genetics

Patricia A. O'Shea, M.D.
Associate Professor of Pathology, Emory University School of Medicine; Pediatric Pathologist, Egleston Children's Hospital at Emory University, Atlanta, Georgia
5. Fetal and Neonatal Pathology; 8. Congenital Defects and Their Causes; 15. The Fetus as Patient: Prenatal Diagnosis and Treatment

Karen Rosene-Montella, M.D.
Assistant Professor of Medicine and of Obstetrics and Gynecology, Brown University School of Medicine; Director, Division of Obstetric and Consultative Medicine, Women and Infants' Hospital of Rhode Island, Providence, Rhode Island
23. Medical Complications of Pregnancy

Don B. Singer, M.D.
Professor of Pathology, Brown University School of Medicine; Pathologist-in-Chief, Women and Infants' Hospital of Rhode Island and Rhode Island Hospital, Providence, Rhode Island
1. The Menstrual Cycle; 3. Human Embryogenesis; 4. The Placenta; 5. Fetal and Neonatal Pathology

Carol A. Wheeler, M.D.
Assistant Professor of Obstetrics and Gynecology, Brown University School of Medicine; Gynecologic Endocrinology Specialist, Division of Reproductive Endocrinology, Women and Infants' Hospital of Rhode Island, Providence, Rhode Island
17. Labor: Normal and Dysfunctional; 21. Family Planning

Preface

The idea for *Human Reproduction: Growth and Development* arose from the faculty of the Brown University School of Medicine, specifically from a course of the same name. This is a section of the year-long Integrated Medical Sciences course for second-year medical students. The course is taught by faculty members from the departments of Obstetrics and Gynecology, Pathology, and Pediatrics. It integrates concepts of pathophysiology, pharmacology, pathology, and clinical medicine. The first half of the book is based on our syllabus for the course, while the second half encompasses material relevant to the core clerkship in obstetrics and gynecology.

There are a number of large, excellent, extensively referenced textbooks of obstetrics currently available. This book is not meant to replace them, and the student is often referred to these more encyclopedic works for further reading. Such textbooks, however, often include a level of detail that may overwhelm students, possibly inhibiting the learning process. This book is intended to provide students with the physiologic, pathologic, and clinical concepts relevant to an understanding of human reproduction. Rather than provide references to back up every statement, we have appended a list of recommended readings at the end of each chapter. Students who would like to learn more about a specific issue, or who need to prepare a report on some aspect of a chapter, are urged to utilize these reading lists.

Two of the faculty members of our course have moved from Brown University. We are grateful to them for taking the time to prepare superb contributions despite the responsibilities of their new positions. Chapters 11 to 22, which are most applicable to the core clerkship, were prepared by faculty members who practice clinical obstetrics, including two nurse midwives who play an important role in teaching medical students and residents in our program.

We would like to express our appreciation to John LaRiviere, who created most of the illustrations in the book, and to the editors at Little, Brown for their patience over the years required for this book to be written.

D.R.C.
R.V.H.
D.B.S.

Human Reproduction

Notice

The indications and dosages of all drugs in this book have been recommended in the medical literature and conform to the practices of the general medical community. The medications described do not necessarily have specific approval by the Food and Drug Administration for use in the diseases and dosages for which they are recommended. The package insert for each drug should be consulted for use and dosage as approved by the FDA. Because standards for usage change, it is advisable to keep abreast of revised recommendations, particularly those concerning new drugs.

The Menstrual Cycle

Don B. Singer and Ray V. Haning, Jr.

The *menstrual cycle* is the biologic phenomenon by which the uterus is prepared each month for receiving and nurturing the conceptus. In all of nature, the relatively large amount of bleeding in the menstrual cycle is unique to primates; other mammals have periods of estrus at irregular intervals throughout the year, sometimes more often and sometimes less often than humans and other primates. In some animals, this cycle is determined by the photoperiod. The related word *menses* (from the Latin *mensis,* or month) suggests the length of the menstrual cycle.

Premenarchal State

In the newborn female, the internal reproductive tract consists of small, slightly coiled fallopian tubes, slender elongated and flattened pink-yellow ovaries, a small uterine fundus, a relatively large cervix, and a minimally rugated vagina. The lining of the uterine cavity is a simple, single layer of cuboidal or minimally elongated endometrial cells. A few glands develop in the stroma below the surface (Fig. 1-1). Glycogen secretion is detectable in fetuses at 8 months' gestation. As the infant grows into childhood, the fundus and body of the uterus remain smaller than the cervix and the endometrium remains simple. As menarche approaches, the uterine fundus and body grow more rapidly than does the cervix and the endometrial tissues become more prominently glandular. These changes are under the influence of estrogen (estradiol-17ß), which is produced by the ovaries. The ovaries, in turn, are stimulated by rhythmically peaking hormones from the pituitary (mainly follicle-stimulating hormone [FSH]) and the

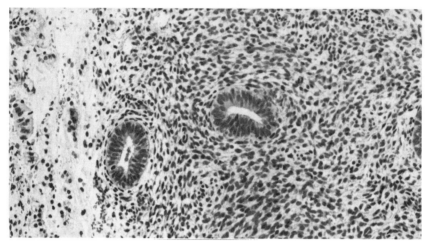

Fig. 1-1. Endometrium from newborn infant. The endometrial glands are small with minimal evidence of proliferative activity. The glands are embedded in a compact, cellular stroma. (Original magnification: x200.)

pituitary is stimulated by hypothalamic hormones. The structures derived from the müllerian ducts (including the oviducts, uterus, endometrium, cervix, and upper third of the vagina) contain estrogen receptors and progesterone receptors.

Menarche

The first menstrual flow is called *menarche* and usually is not associated with ovulation. The anatomic changes that take place in the endometrium are profound as are the ovarian hormonal changes. The ovary, uterus, cervix, and vagina and the secondary sexual structures all begin to manifest maturational changes.

The average age of menarche in the United States is 12.5 years (Table 1-1). This age is younger than in previous times in this country. In other countries where nutrition and socioeconomic factors are not as favorable, menarche occurs in older individuals. Menarche should be distinguished from *puberty*. Puberty implies a broad range of changes, many of which precede menarche by 2 to 3 years and many of which follow menarche by 5 to 8 years. Puberty is due to gradually maturing hormonal secretions.

Although menarche usually begins without ovulation, a pubescent girl can become pregnant without experiencing menarche. Many obstetricians have attended patients whose first ovulation was followed by fertilization. Also, the first menstrual flow is often followed by anovulatory cycles. The fluctuations of estrogen (in the absence of progesterone) may or may not lead to bleeding. Such cycles are irregular both in duration and amount of menstrual flow.

Table 1-1. Menstrual function: national average data

	Average	Range
Age at menarche	12.5 yr	10–16 yr
Duration of menstrual cycle	28 d	22–35 d
Duration of flow	5 d	2–8 d
Amount of flow	40 ml	15–75 ml
Age at menopause	51 y*	42–54 yr

*Median age

The Average Menstrual Cycle

The average length of the menstrual cycle is 28 days, with a range of 22 to 35 days. The *preovulatory phase* of the cycle is more variable than the postovulatory phase. That is, the preovulatory phase can be as short as 7 to 8 days or as long as 21 to 22 days, whereas the postovulatory phase is almost consistently 12 ± 2 days (Fig. 1-2). Cycles in an individual may vary in length from month to month by 2 to 5 days. The duration of menstrual bleeding averages 5 ± 3 days. The amount of blood loss is 15 to 75 ml.

The physiologic and anatomic events of the menstrual cycle are as follows. With increased FSH from the pituitary, the ovarian stroma surrounding the developing ovum proliferates and a follicle with a cavity is formed. The granulosa cells become more prominent and the theca interna also thickens. Estradiol-17ß production is markedly elevated within the follicle. Estrogen is a mitogen for certain müllerian tissues, i.e., it causes proliferation. In the uterus, the endometrial glands and stroma respond to the increased estrogen by undergoing mitotic division and proliferation. The endometrium thickens two- to threefold and the endometrial glands coil and become much more prominent. Mitoses are scattered among the glandular cells and also among the stromal cells. By 10 days the glands are elongated and tortuous. The endometrial cells develop a low columnar appearance. By 12 days, the lining cells are pseudostratified (Fig. 1-3).

Ovulation occurs at midcycle (14–15 days) and marks the end of the preovulatory or proliferative phase. At this time an ovum, with its surrounding supporting granulosa and zona pellucida, has eroded through the surface of the ovary and is expelled into the abdominal cavity close to the fimbriated end of the oviduct. The recruitment of a particular oocyte for ovulation is not well understood but probably begins with a luteinizing hormone (LH) surge during the previous month (see Chap. 2).

The four possible signs of ovulation are midcycle pain, a rise in basal body temperature of 0.5 to 1.5°F, intermenstrual cervical-vaginal bleeding, and cervical-vaginal mucorrhea. In about 20 percent of women, the midmonth event is associated with lower abdominal or pelvic pain *(mittelschmerz)* localized to the side of the ovulating ovary.

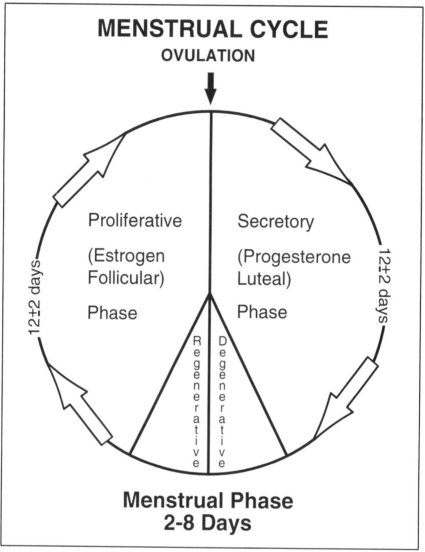

Fig. 1-2. Diagram of the menstrual cycle. The regeneration of endometrium begins about 2 to 4 days after the beginning of menstrual flow and is part of the proliferative phase. This phase is also called the estrogen, or follicular, phase, since the ovarian follicular cells secrete estrogen, a potent mitogen for the endometrium. The proliferative phase is represented here as being equal in duration to the secretory phase. In many women, the proliferative phase may vary considerably in duration, whereas the secretory phase is quite consistent. The secretory phase begins with ovulation. It is also called the progesterone phase or the luteal phase, since the ovarian follicle's cells become larger due to cytoplasmic accumulation of progesterone-rich lipid.

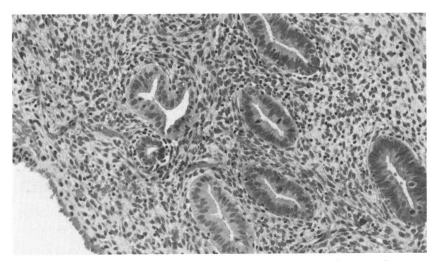

Fig. 1-3. Late proliferative endometrium with numerous mitotic figures and pseudostratification of glandular cells. This is from the twelfth day of the menstrual cycle. (Original magnification: X200.)

Ovulation is a dramatic physiologic event that is preceded by a few days of increasing secretion of LH from the pituitary. The surge of LH causes the granulosa to switch from predominantly estrogen production to a mixed production of estrogen and progesterone. The switch signals the beginning of the *postovulatory* (secretory, luteal, or progesterone) phase of the menstrual cycle (see Fig. 1-2). The granulosa cells accumulate abundant lipid, become golden yellow, and swell up to form the prominent corpus luteum of the ovary.

In response to the addition of progesterone to the hormonal mix, the earliest change in the endometrial glandular cell is the formation of giant mitochondria and a nucleolar channel system. These are visible only by electron microscopy and have no practical application in evaluating the menstrual cycle in clinical situations.

Within a day or two following ovulation, subnuclear, epibasal vacuoles form in an irregular distribution throughout the endometrial glandular tissue. By day 17 to 18, which is postovulatory day 2 to 3, the subnuclear vacuoles are prominent and regular in distribution (Fig. 1-4). This is so reliable a finding that with endometrial biopsy and microscopic examination, it is clinically used as a sure sign that ovulation has occurred.

Over the next 2 or 3 days, the secretory vacuoles, which are loaded with glycogen, fill the apical portion of the cytoplasm in each endometrial glandular cell. By day 20 of the cycle, secretion is quite prominent and it becomes maximal on day 21 (Fig. 1-5). This is the day on which the endometrium is said to be most receptive to the implantation of the conceptus (blastocyst).

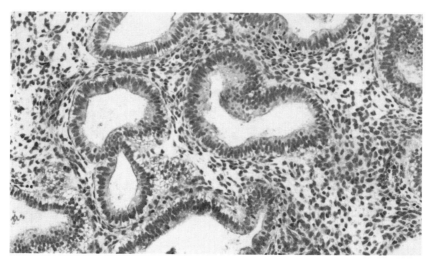

Fig. 1-4. Postovulatory (secretory) phase is heralded by vacuoles forming between the endometrial gland nuclei and the basal portion of the cell. These are secretions induced by progesterone production in the ovarian follicle after the ovum has been expelled. (Original magnification: X200.)

Meanwhile, the stromal cells have changed from spindly shapes to cells with rounded or polygonal cytoplasms and the interstitium becomes more and more edematous. By day 22 to 23 (postovulatory day 7–8), stromal edema is maximal (Fig. 1-6). In fact, edema is such a characteristic feature of day 22 to 23 that many women notice more tightly fitting shoes and rings and they sometimes complain that their contact lenses pop out, presumably due to corneal edema. Atrial natriuretic peptide drops by 40 percent from postmenstrual levels during the luteal or secretory phase of the cycle. This may help account for some of the edema and also compensate for the natriuretic effect of the rising progesterone levels. The glands appear serrated in longitudinal profile by day 24 to 25 (Fig. 1-7). The arteries begin to coil or spiral. The stroma undergoes predecidual change, particularly around the spiral arteries. (In older texts this was called *pseudodecidua* to differentiate it from *decidua,* which is the endometrial stroma of pregnancy.) By day 26 or 27 of the cycle, a few leukocytes invade the stroma and glands. The secretions are expelled from the gland lumens with partial collapse of their walls (Fig. 1-8).

On day 28, breakdown of the stroma and glands is marked and menstrual flow is set to begin. This is the *degenerative phase* that continues during the *menstrual phase.* On day 1 of the cycle, the inflamed, necrotic, bloody, and degenerated superficial endometrium sloughs and is expelled via the vagina. The basal endometrium and portions of the middle spongy layers may remain relatively intact. The superficial layer of the endometrium and fluid blood form the components of the menstrual flow. The flow con-

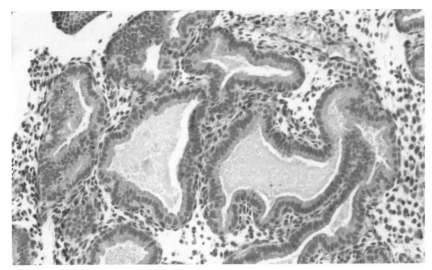

Fig. 1-5. The glandular lumens are filled with glycogen-rich secretions and the stroma is edematous. This stage corresponds to day 21 of the menstrual cycle or the sixth to seventh postovulatory day. (Original magnification: X200.)

sists mostly of liquid and unclottable blood in volumes ranging from 15 to 75 ml. The volume increases with age.

The basis for the inflammation and degenerative changes in days 26 to 28, i.e., the last 2 to 3 days of the cycle, and days 1 to 3, the first 3 days of the next cycle, are a combination of changes in the coiled arteries and cytokines in the endometrium. The coiled vessels generally extend to the middle of the spongy layer of endometrium during the lush secretory phase. Under the influence of interleukin-1, which is produced by macrophages and by stromal cells in the predecidua, increased prostaglandin forms. The prostaglandins induce constriction of the spiral arterioles with resulting ischemia of tissues, probably including ischemia of the vessel walls themselves. The phase of constriction is followed by waves of relaxation with filling of the damaged vessels that causes their walls to give way. Hemorrhage is the result. The blood fails to coagulate because the tissues contain plasminogen activators with fibrinolytic activity.

Gonadotropin-releasing hormone from the hypothalamus stimulates secretion of FSH by the pituitary. The highest values of FSH occur during the midproliferative phase (day 8–10) and correspond to increased estradiol-17ß levels. Estradiol-17ß promotes production of both estrogen and progesterone receptors. Then the pituitary releases large amounts of LH, which causes the ovary to produce progesterone. Progesterone inhibits estrogen receptors in the main target tissue, the endometrium. The sequence leading to menstrual flow begins with decline of LH, involution of the corpus luteum, withdrawal of the ovarian hormones (particularly progesterone), and the increased production of prostaglandins and cytokines in

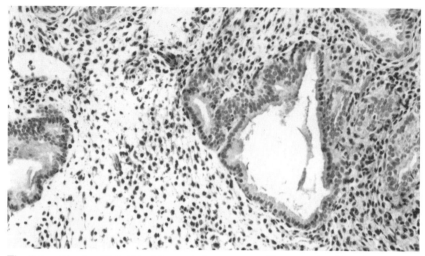

Fig. 1-6. The day 22 to 23 of the cycle is represented by a maximally edematous stroma and dilated glands. The secretions in the lumens of the glands are artifactually missing. (Original magnification: X200.)

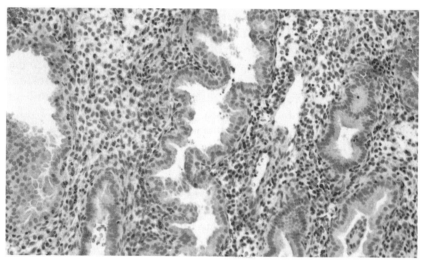

Fig. 1-7. The day 24 to 25 of the menstrual cycle is represented by elongated and serrated glands. The stroma is no longer edematous but cells show early enlargement. (Original magnification: X200.)

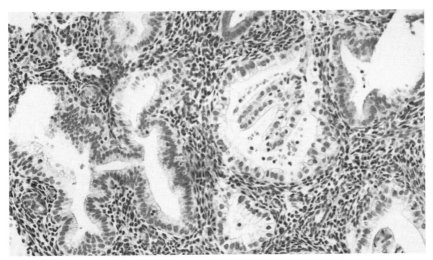

Fig. 1-8. Early menstrual endometrium with collapsed lumens and degenerating cells. Glandular cells are fading away and leukocytes are scattered in the glands and stroma. (Original magnification: ×200.)

the endometrial stroma. The results are degenerative changes in the endometrial glands, stroma, and vessels that progress to necrosis and bleeding.

The regulation of the menstrual cycle can be influenced by environment. College roommates tend to have coordinated cycles after living together for a few months. Perhaps pheromones have a role in such coordination.

Effect of Pregnancy

If the ovarian source of progesterone, the corpus luteum, remains active, for example under the influence of human chorionic gonadotropin (hCG) from the trophoblast of an implanted conceptus, the degenerative changes in the last 2 to 3 days of the cycle do not take place and menstruation does not occur. Therefore, one may infer that menstruation represents failed fertility.

The effect of hCG is profound. The corpus luteum is sustained and, in fact, enlarges so that large amounts of progesterone are produced. The predecidual changes of the stroma thus become accentuated and converted to prominent decidua. Some of the endometrial glands become crowded by the enlarging decidual cells and after a week or two, they become attenuated and compressed. In other endometrial glands the nuclei enlarge and the cytoplasm is ballooned with clear secretions. Such glands are often crowded together in a haphazard pattern and appear quite prominent. These changes have been mistaken for the anaplasia of malignancy but should be recognized as a physiologic change of pregnancy. This alteration of endometrium is called the *Arias-Stella reaction*.

After delivery, postpartum regeneration of endometrium progresses from the residual basal layer in as little as 3 weeks. The first postpartum ovulation occurs after 7 to 8 weeks, providing it is not suppressed by breast-feeding or exogenous hormones.

Effect of Oral Contraceptives

Oral contraceptives are used to suppress ovulation. They usually contain synthetic estrogens and progesterones. In some preparations, both hormones are combined uniformly in each pill; in others, the concentrations of the two hormones are varied to simulate the natural cycle. In any case, the pituitary FSH and LH are suppressed and the ovarian follicle does not develop. The synthetic hormones stimulate the endometrium, which responds much as in the natural cycle. Withdrawal of the pills results in menstruation. The special feature of the combination pill is that cyclic changes in the endometrial glands and stroma are telescoped in time. Thus, at 8 to 9 days, proliferative changes are mingled with early secretory changes. Histologically, glands may show both mitotic (proliferative) activity and glycogen secretions at various positions in the endometrial cells. The stroma may show prominent predecidual change. By day 18 to 21, the stroma often resembles the decidua of pregnancy. In the usual regimen, the hormones are abruptly withdrawn on day 22 and degenerative changes quickly follow, resulting in menstrual flow.

After several cycles, glands tend to remain small with minimal secretions and small volumes of menstrual blood. Adverse effects of contraceptive pills are uncommon. Rarely, suppression of maturation of oocytes results in small ovaries with stromal fibrosis. Another rare complication is irreversible atrophy of the endometrium. The fallopian tubes may become atrophic. The vaginal mucosa can become thinned and somewhat dry with resultant dyspareunia. Prolactin-secreting pituitary microadenomata have been reported in a few women who used contraceptive pills.

The oral abortifacient, mifepristone (RU-486), developed in France, acts by competitively binding to progesterone receptors in the endometrium and stroma. The effect is the same as shutting off progesterone, which is known to cause failure of an established pregnancy in the first few weeks after conception.

Premenstrual Syndrome

Many women have varying degrees of discomfort, anxiety, and pain in the days preceding menstrual flow. Specific symptoms and signs include breast tenderness and swelling, constipation, headache, irritability, and edema. Women with acne note accentuation of the lesions. Most of these symptoms are due to the physiologic effects of progesterone on hormone receptors in the breasts, intestine, brain, kidney, and skin. Just before onset and during menses, elaboration of prostaglandins by the endometrium is responsible for acute onset of headaches, uterine cramps, and diarrhea in some women. There is no evidence of endocrine abnormality in women with unusually pronounced symptoms.

Abnormal Menstrual Cycles

An *anovulatory cycle* is defined as a cycle terminating in a menstrual flow in the absence of ovulation. With menarche, adjustments to the hormonal changes of puberty are still unstable and anovulatory cycles are common. Anovulatory cycles may also be found with pathologic hormonal conditions. Exogenous estrogen and progesterone inhibit ovulation and fluctuations in these hormones may lead to cyclic changes including menstrual blood flow.

Female athletes, especially long-distance runners, often do not ovulate or menstruate. The same is true of those suffering from anorexia and bulimia. The endometrium in these conditions remains thin and unstimulated.

If a cycle is unattended by menstrual flow in a woman with normal or increased amounts of estrogen production, the endometrium continues to proliferate and may become quite bulky. The next episode of estrogen withdrawal then leads to a copious menstruation and a prolonged menstrual phase with bleeding lasting up to 7 to 10 days.

Progesterone production may be decreased, resulting in disordered and generally hyposecretory endometrium. This has been called *luteal phase deficiency* and is considered to be the cause of infertility or spontaneous abortion in some women. The endometrium is more than 3 days retarded in its secretory phase; the histology may be disordered with proliferative and secretory changes side by side. Irregular shedding may result in prolonged menstrual flow.

Menorrhagia is bleeding at menstruation in excess of 80 ml after a normal ovulation. About 10 to 15 percent of women have occasional menorrhagia. The incidence is slightly higher in Asia. Abnormal clotting mechanisms or platelet functions are sometimes involved. Menorrhagia may be associated with leiomyomas (particularly those with a submucosal location), endometrial polyps, or intrauterine contraceptive devices.

Metrorrhagia is uterine bleeding in the middle of a cycle. Lesions such as endometrial or endocervical polyps and submucosal leiomyomas may cause metrorrhagia. Two important causes of abnormal uterine bleeding are pregnancy and malignant tumors of the uterus or cervix.

Dysmenorrhea is discomfort or pain during menstruation. Most cases are probably due to hypercontractility of uterine muscle. Pain is referred to the lower back, legs, pelvis, and lower abdomen. Prostaglandins are the driving force for these contractions and therefore dysmenorrhea may be relieved by inhibitors of prostaglandin production. Another major cause of pain during

during menses is endometriosis. Islands of endometrium form in pelvic and abdominal serosal surfaces. Proposed mechanisms are metaplasia of serosal epithelium or, alternatively, retrograde menstrual flow. These foci respond to cycling hormones and bleed at menstruation, just as does the normal uterine endometrium. Peritoneal serosal hemorrhages, even though small and localized, can result in considerable pain and discomfort.

Vaginal bleeding can occur in newborn girls. Maternal hormones stimulate proliferation of the fetal endometrium. When the baby is born, withdrawal of the placental hormones induces endometrial degeneration and bleeding just as in menses. Vaginal bleeding in older infants and children is most often due to trauma. Tumors such as sarcoma botryoides should be ruled out.

Postmenopausal vaginal bleeding is a cause for thorough workup without delay. Submucosal leiomyomas are uncommon causes of such bleeding since these tumors tend to regress after menopause. More common are other benign conditions such as endometrial or endocervical polyps or trauma to the vagina or cervix. Adenomatous or cystic endometrial hyperplasia results in irregular shedding with associated bleeding. Endometrial carcinomas and sarcomas, tumors of the oviduct, and cervical and vaginal tumors are all to be considered in postmenopausal women with vaginal bleeding.

Sexuality During the Menstrual Cycle
Sexual arousal at specific times during the menstrual cycle is quite variable. In some women, arousal peaks during the proliferative phase, whereas in others, it peaks during the secretory phase. In a minority, arousal is achieved during menstruation. In most studies of these phenomena, psychosocial influences are at work. Arousal during actual menstrual flow may be suppressed by cultural taboos. In most studies, sexual arousal has been shown to peak at ovulation with obvious advantages for procreation.

Menopause
Menopause is the individual's last episode of menstrual bleeding. About half of the female population experiences menopause between 45 and 50 years of age. Approximately 25 percent have menopause before age 45 and about 25 percent have menopause after age 50. Rarely, menopause occurs as late as 56 or 57 years. Just as menarche is a sharply demarcated event in puberty, so menopause is a sharply demarcated event during the *climacteric.*

The climacteric is characterized by unpredictable concentrations of ovarian hormones. The pituitary response remains appropriate to the hormonal status alternating between normal blood levels and elevated blood levels.

The resulting symptoms are most often associated with the *hot flash*, which is characterized by an abrupt sensation of heat in the face, scalp, and neck followed by sweats (including night sweats) and a reduction of the core body temperature of 1.0 to 1.5°F. LH-releasing hormone agonists may produce these symptoms and signs while inhibiting production of estrogen. The climacteric is of variable duration, usually a few years, but may be as abrupt as a few months to as long as 10 to 11 years.

If menopause occurs in women younger than 38 years, it is considered to be premature. A variety of ovarian lesions may be responsible. Hypersecretion of FSH is the hallmark of ovarian failure and is used clinically in its diagnosis.

Changes in the Cervix and Vagina During Menstrual Cycles

During the follicular phase, when estrogen production reaches its peak, cervical glands become tortuous and mucus secretions increase in volume and viscosity. At ovulation and during the luteal phase, these changes in the cervical glands regress. The mucus becomes less viscous. At about 12 to 14 days, the mucus is most susceptible to penetration by sperm. *Spinnbarkeit* refers to the stringy nature of the cervical mucus at this phase of the cycle, which lasts for about 3 days.

Ferning is noted in the cervical mucus from about 7 to 18 days. Ferning is produced by making a smear of cervical mucus on a glass slide and allowing it to dry in air. The microscopic pattern is that of a fern leaf. During the mid- and late-secretory phase, when progesterone predominates, the mucus has a beading pattern when similar preparations are made.

Estrogen causes thickening of the vaginal squamous epithelium. The superficial cells become flattened and their nuclei become pyknotic. A smear of vaginal mucosa on a glass slide will show a large majority of flattened superficial cells (80–90 percent) during the estrogen-rich proliferative phase. During the secretory (luteal, progesterone) phase of the cycle, a fair number of more rounded cells with vesicular nuclei occupy the smear. The proportion of the superficial flattened cells to the rounded parabasal and basal cells has been used in a common cytologic test called the *estrogen index*. It is helpful in cases of abnormal menses or infertility. In fact the Pap smear, widely used to detect cervical cancer, was a spinoff from George Papanicolaou's elegant physiologic-histologic correlative studies on the changes in vaginal epithelium during the menstrual cycle.

During pregnancy, the vaginal epithelium is maintained in a mixed parabasal-superficial cell pattern. The cervix develops a thick tenacious mucus that plugs the external cervical os. The contraceptive pill and pregnancy are equally effective in producing a microglandular hyperplasia in the endocervical epithelium.

Recommended Reading

Arias-Stella, J. Atypical endometrial changes associated with the presence of chorionic tissue. *Arch. Pathol.* 58:112–128, 1954.

Asso, D. *The Real Menstrual Cycle.* Chichester: Wiley, 1983.

Baird, D., and Michie, E. *Mechanism of Menstrual Bleeding.* New York: Raven, 1985.

Bider, D., et al. Endocrinologic basis of hot flashes. *Obstet. Gynecol. Survey.* 44:495–499, 1989.

Chang hai, H., et al. Pharmacokinetic study of orally administered RU 486 in non-pregnant women. *Contraception.* 40:449–460, 1989.

Cunningham, F., MacDonald, P., and Gant, N. *Williams Obstetrics.* Norwalk: Appleton & Lange, 1989.

Cutler, W., and Garcia, C.-R. *The Medical Management of Menopause and Premenopause. Their Endocrinologic Basis.* Philadelphia: Lippincott, 1984.

Fox, H., and Buckley, C. *Pathology for Gynecologists.* Baltimore: University Park Press, 1982.

Gabbe, S. G., Niebyl, J. R., and Simpson, J. L. *Obstetrics: Normal and Problem Pregnancies* (2nd ed.). New York: Churchill-Livingstone, 1991.

Gise, L., Kase, N., and Berkowitz, R. *The Premenstrual Syndromes.* New York: Churchill-Livingstone, 1988.

Golub, S. *Menarche: The Transition from Girl to Woman.* Lexington, MA: Lexington Books, DC Heath, 1983.

Gompel, C., and Silverberg, S. *Pathology in Gynecology and Obstetrics.* Philadelphia: Lippincott, 1985.

Jensen, L., Svanegaard, J., and Husby, H. Atrial natriuretic peptide during menstrual cycle. *Am. J. Ob. Gyn.* 161:951–952, 1989.

McClennan, C., and Rydell, A. Extent of endometrial shedding during normal menstruation. *Obstet. Gynecol.* 26:605–610, 1965.

Naeye, R. L. Disorders of the placenta, fetus, and neonate: Diagnosis and clinical significance. St. Louis: Mosby, 1992. P. 2.

Papanicolaou, G., Traut, H., and Marchetti, A. *The Epithelia of Woman's Reproductive Organs: A Correlative Study of Cyclic Changes.* New York: Commonwealth Fund, 1948.

Sloane, E. Premenstrual Syndrome. In *Biology of Women.* New York: Wiley, 1985.

Ushiroyama, T. Hypergonadotropinemia with estradiol secretion in peri- and postmenopausal period. *Acta. Obstet. Gynecol. Scand.* 68:139–143, 1989.

van Eijkeren, et al. Menorrhagia: A review. *Obstet. Gynecol. Survey.* 44:421–429, 1989.

Velasco, E. Gonadotrophins and prolactin serum levels during the perimenopausal period: Correlation with diverse factors. *Fertil. Steril.* 53:56–60, 1990.

Vollman, R. *The Menstrual Cycle.* Philadelphia: Saunders, 1977.

2

Gametogenesis, Fertilization, and Implantation

Gary Frishman

Gametogenesis, the formation of germ cells, along with their subsequent combination and integration via fertilization, are integral to the existence and survival of the human race. In these processes, the genetic material of each individual is duplicated and packaged for storage and transport, which may take place anywhere from months to decades later. The sperm and egg must journey to the fallopian tube where they meet and fertilization occurs. After fusion of the parents' respective DNA, the early embryo, smaller than a pinhead, must journey to the mother's uterus and successfully implant there. This chapter will follow this amazing journey and describe the events that culminate in the propagation of our species.

Gametogenesis

Although the development of reproductive potential is classically associated with puberty, the process of gametogenesis is initiated much earlier. Primitive germ cells *(gametes)* are detectable in the male and female embryo as early as the end of the third week of development. The production of gametes serves to first replicate and then reduce the normal genetic complement. Although the gametes start out with 46 chromosomes (diploid), they ultimately have only 23 (haploid). Of these 23 chromosomes, 22 are autosomes and one is a sex chromosome (either X or Y).

Mitosis and Meiosis

Mitosis and meiosis are the two processes that are integral to gametogenesis and all reproduction. *Mitosis* produces identical (duplicate) chromosomal components of the parent's DNA. *Meiosis*, on the other hand, produces haploid daughter cells with random combinations of chromosomes. The process of meiosis allows for an exchange of genes and ensures a random recombination of genetic material.

There are striking differences between men and women in gametogenesis that are reflected in the processes of mitosis and meiosis. In spermatogenesis, the mitotic divisions of male gametes occur throughout the male's reproductive life. This process contrasts with the mitotic divisions in the production of female gametes (oogenesis), which peak during fetal life and cease by birth.

The first meiotic division transforms primary gametes to secondary gametes and yields spermatocytes in the male (Fig. 2-1A) and oocytes in the female (Fig. 2-1B). This event in the female occurs only during ovulatory menstrual cycles. It is initiated by the midcycle LH surge, and results in the extrusion of the first polar body. Polar bodies are nonfunctional gametes that result from divisions of the oocyte. As such, although each primary spermatocyte yields four viable sperm, each primary oocyte results in only one viable ovum.

The second meiotic division signals the end of a cycle of meiosis and in females occurs only after extrusion of the second polar body (coinciding with penetration of the sperm). In the male, the second meiotic division transforms secondary spermatocytes to spermatids and is an ongoing event that takes place as long as spermatogenesis is occurring.

The specific order of and the gender-related differences in the steps involved in gametogenesis can have major implications. For example, an error in meiosis I division in the male will ultimately yield four abnormal spermatids, whereas an error in the meiosis II division will result in only two abnormal gametes, with the other two spermatids being completely normal. This difference is of significant consequences for reproductive prognosis and genetic counselling since an error in meiosis I will result in a chromosomally abnormal conceptus 100 percent of the time, whereas a couple with an error in meiosis II have a 50 percent chance of normal chromosomes. The study and analysis of these and other chromosomal aberrations have evolved from the primitive cytogenetic applications used in the 1950s, to extremely sophisticated techniques including high-resolution banding chromosomal analysis and molecular biology. These processes have enabled the exact pinpointing of the locations of many chromosomal-based disorders and have paved the way for the next stages of research. These areas potentially include genetic testing of the embryo prior to implantation with eventual targeted treatment to correct or replace any chromosomal defects.

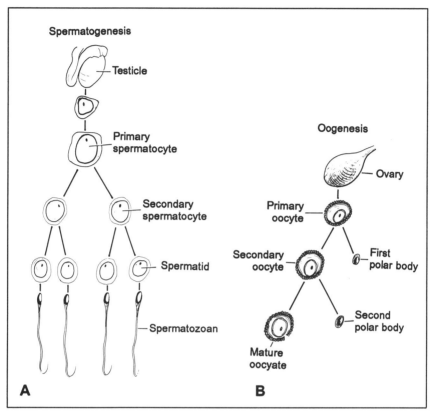

Fig. 2-1. Gametogenesis: (A) spermatogenesis and (B) oogenesis.

Amount and Timing of Gamete Production

Another conspicuous distinction between the sexes is illustrated in the number and timing of gametes produced. In adult males, the normal semen specimen contains between 20 and 200 million sperm per milliliter of seminal fluid. Given a volume of 2 to 6 ml, up to 1 billion sperm are contained in one normal ejaculate. This number is remarkably large given the fact that the only goal of this vast quantity of sperm is to fertilize a single egg.

In the female, peak oogenesis occurs when a female fetus has reached the gestational age of 20 weeks after the last menstrual period and is still in her mother's uterus. Approximately 7 million primary oocytes are present at that time. This number rapidly declines via atresia (degeneration) so that at birth there are 2 million and at puberty there are 400,000 primary oocytes. Despite this relatively large pool of remaining follicles, less than 500 oocytes actually ovulate. The rest are either never recruited or lost through atresia.

In addition to the diminishing total complement of primary oocytes, post-natal aging of these primary oocytes also occurs. In association with this phenomenon, the risk of having an abnormal genetic transmission dramatically increases with age, especially the trisomies 13, 18, and 21, 47 XXX, and 47 XXY. Because of this elevated risk, pregnant women are usually offered genetic testing, such as an amniocentesis, on reaching age 35.

In contrast to the initially finite and subsequently diminishing number of eggs in females, males continue to produce sperm and remain potentially fertile throughout their life. However, there is a 30 percent decrease in sperm production between the ages of 50 and 80 years. Other factors, such as illness or medication, may also affect fertility adversely.

It takes approximately 70 days for an undifferentiated *spermatogonium* (primitive sperm cell) to make the transition to a motile sperm. Of this time, 50 days are spent in the seminiferous tubules with transport through the epididymis to the ejaculatory duct requiring up to an additional 21 days.

The amount of time required for gamete maturation in the male is clearly defined; however, the amount of time required for gamete maturation in the female is not as well understood. Although it has been classically taught that oocyte maturation requires only 2 weeks (occurring during the follicular phase of the menstrual cycle), research suggests that the initial stages of recruitment may begin well before this. In these investigations, ovaries that were surgically removed from women at different stages of their menstrual cycle were meticulously examined. These ovaries contained primary oocytes in the early stages of development that were believed to be recruited during the luteal phase of the preceding menstrual cycle. This activation of the next cycle's follicle may be precipitated by the same luteinizing hormone (LH) surge that initiates ovulation.

Reproductive Tract Anatomy and Function

The Male Reproductive Tract

In males, as in females, the production of gametes is gonadotropin-dependent. In the testis, the Leydig cells (Fig. 2-2) produce testosterone in response to the positive stimulation of LH, via a cyclic adenosine monophosphate (cAMP)–dependent process. Testosterone and follicle-stimulating hormone (FSH), in turn, are the principal regulators of the seminiferous tubules. FSH also binds to the Leydig cells, where it increases the number of LH receptors.

The seminiferous tubules (Fig. 2-3), which make up approximately 75 percent of the testis' volume, are ducts where sperm are developed. These tubules are lined by spermatogonia, which become primary spermatocytes via a mitotic division and subsequently produce secondary spermatocytes via a meiotic division. These haploid cells then mature into spermatids and eventually sperm.

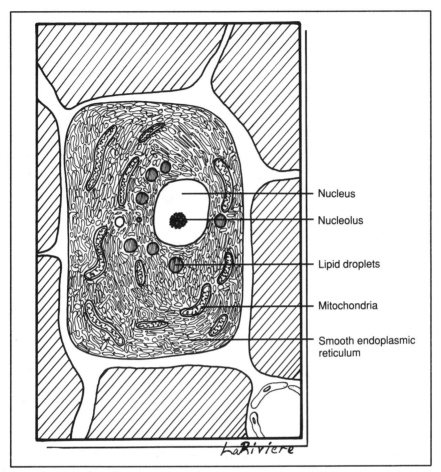

Fig. 2-2. Leydig cell.

Sertoli's cells, like the Leydig cells, are specialized cells that exist only in the male reproductive tract. They rest on the basal lamina of the seminiferous tubules, sealing the tubules and maintaining the testicular equivalent of the blood-brain barrier that is present in the CNS. Under the direction of FSH, Sertoli's cells secrete androgen-binding proteins (ABP) into the tubule lumen. By binding testosterone and dihydrotestosterone, ABP increases the local androgen concentration in the seminiferous epithelium and epididymis (a key reservoir for the sperm); this is a critical step for spermatogenesis and sperm maturation.

In the epididymis, through mechanisms that are not well understood, the sperm undergo significant functional alterations in their proteins along with changes in cAMP and other energy metabolisms. During their passage

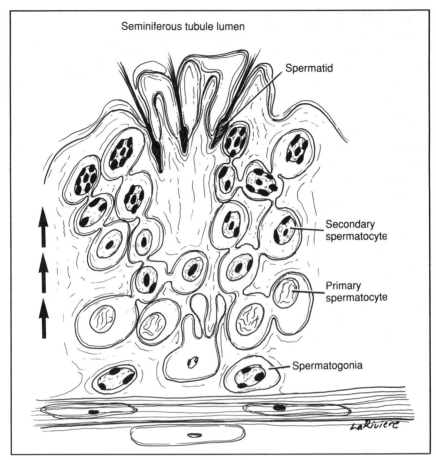

Fig. 2-3. Seminiferous tubule.

through the epididymis, the sperm acquire their motility; this is most likely related to exposure to the fluid of the epididymal lumen. This fluid changes throughout its path in electrolyte content, protein composition, and osmolarity. Proteins within the epididymal fluid include forward motility protein, sperm survival factor, and progressive motility sustaining factor. Sperm motility may be mediated via a cAMP-dependent action of the mitochondria in the midpiece of the sperm (Fig. 2-4) on the microtubules in the tail of the sperm.

The male's ejaculate is comprised not only of sperm provided by the testes and epididymis, but also of other constituents. The seminal vesicles and prostate provide many components including prostaglandins, ascorbic acid, fructose, amino acids, and alkaline and acid phosphatases. These components buffer the acid pH of the vagina, help stimulate uterine contractions to propel the sperm to the fallopian tubes, nourish the sperm, and provide a host of other functions.

Critical to the sperm's ability to fertilize an egg is the process of capacitation. This is a reversible calcium-dependent process that initiates a decrease in the stability of the plasma and outer acrosomal membranes. These membranes eventually break down, releasing enzymes that are essential for sperm penetration and the increased flagellar activity (hypermotility) associated with capacitation. Although capacitation normally occurs in the female reproductive tract, it can be elicited in the laboratory after incubation in media and is dependent on neither contact with an oocyte nor exposure to the female reproductive tract.

The Female Reproductive Tract

There are many apparent barriers to sperm viability and oocyte fertilization that must be overcome. The vagina normally maintains an acid environment that is hostile to sperm but serves as a barrier to foreign bacteria. The alkaline pH of the seminal fluid acts to buffer this acidity and foster the sperm's ability to survive. The expulsion of semen from the vagina that might occur following withdrawal of the penis is partially prevented by vaginal rugae (folds), which prolong the contact of sperm with the cervix and increase the chance of sperm entry.

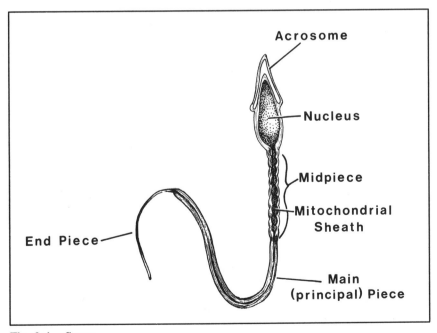

Fig. 2-4. Sperm.

After ejaculation, the seminal plasma is left behind in the vagina with only sperm making their way into the cervix. Sperm can enter the cervical mucus within 90 seconds. Having made their way into the cervix, sperm are nourished by vital endocervical glands (Fig. 2-5), prolonging their viability for up to 72 hours. Although sperm have been present for longer than this time period, their ability to fertilize an occyte may be diminished.

Sperm may be found in the fallopian tube within 5 minutes of deposition in the vagina. The known inability of sperm to traverse this distance unassisted in such a short time span led to a search for other factors. Intrauterine sperm transport is facilitated by uterine contractions, which may be stimulated by female orgasm, oxytocin release, and seminal prostaglandins. In the fallopian tube, peristaltic movements of the oviduct propel the sperm from the uterus to the ampullary portion of the tube, where fertilization takes place. Despite the hundreds of millions of sperm deposited

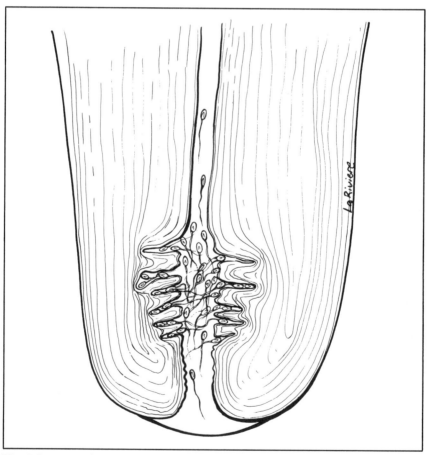

Fig. 2-5. Sperm in the endocervical glands.

in the vagina, only several hundred achieve close proximity to the oocyte in the fallopian tube.

Ovulation and Fertilization

Ovulation

In contrast to what was previously thought, the egress of the oocyte from the follicular cyst is not an explosive phenomenon. However, there are smooth muscle fibers that are present in the ovary, which along with prostaglandins may contribute to ovum release. On release, the normal egg is surrounded by a gelatinous mass of cumulus cells that are critical for ovum retrieval and handling by the fallopian tube. Clinical investigations have demonstrated the presence of mucus strands, around the time of ovulation, that link the ovary to the fimbria. These connecting bridges may play a part in ovum pick-up, and may enhance the function of the fimbria's cilia by guiding the oocyte to the fallopian tube and enabling the fimbria to capture it.

After ovulation, the oocyte takes approximately 30 hours to reach the isthmic-ampullary junction, where it remains for another 30 hours. Transport through the isthmic portion of the fallopian tube to the uterus is then relatively rapid by comparison. In contrast to the life span of a sperm, the viability of the egg is probably at most 24 hours.

Penetration of the Cumulus Mass and Egg

To penetrate the egg, sperm must pass between the granulosa cells of the cumulus mass (Fig. 2-6). These granulosa cells substantially increase the mass of the oocyte and are integral for pick-up and transport of the oocyte by the fallopian tube. In penetrating the granulosa cell mass, the sperm are aided by the key acrosomal enzyme, hyaluronidase. Hyaluronidase, along with the other proteases released from the acrosome, assist the sperm most likely by weakening the matrix that binds the granulosa cells. This weakening, combined with the sperm hypermotility that is associated with capacitation, enables a sperm to reach the egg itself. The sperm, aided by the enzyme acrosin, then digest a pathway through the ovum's zona pellucida.

Events Within the Egg Following Sperm Penetration

The cortical reaction is the critical response of the oocyte that prevents more than one sperm from penetrating it (polyspermy). This process, involving exocytosis of cortical granules into the perivitelline space, is propagated circumferentially from the point of sperm entry through the zona pellucida and is completed within minutes. These granules are not seen on the oocyte until the time of ovulation. After the cortical reaction is

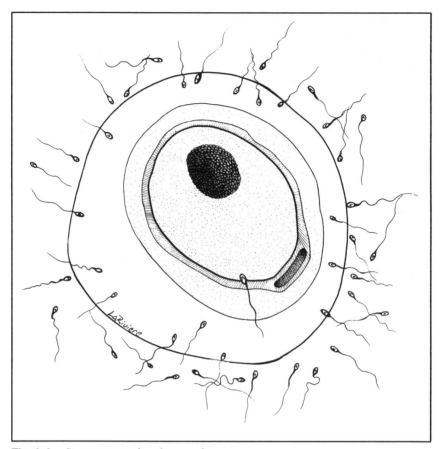

Fig. 2-6. Sperm penetrating the cumulus mass.

completed, acrosomal enzymes are unable to digest a path through the reacted zone.

Once the sperm has entered the perivitelline space, gamete membrane fusion occurs. During this process, the sperm nucleus swells and its membrane breaks down with the unravelling, or decondensation, of the sperm's genetic material. The tail, mitochondria, and all components other than the genetic material of the sperm are absorbed by the ovum with only the sperm's DNA being preserved. Mitochondrial DNA is provided exclusively by the oocyte while the sperm essentially functions as a vehicle to deliver the nuclear genetic material contained within it.

Completion of meiosis in the oocyte then occurs with expulsion of the second polar body. This polar body can be differentiated from the first because of an absence of any cortical granules. Two pronuclei form, one from the nuclear material of each gamete, and contain the DNA of the sperm or the ovum. The male pronucleus is formed near the site of penetration. With normal fertilization, one male and one female pronucleus are produced. These pronuclei are formed simultaneously and usually come together soon thereafter. If more than one sperm penetrates the oocyte, abnormal fertilization occurs and more than two pronuclei are present.

Syngamy is the conjugation of gametes in fertilization. This association of maternal and paternal chromosomes marks the completion of fertilization and the development of the new genome. The resulting zygote soon thereafter undergoes its first cleavage and continues its migration towards the uterus.

Ovum Transport and Implantation

The cilia of the fallopian tube beat towards the uterus and, along with muscular contractions, help transport the egg. The fertilized egg divides and becomes multicellular (Fig. 2-7). It reaches the uterus approximately 4 to 5 days after ovulation, and implantation occurs on approximately the sixth postovulatory day (Fig. 2-8). Implantation is dependent on a suitable

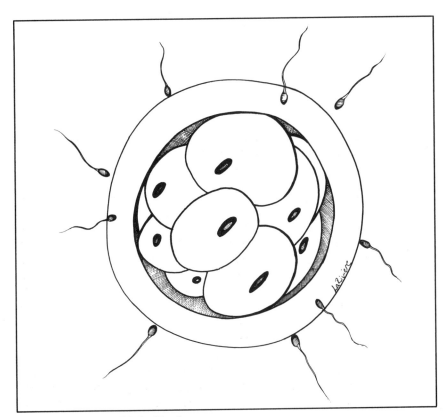

Fig. 2-7. Multicellular fertilized egg.

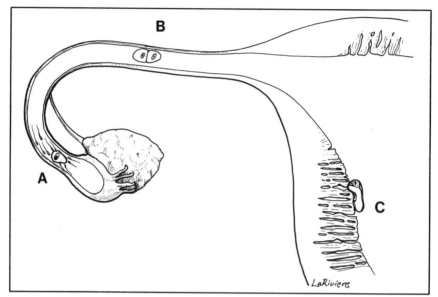

Fig. 2-8. Oocyte migration. (A) Oocyte immediately following ovulation, after tubal pick-up prior to fertilization. (B) Fertilized oocyte being transported to uterus. (C) Embryo undergoing implantation into secretory endometrium of uterus.

endometrial lining that reflects an adequate local estrogen-progesterone ratio. The key hormone progesterone is produced principally from the corpus luteum, which evolves from the follicular cyst. A deficiency in the production of progesterone from the corpus luteum (luteal phase defect) may precipitate a failure in implantation, resulting in a miscarriage. Secretions originating in the endometrial glands are also critical for embryo nourishment and survival.

When these numerous events involved in the production, reduction, packaging, combination, transport, and implantation of genetic material occur successfully, the first steps are taken toward the birth of a unique newborn infant.

Recommended Reading

Speroff, L., Glass, R. H., and Kase, N. G.: *Clinical Gynecologic Endocrinology and Infertility* (5th ed.). Baltimore: Williams & Wilkins, 1994. Pp. 93–102, 231–250, and 873–876.

Wilson, J. D., and Foster, D. W. (eds.). *Williams Textbook of Endocrinology* (8th ed.). Philadelphia: Saunders, 1992. Pp. 809–811, 866–867.

3

Human Embryogenesis

Don B. Singer

The embryonic period begins with fertilization of the ovum by the sperm. In natural human conception, fertilization occurs in the oviduct within 1 to 2 days after ovulation or about 2 weeks following the start of the last menstrual period (LMP). In the embryologic literature the day of fertilization is the starting point for developmental age, whereas in the obstetric literature, the first day of the LMP is the starting point of the "gestational age." Thus embryonic developmental age is always 2 weeks shorter than obstetric gestational age.

The conventional duration of embryogenesis is 8 completed weeks or 56 days. This is 10 weeks or 70 completed days dating from the start of the LMP. On day 57 (day 71 after the start of the LMP), the conceptus becomes a fetus. Biologic variation plays a role in this process. That is to say, some individual embryos may be either accelerated or retarded in development at the end of 56 days. In addition, certain developmental processes normally continue well beyond 56 days in forms similar to those of embryogenesis. For example, nephrons continue to form through 35 to 36 weeks following conception, nerves continue to myelinate for the first 2 years of life, and alveoli in the lung continue to form through 8 years.

The diagnosis of pregnancy is established biochemically by measuring human chorionic gonadotropin (hCG) in the mother's serum or her urine. This substance is the product of the trophoblast that forms from the embryo as it implants in the endometrium. To date, no test can be used to diagnose conception before the event of implantation (4–7 days after fertilization) although the preimplantation embryo synthesizes unique hormones. Sufficient quantities of hCG (20–50 mIU) are produced to be measured by sensitive techniques by about the seventh day of development or

21 days after the start of the LMP. This is 1 week *before* the next expected episode of menstrual bleeding.

Embryogenesis for humans is described in 23 developmental milestones, or stages. Streeter referred to these as "horizons" in his classic comparative studies of embryos from mammals, birds, and reptiles. Working with human embryos, O'Rahilly established the current term "stages." The descriptions that follow are mainly of external features. Embryogenesis of internal organ systems is concurrent with external features but is not detailed in this chapter.

Week 1 (Stages 1–4)

Fertilization and formation of the unicellular *zygote* constitute stage 1 (Fig. 3-1). The contact with and penetration of the ovum *(female gamete)* by the sperm *(male gamete)* takes place in the middle of the oviduct or in its ampulla. Each of the two gametes has a haploid complement of chromosomes. As stage 1 progresses, the nuclear chromosomal elements fuse and the resulting zygote possesses 46 chromosomes. This process takes about 24 hours. Forty-four of the chromosomes are autosomes: 22 from the father and 22 from the mother. Two are sex chromosomes, one each from the father and mother. The ovum's (mother's) sex chromosome is always an X, whereas the sperm's (father's) sex chromosome by random selection of a particular haploid sperm may be an X from an X-bearing sperm or a Y from a Y-bearing sperm. The sex of the zygote is determined at the moment of conception.

Stage 2 begins with a series of cell divisions. The first division into two cells takes about 24 hours. Subsequent divisions take progressively less time. By about 72 to 80 hours after conception, a ball of 12 to 16 cells has formed and is called a *morula* (mulberry) because of the knobby appearance of its surface. By this time the conceptus has reached the uterine cavity. With each cell division the total mass remains relatively constant; that is, a single cell in each succeeding generation is about one-half the size of its parent cell. The fate of a given cell is not exactly determined. The progeny may become skin cells or brain cells. This depends on a precursor cell's location and the fate of its neighboring cells. Some cells will migrate, others remain stationary. Some cells live to proliferate and differentiate while other cells die.

Stage 3 begins with fluid-filled spaces that develop between cells in the morula. These cavities coalesce into one large space while the conceptus becomes a *blastocyst*. At about 96 to 120 hours after conception, the blastocyst plants itself in the endometrium. This is stage 4. This stage occurs about 18 to 20 days after the LMP when the secretory endometrium is beginning to be most receptive to implantation and to nurturing the conceptus.

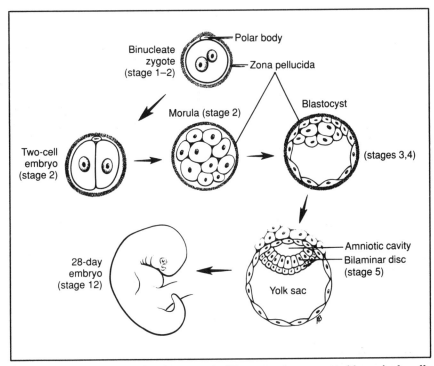

Fig. 3-1. Stages 1 to 12 of embryogenesis. The zygote is represented by a single cell (stage 1) that has already divided its nucleus into two. A single polar body is shown at the edge of the cell. The cytoplasm then divides and two distinct cells are formed. (Note that the two-cell embryo is still surrounded by a zona pellucida that becomes thinner in subsequent stages and finally disappears during the latter part of the first week.) Stage 2 is the multicellular morula. Although there are upwards of 12 to 16 cells, the total mass of the embryo is not much larger than the one-cell zygote or the two-cell embryo. The morula begins to hollow its center to form a small cystic cavity. Stage 3 is the blastocyst. As the zona pellucida disappears, the blastocyst implants in the endometrium (stage 4). The next figure is the bilaminar embryo with the smaller amniotic cavity partially lined by epiblast, or ectoderm, and the larger yolk sac lined by hypoblast, or endoderm. An outer layer of cells represents cytotrophoblast and a mound of cells at the top of the figure represents the syncytiotrophoblast (stage 5). The embryo shown is in stage 12 at about 28 days of development.

Week 2 (Stage 5)

The outer cells forming the shell of the blastocyst form the layer called *trophoblast.* The trophoblast then develops a second layer and the two are named *cytotrophoblast* and *syncytial trophoblast* (Fig. 3-2). Cells intermediate between these two layers have invasive properties and generally do not form a layer but appear as individual cells migrating through the endometrium. These cells are called *intermediate trophoblast.* The inner cell

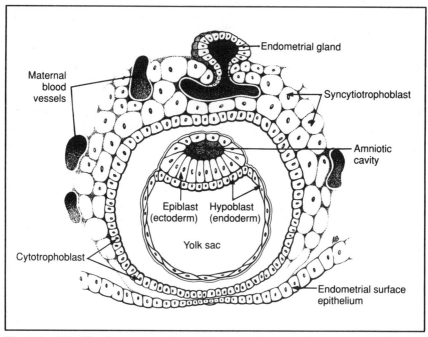

Fig. 3-2. The bilaminar embryo (stage 5) is shown implanted in the endometrium. (Modified from Kalousek, D. K., and Neave, C. Pathology of Abortion, the Embryo and the Previable Fetus. In J. S. Wigglesworth and D. B. Singer [eds.], *Textbook of Fetal and Perinatal Pathology.* Boston: Blackwell, 1991.)

mass of the blastocyst becomes organized into a two-layered disc, the *bilaminar embryonic disc* (stage 5). The disc separates the cavity of the blastocyst into two cavities: the smaller amniotic sac and the larger yolk sac. The layer of cells in the bilaminar disc forming the floor of the amniotic sac is the *epiblast,* or *ectoderm.* The layer forming the floor of the yolk sac is the *hypoblast,* or *endoderm.* Thus, since there are two layers of trophoblast, two sacs, and two layers in the embryonic disc, Crowley has suggested that the second week of development is the "period of twos."

Week 3 (Stages 6–9)

The *primitive streak,* an important and pivotal structure in the embryo, develops during the third week (stage 6) (Fig. 3-3). It forms from a linear condensation of proliferating ectodermal cells at the caudal end of the disc, and expands in all directions by proliferation of cells between the endoderm and ectoderm to form the *mesoderm. Gastrulation* is the term applied to the process by which the three germ layers become fully developed. This process coincides with folding of the embryonic tissues to form a tube within a tube.

While polarity is said to exist in the fertilized ovum, *laterality* of the embryo (and caudal and cephalad ends) is most obvious after formation of the primitive streak. At the cephalad end of the streak, the *primitive knot,* another proliferation of cells, becomes attached to the endoderm and is the precursor of the notochord. Just cephalad to the primitive knot, the ectoderm and the endoderm fuse to form the buccopharyngeal membrane, while at the caudal end of the primitive streak, the comparable fusion of ectoderm and endoderm forms the cloacal membrane (stage 7).

Meanwhile, the ectodermal cells close to the notochord proliferate to form the *neural plate,* which very soon has a longitudinal depression, the *neural groove.* As this deepens, the lateral edges of the neural plate proliferate to form folds that eventually fuse dorsally (stage 8). This fusion begins in a region destined to become the neck and progresses cranially and caudally during the fourth week of development, creating the *neural tube.* This gives rise to the central nervous system and the whole process is called *neurulation* (Fig. 3-4).

At the same time, the paraxial mesoderm becomes segmented into somites from which bones, cartilage, ligaments, and skeletal muscles form.

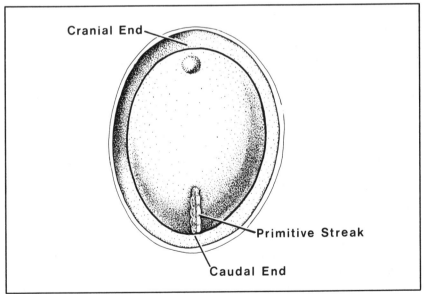

Fig. 3-3.   The slightly elongated disc-shaped embryo of the third week is viewed from the dorsal aspect. The primitive streak is represented by a proliferation of condensed ectodermal cells. The embryo's caudal end, cranial end, and right and left sides are now clearly defined (stage 6).

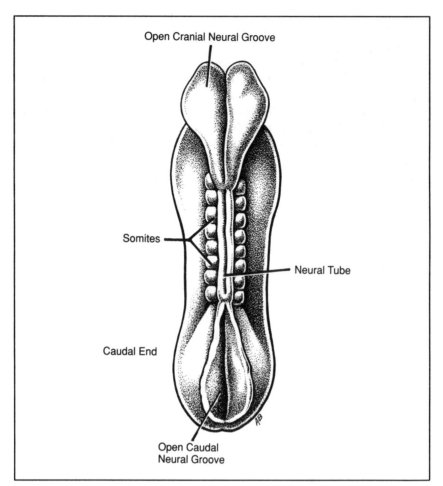

Fig. 3-4. The embryo of stages 9 to 10. The actual length of such an embryo is 2 to 3 mm. (Modified from Kalousek, D. K., and Neave, C. Pathology of Abortion, the Embryo and the Previable Fetus. In J. S. Wigglesworth and D. B. Singer [eds.], *Textbook of Fetal and Perinatal Pathology.* Boston: Blackwell, 1991.)

Mesoderm lateral to the somites gives rise to the urogenital system and the lateral-most mesoderm forms the cardiovascular system, the pericardial, pleural, and peritoneal cavities (stage 9).

In the placenta, chorionic villi develop from the trophoblast cords. The villi become vascularized and cytotrophoblast forms a sac. The whole structure is the chorionic vesicle.

Thus, the third week of development has been called the "period of threes" perhaps because the three germ layers are well developed (i.e., gastrulation); and neurulation and the formation of a chorionic sac are important events.

Weeks 4–5 (Stages 10–15)

At the beginning of the fourth week, at 22 to 24 days, the embryo measures 2 to 3 mm, and has a rostral opening of the neural tube (stage 10) (see Fig. 3-4). The rostral and caudal ends begin to curl, producing a "C"-shaped embryo (stage 11). The ventral cardiac bulge becomes visible, followed by the upper limb buds and the otic pits. The short body stalk connects the lower ventral aspect of the embryo to the placenta (stage 12) (see Fig. 3-1). The body stalk by this time contains the umbilical vein and two umbilical arteries. At about 30 days, the embryo measures 5 to 6 mm (about the diameter of an English pea or a pencil's eraser).

Rapid head growth characterizes the next few days. The lower limb buds appear and four branchial arches are visible on the ventral aspect of the rostral end (stage 13).

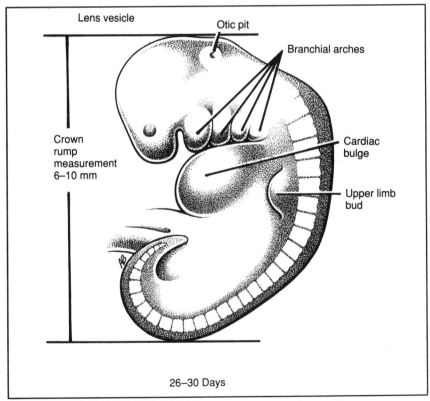

Fig. 3-5. The embryo of the fourth week. It measures 6 to 10 mm from crown to rump (stage 13). (Modified from Kalousek, D. K., and Neave, C. Pathology of Abortion, the Embryo and the Previable Fetus. In J. S. Wigglesworth and D. B. Singer [eds.], *Textbook of Fetal and Perinatal Pathology.* Boston: Blackwell, 1991.)

The limb buds elongate and the lens vesicle appears next (stage 14) (Fig. 3-5). Nasal pits and further development of the distal ends of the limb buds mark stage 15 (Fig. 3-6).

Weeks 6–8 (Stages 16–23)

At about 36 to 38 days, the embryo measures 10 to 15 mm. Retinal pigment becomes visible (stage 16) followed by visible finger rays (stage 17). Later in the sixth week, the upper lip forms and the eyes move toward the anterior aspect of the face. Elbows and toe rays become visible at about 42 to 44 days (stage 18) (Fig. 3-7). The rapidly growing intestine protrudes into the umbilical cord during the seventh week. At the beginning of the eighth week, the fingers are visible but still fused; by the end of the week

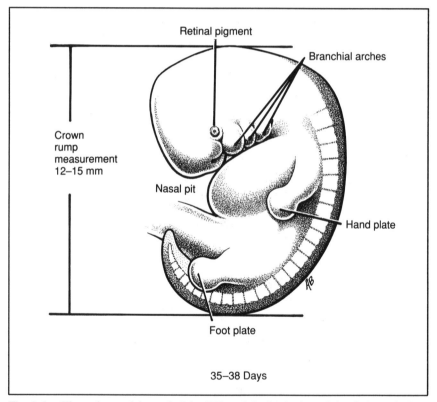

Fig. 3-6. The embryo of the end of the fifth and the beginning of the sixth week. It measures 12 to 15 mm from crown to rump. Retinal pigment and finger rays mark this stage (stage 15–16). (Modified from Kalousek, D. K., and Neave, C. Pathology of Abortion, the Embryo and the Previable Fetus. In J. S. Wigglesworth and D. B. Singer [eds.], *Textbook of Fetal and Perinatal Pathology.* Boston: Blackwell, 1991.)

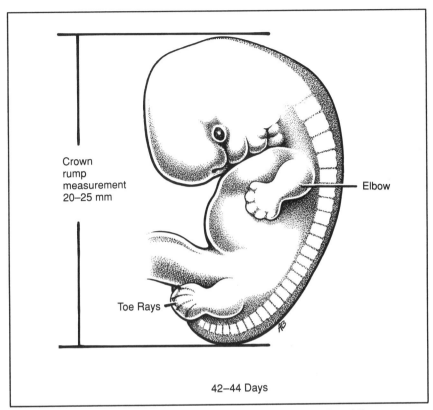

Crown
rump
measurement
20–25 mm

Elbow

Toe Rays

42–44 Days

Fig. 3-7. The embryo of 42 to 44 days (stage 18) with well-developed finger rays and toe rays beginning to form. The elbow is now visible. (Modified from Kalousek, D. K., and Neave, C. Pathology of Abortion, the Embryo and the Previable Fetus. In J. S. Wigglesworth and D. B. Singer [eds.], Textbook of Fetal and Perinatal Pathology. Boston: Blackwell, 1991.)

(55–56 days) they become separated. The embryo has grown to about 30 mm (Fig. 3-8). This marks the end of the embryonic period. Most of the organs are formed although elements of embryonic tissue will persist well into the fetal period, most prominently in the nephrogenic zone of the kidney and the germinal matrix of the brain.

Abnormal Embryos

The great embryologist and morphologist, Frank Mall, observed early in the 20th century that embryonic abnormalities were far more frequent than were congenital anomalies in fetuses or neonates at term gestation. Specific anomalies are not readily detected in early embryos but generally

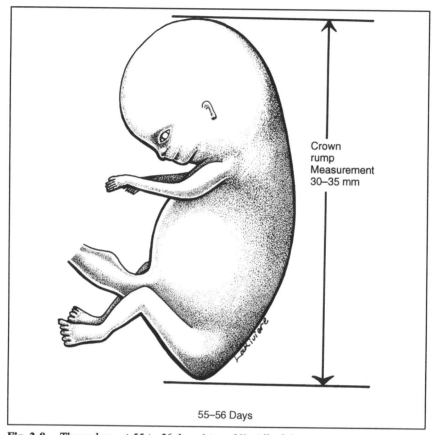

Crown
rump
Measurement
30–35 mm

55–56 Days

Fig. 3-8. The embryo at 55 to 56 days (stage 23). All of the organs are present. Macroscopic form and position are as they will be throughout most of fetal life. (Modified from Kalousek, D. K., and Neave, C. Pathology of Abortion, the Embryo and the Previable Fetus. In J. S. Wigglesworth and D. B. Singer [eds.], *Textbook of Fetal and Perinatal Pathology.* Boston: Blackwell, 1991.)

disorganized growth is recognized. The vast majority (about 85%) of conceptuses spontaneously aborted in the first 8 to 10 weeks of gestation are abnormal. These have been classified in four groups: Growth Disorganization, 1 through 4 (GD1, GD2, GD3, GD4) (B. J. Poland, et al.):

GD1: A chorionic vesicle without an umbilical cord remnant or embryo is certainly abnormal; this has commonly been called a "blighted ovum" but is better termed descriptively, i.e., an "empty chorionic vesicle" or "unembryonic sac" (Kalousek and Neave).

GD2: A nodular embryo with no recognizable external structures, 1 to 4 mm in maximum dimension within a chorionic sac.

GD3: A cylindrical embryo up to 10 mm in length with retinal pigment but no other distinct structures, i.e., no limb buds, no branchial arches, etc.

GD4: A stunted embryo, usually more than 10 mm long, but with major distortion of shape. Head, trunk, and limb buds may be recognized, but the length is usually less than expected for the gestational age, and development of structures such as the limbs is retarded or distorted relative to other structures.

Among spontaneously aborted embryos, abnormal chromosomal makeup, mainly from meiotic nondisjunction, is detected in about 60 percent (Boué, et al.). Triploidy, trisomy 16, trisomy 13, and monosomy X are among the more frequently occurring chromosomal abnormalities in aborted embryos.

Recommended Reading

Boué, J., Boué, A., and Lazar, F. Retrospective and prospective studies of 1500 karyotyped spontaneous abortions. *Teratology* 12:11–26, 1975.

Crowley, L. V. *An Introduction to Clinical Embryology.* Chicago: Year Book, 1974.

Dimmick, J. E., and Kalousek, D. K. *Developmental Pathology of the Embryo and Fetus.* Philadelphia: Lippincott, 1992.

Edelman, G. M. *Topobiology: An Introduction to Molecular Embryology.* New York: Basic Books, 1988.

Kalousek, D. K., Fitch, N., and Paradice, B. A. *Pathology of the Human Embryo and Previable Fetus. An Atlas.* New York: Springer, 1990.

Kalousek, D. K., and Neave, C. Pathology of Abortion, the Embryo and the Previable Fetus. In J. S. Wigglesworth and D. B. Singer (eds.), *Textbook of Fetal and Perinatal Pathology.* Boston: Blackwell, 1991. P. 141.

Mall, F. P. A study of the causes underlying the origin of human monsters. *J. Morphol.* 19:3–368, 1908.

Mall, F. P. On the frequence of localized anomalies in human embryos and infants at birth. *Am. J. Anat.* 22:49–72, 1917.

Moore, K. L. *The Developing Human. Clinically Oriented Embryology* (4th ed.). Philadelphia: Saunders, 1988.

O'Rahilly, R., and Müller, F. *Human Embryology and Teratology.* New York: Wiley, 1992.

Poland, B. J., et al. Spontaneous abortion: A study of 1961 women and their conceptuses. *Acta. Obstet. Gynecol. Scand.,* 102:5–32, 1981.

Streeter, G. L. Developmental horizons in human embryos: Description of age group XI, 13 to 20 somites and age group XII, 21 to 29 somites. *Contrib. Embryol. Carnegie Inst.,* 30:211, 1942.

4

The Placenta

Don B. Singer

The placenta at 40 weeks' gestation is usually a rounded or oval disc that weighs 450 to 550 g and measures about 20 x 20 x 2.5 cm. The umbilical cord is 40 to 70 cm long, 1.0 to 2.0 cm in diameter, and is most often inserted close to the center of the fetal surface of the placenta. The vessels spread from the umbilical cord to the chorionic plate (fetal side of the placenta) in a radial fashion with branches dipping into the stem villi along each radial arm (Figs. 4-1, 4-2). Arteries always cross over veins on the placental surface. Venous blood in the fetal-placental circulation is more oxygenated than arterial blood but neither venous nor arterial blood is bright red since its partial pressure of oxygen may be on the order of 25 to 35 mm Hg.

From the fetal perspective, the amnion covers the chorion and the chorion covers the villous tissue of the placenta. The amnionic and chorionic sacs surround the fetus (amnion within chorion, sac within sac, the fetus on the inside of the "double sac"). The umbilical cord is attached to the abdomen of the fetus. The umbilical arteries arise from the hypogastric branches of the fetal internal iliac arteries. The umbilical vein is continuous with the ductus venosus, which drains directly into the inferior vena cava after traversing the liver.

Placental Formation

The placenta, its membranes, and the umbilical cord are derived from the embryo. No part is of maternal origin. Delicate cellular fronds or cords grow from the surface of the spherical blastocyst. The appearance can be compared to that of a new tennis ball with abundant fuzz (Fig. 4-3). The

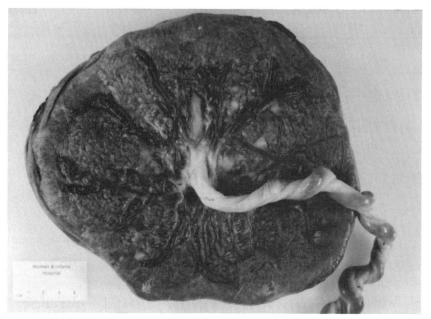

Fig. 4-1. The placenta at term as seen from the fetal side. It has a diameter of about 20 cm, a thickness of 2.5 cm, and it weighs about 500 gm. The umbilical cord is centrally placed and measures 42 X 1.2 cm. Fetal vessels emerge from the umbilical cord and spread radially over the surface of the placenta, with arteries crossing over veins. The placental membranes have been removed.

layer formed by the cords is called the *trophoblast. Intermediate trophoblast* are large mononuclear polygonal cells that have invasive capacity. They penetrate the maternal endometrium and maternal vessels, eventually replacing the endothelium (Fig. 4-4). Maternal blood then bathes the trophoblast cords and nourishes the blastocyst. The invasion of endometrium by the intermediate trophoblast establishes both an anchor and a blood supply for the developing conceptus. The invasion during the first week of gestation is the first of two such waves; the second invasion commences at around 18 to 21 weeks of gestation.

Inside the blastocyst, the embryo proper begins to form. Its ectoderm is continuous with the *amnionic sac* and its endoderm is continuous with the *yolk sac* (see Fig. 3-2). The outer trophoblast layer forms the *chorionic sac* or *chorionic vesicle.* This is a large sac that surrounds the amnionic sac, the yolk sac, and the embryo proper. Extraembryonic mesoderm makes up the connective tissue that holds the chorionic vesicle together.

The chorionic vesicle is large relative to the amnionic sac, the yolk sac, and the embryo. The embryo and the amnionic sac rapidly enlarge while the yolk sac begins to shrink, eventually leaving only a nubbin of a calcified

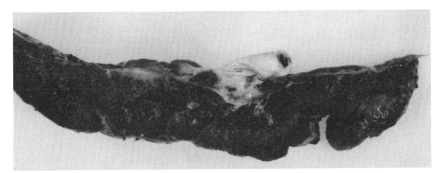

Fig. 4-2. Cross section of the placenta from Fig. 4-1 showing disc shape. Branches of the umbilical arteries and veins course through the chorionic plate. The amnion covers the fetal surface of the chorionic plate. Villous tissue makes up the bulk of the tissue beneath the chorionic plate.

remnant embedded in the amnion. The chorionic vesicle also grows but at a slower rate than the amnion. The amnionic sac finally fills the chorionic vesicle and fuses with it at about 6 to 8 weeks of gestation.

Stem villi

The *stem villi* develop from the thickened cords of trophoblast embedded in the maternal endometrium. Just as roots anchor a tree in the earth, the stem villi anchor the developing placenta in the nourishing maternal endometrial tissues. As these stem villi grow and root, tendrils form as *primary, secondary,* and *tertiary villi.* These villi are the functional units of the placenta. They are lined on their outer surface by trophoblast (Fig. 4-5). The cores of the villi are composed of connective tissue derived from the extra-embryonic mesoderm. Fibrocytes are plump and numerous in early stages of villous development. Fetal vessels occupy the cores of the villi. These are distal branches of the umbilical arteries and distal tributaries of the umbilical vein with a capillary bed between them. The vessels form in the central portions of villous connective tissue. Placental *macrophages,* also known as *Hofbauer cells,* are present.

Cytotrophoblast and Syncytiotrophoblast

The villus surface is specialized and is composed of two cell layers. The *cytotrophoblast* is the inner lining and the *syncytiotrophoblast* is the outer lining (see Fig. 4-5). Cytotrophoblast cells contain few organelles. Their primary function is proliferation and maturation to form syncytiotrophoblast. Cytotrophoblast also produces small amounts of human chorionic gonadotropin (hCG) and other placental hormones. The syncytiotrophoblast is a layer of highly specialized cells on the outer surface of each villus (see Fig. 4-5). The syncytiotrophoblast is designed for absorptive and secretory functions. Microvilli line the surfaces of these cells, which are bathed in

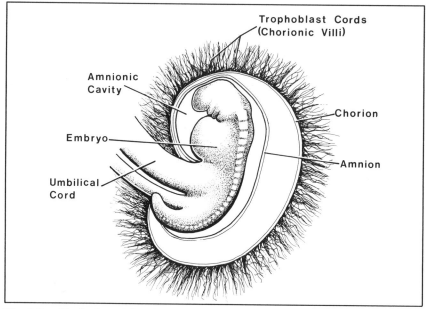

Fig. 4-3. Chorionic vesicle with cords of trophoblast covering the entire surface. Only those that attach to the endometrium will proliferate to form the definitive placenta. Remaining cords will involute and become incorporated in the chorionic sac. This is an embryo at about 24 days after conception. The yolk sac is not shown.

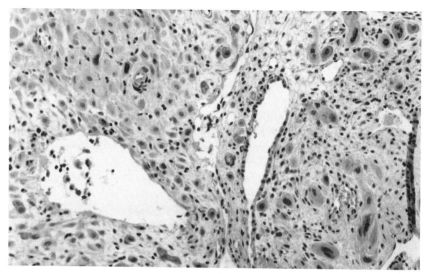

Fig. 4-4. Microscopic view of decidualized endometrium with intermediate trophoblast. The large prominent cells are invading the stroma and maternal vessels. This is how the implanting conceptus anchors itself to the maternal tissues and establishes contact with the maternal blood.

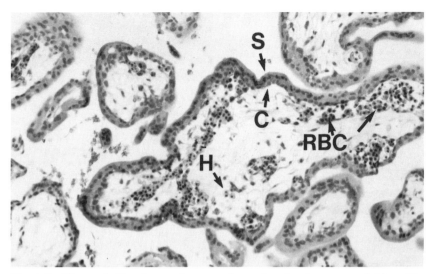

Fig. 4-5. Placental villus from early stage of gestation showing cytotrophoblast *(C)* and syncytiotrophoblast *(S)*. The villous core is composed of vascular mesenchymal tissue. The fetal red blood cells *(RBC)* are nucleated, a feature common in the first 8 to 10 weeks of development. Hofbauer cells *(H)* are the fetal villous macrophages.

the maternal circulation (Fig. 4-6A). Prominent profiles of rough endoplasmic reticulum in the cytoplasm indicate an active synthesizing process (Fig. 4-6B). Microbodies represent digestive function and degenerative change. Dense core granules are packets of polypeptide hormones. Nuclei of syncytiotrophoblast are irregular in outline and contrast to the rounded vesicular (open) nuclei of cytotrophoblast. The basal lamina is composed of type IV collagen and is permeable to many substances that cross freely into and out of the fetal blood vessels.

Throughout the first 10 to 15 weeks of gestation, the cytotrophoblast and syncytiotrophoblast have equal numbers of cells. The cytotrophoblast layer becomes progressively depleted and leaves a few scattered cells lying inside the rim of syncytiotrophoblast. Meanwhile, the syncytiotrophoblast has become more cellular. Its cells fuse together to form the syncytial masses from which it derives its name. As gestation progresses, this process becomes more and more pronounced. Cytotrophoblast cells are sparse in the last 4 to 8 weeks of pregnancy. Syncytial knots leave stretches of the villous surface where one finds no discernible cells. However, the surface is covered by a thinned layer of cytoplasm with a few microvilli still visible.

Meanwhile, the vessels of the villus core have dilated, increased in number due to branching, and pushed toward the surface just inside the synctial cells, i.e., close to the surface of the villus. This is the *synctiovascular membrane,* and it facilitates the transfer of solutes and gases between the

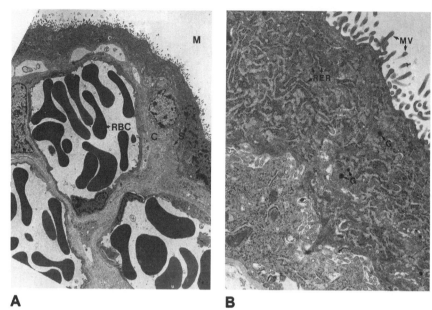

Fig. 4-6. (A) Electron micrograph of villus structure. The cytotrophoblast *(C)* has few organelles while the syncytiotrophoblast *(S)* is metabolically active. The fetal blood *(RBC)* is separated from the maternal blood space *(M)* by endothelium, capillary basement membrane, trophoblast basement membrane, and trophoblast cells. (B) The microvilli *(MV)* increase the surface of syncytiotrophoblast exposed to the maternal blood for both absorption and secretion. The profiles of rough endoplasmic reticulum *(RER)* indicate active metabolism and the dark granules *(G)* may be polypeptide hormone in secretory granules.

maternal and fetal circulations (Fig. 4-7). The syncytiovascular membrane and the syncytial knots are also clear signs of maturation of the placenta. Another feature of maturation is development of very small villi, especially those found just beneath the placenta's fetal surface. The change to this mature appearance accelerates in the last 3 to 4 weeks of gestation.

Placental Circulation

The umbilical vessels spread over the amnionic surface of the placenta (Fig. 4-8). They penetrate the stem villi and then the chorionic villi. As explained above, the stem vessels branch into the tendrils of the chorionic villi and become capillary in their structure. At first, they are centrally located within villi, separated from the maternal blood by a fairly wide expanse of tissue, including the villous connective tissue core and both the cytotrophoblast and the syncytiotrophoblast. As maturation progresses, the vessels increase in number and become peripherally located in the smaller and smaller villi, increasing the surface area and facilitating exchange between fetus and mother.

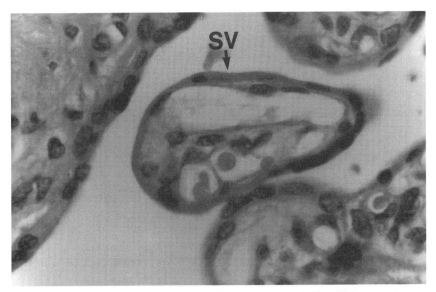

Fig. 4-7. Villus from late stage of gestation with sinusoidal dilatation of the fetal blood vessels. Syncytiotrophoblast cells have thinned and their nuclei coalesce to form knots. The thinned cytoplasm of the syncytiotrophoblast reduces the distance between fetal and maternal bloodstreams. This is the syncytiovascular membrane *(SV)*.

Intervillus Circulation

The maternal endometrial vessels continue to be invaded by the expanding tendrils of chorionic villi as the placenta spreads laterally. Maternal decidual arteries and arterioles are coiled. The parts that are invaded by trophoblasts lose muscle from their walls. They become sinusoidal and lake-like. The coiled arteries and arterioles proximal to these dilated sinusoidal channels are under arterial pressure. The result is the introduction of blood under great pressure into the sinusoids. This pressure produces a fountain-like effect that sprays the maternal blood into the placenta (Fig. 4-8). The blood percolates around the chorionic villi and enters maternal venous channels. As mentioned above, the first wave of trophoblast invasion into maternal vessels takes place at implantation and for the first several weeks thereafter as the placenta spreads laterally. A second wave of trophoblast invades deeper maternal vessels between 18 and 21 weeks. This invasion establishes a larger sinusoidal component to the vascular supply.

Chorionic and Amnionic Sacs

The trophoblast shell does not persist around the entire surface of the chorionic vesicle after the first few weeks of gestation. Most of the trophoblast involutes except for that which becomes the placenta proper. The

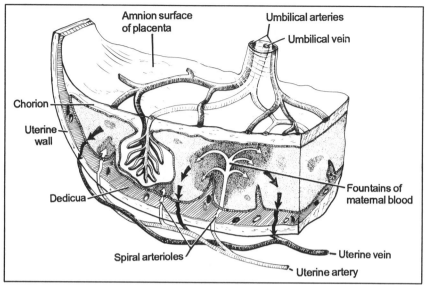

Fig. 4-8. Diagram of the surface of the placenta, showing the vascular relationships. Branches of the two umbilical (fetal) arteries cross over branches of the umbilical (fetal) vein. The villus tree of the placenta is shown on the left and the fountains of maternal blood *(curved arrows)* are shown on the right.

involuted cords become fibrotic remnants in the chorionic membrane. The amnionic sac, after fusing with the chorionic sac, continues to expand as more amnionic fluid forms and the fetal size increases. The amnionic epithelium is cuboidal (Fig. 4-9). The amnion is the surface facing the fetus while the chorion is fused to it on the outside and faces the decidual layer of the uterus. The decidua at the base of the placenta is called *decidua basalis*. The decidua away from the implanted placenta is known as *decidua capsularis*. Decidua is of maternal origin.

Further Features of Placental Maturation

As the pregnancy approaches 36 to 38 weeks, fibrin forms where maternal blood is in contact with placental tissue. In the case of perivillous fibrin, syncytiotrophoblast may grow over the fibrin mass. Fibrin may also form a layer of varying thickness beneath the chorionic plate of the placental disc or between the placental villi and the maternal decidua.

Another feature of maturation is calcification. The mechanism for the calcification is not clearly understood, but it usually has no pathologic significance. The maternal surface of the placenta may be thoroughly crusted with dense calcium deposits especially after 40 to 42 weeks' gestation.

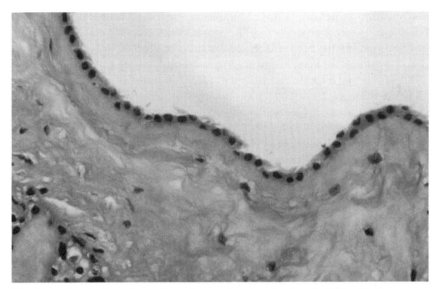

Fig. 4-9.   Amnionic surface of membranes showing simple cuboidal epithelium. This surface has secretory and absorptive function since the amnionic fluid changes completely once every 24 to 36 hours.

Variations of Placental Structure

The amnion and chorion covering the fetal surface of the placenta usually extend to the edges of the placenta circumferentially. When they extend only partially toward the edge of the disc, the configuration is designated *circummarginate* placenta. This configuration has little or no significance. The portion of the placenta uncovered by amnion and chorion is apparently embedded in the decidua. When the circummarginate placental configuration has an added feature, namely a ridge of fibrin around the circumference, the designation is *circumvallate* placenta. This, too, is of questionable significance but is sometimes associated with premature delivery. That portion of the placenta that is not covered by membranes is called *extrachorial* placenta.

Sometimes the umbilical cord inserts at the edge of the placenta; i.e., it has a marginal insertion. This variant reminded anatomists from an older era of a battledore (badminton racquet), thus the term *battledore* placenta. It has little significance although the cord is seemingly more vulnerable to avulsion. Another variant of umbilical cord insertion is the *velamentous* cord. In this configuration, the umbilical cord ends in a membrane formed from the amnion and chorion. Only membrane surrounds the bare umbilical vessels in the remainder of their course to the surface of the placenta. Velamentous cord insertion is potentially dangerous since the vessels in the membranes are unprotected by *Wharton's jelly* (the turgid substance that cushions the vessels in the umbilical cord and protects them from being compressed or twisted). The vessels thus are vulnerable to tearing or compression although these are uncommon events.

If the spherical distribution of trophoblast cords in the early development of the placenta do not fully involute, remnants develop into placental tissue that may be separated by varying distances from the main placental mass. They are, of necessity, always connected to the main placental mass by branches of the placental vessels and by membranes. Such lobules or lobes are called *accessory lobes* or *succenturiate lobes.* They may be attached close to the edge of the main placental mass or may be connected by a broad isthmus of placental tissue to the main placental mass. A bilobed placenta is one in which both the accessory lobe and the main placental mass (the one with the umbilical cord attached) are of approximately equal size (Fig. 4-10). In the Rhesus monkey the placenta is usually bilobed with the accessory lobe only slightly smaller than the main placental mass.

Multiple Births

The placentas in twins may take any of several forms. If a single ovum is fertilized by a single sperm, and the zygote, or developing embryo, then divides, this produces *monozygotic* (identical) twins. If two ova are fertilized

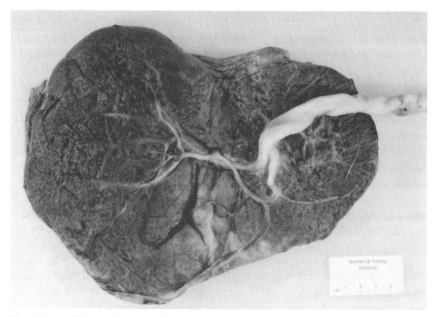

Fig. 4-10. Bilobed placenta with vessels reaching the second lobe by crossing through connecting membranes of amnion and chorion.

by two sperm, *dizygotic* (fraternal) twins are formed. In either case, one or two placental discs may form (Fig. 4-11). This is so because if the monozygotic twin embryos separate early, e.g., before implantation, two placental discs can form even though the twins are identical. Similarly, two dizygotic embryos usually implant separately and form two placentas. On the other hand, if the monozygotic twins separate a bit later, even after implantation, a single placental disc may form. Depending on how much later, the sacs and membranes surrounding each of the twins may differ. Separate chorions and amnions may surround each twin, even though the placenta is single and the twins are identical. In this situation, two placental discs probably become fused. The chorionic vesicles and amnions may also fuse but the separate sacs can be easily distinguished from one another by microscopic examination.

Dizygotic fraternal twins that implant close to each other may also have a single placental disc that forms by fusion. Dizygotic twins always have separate chorionic and amnionic sacs even if the discs or the sacs themselves become fused. If monozygotic identical twins separate later, e.g., several days after implantation, the disc will be single and they may share a single chorionic sac but yet have two separate amnions since the amnionic sac forms later than does the chorionic vesicle. In this instance, the dividing membrane between the twins will consist only of amnion apposed to amnion.

If the monozygotic embryo divides into two still later, e.g., inside a single amnion and a single chorion, this is called *monochorionic-monoamnionic* placentation. Danger lies in the fact that both twins share a single cavity and as they tumble and twist in the cavity, their umbilical cords may become entangled and knotted with compressed vessels and disastrous results. The umbilical circulation of one or both twins may be interrupted. If the monozygotic embryo divides still later, not only will the placentas and sacs be single, the twins themselves may be fused together in various forms of *conjoined* twins.

With triplets or quadruplets or higher multiples of concurrent conceptuses, combinations of the sacs and placentas described for twins are found. Examination of the placentas may become quite detailed and complex.

Infections

Infectious diseases can reach the placenta, its membranes, or the fetus by three routes. The first is the *transcervical* route, through which bacteria (and sometimes viruses) penetrate the cervical mucus to reach the amnion at the internal cervical os. The second route is through the mother's bloodstream and is designated *transplacental*. Bacteria, viruses, and protozoa may use this route. The third route is a combination of both the above in that organisms propagate through the cervix but instead of invading the amnion, they invade the decidua until they reach the implanted placenta.

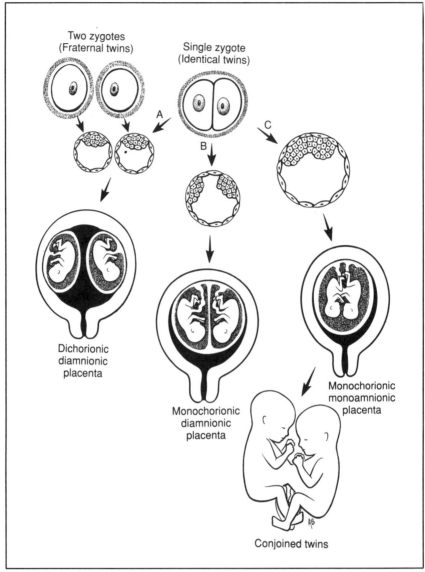

Fig. 4-11. Twinning. On the left, two separate oocytes are fertilized by two separate sperm. This dizygous, or fraternal, twinning results in two separate vesicles. The placentas may, however, fuse to form a single disc. This is dichorionic diamnionic placentation. On the right, a single ovum has been fertilized by a single sperm and divides into two thereafter. This is monozygotic, or identical, twinning. If the zygote divides early, i.e., at the two-cell stage, the nature of the placenta is the same as for dizygotic twins (path *A*). Later division into two embryos results in either (path *B*) monochorionic diamnionic or (path *C*) monochorionic monoamnionic placental sacs. In the very late division into two embryos, the fetuses are joined together (conjoined twins).

Numerically, the most significant of the infectious processes involving the placenta is transcervical infection, also known as the *amnionic sac infection syndrome.* Enteric or vaginal bacteria (e.g., coagulase-negative *Staphylococci,* group B *Streptococcus, Escherichia coli*) invade the attenuated chorionic-amnionic membrane, which at the internal cervical os has no significant nourishment from surrounding maternal tissues. The membranes need not be ruptured to allow bacterial entry.

Once inside the sac, organisms infect the amnionic fluid. This fluid has bacteriostatic properties between 20 and 36 weeks of gestation, but these properties can be overwhelmed by virulent organisms. The infected fluid elicits both a maternal and a fetal inflammatory response. The mother is usually asymptomatic but may develop fever and even septicemia. The fetus develops pneumonia (due to the aspirated infected amnionic fluid) and septicemia from invasion of the bloodstream. The fetal defenses against these infections are less effective than are the defenses of older infants (see Chap. 5).

The inflammatory response in the amnion and chorion consist mostly of maternal leukocytes that migrate to the sac from the surrounding decidua or in the placental disc from the maternal sinusoids. The maternal inflammatory cells, mostly neutrophils, are trapped temporarily beneath the chorionic plate of the placenta. These cells then migrate through the chorion and amnion (Fig. 4-12). The fetal response is noted in the chorionic plate and in the umbilical cord where a fetal vasculitis may be prominent (Fig. 4-13).

Villitis is the result of the fetal inflammatory response to *transplacental infections,* mostly viruses. The acronym TORCH is a useful reminder for some of these organisms; *TO* is for toxoplasmosis (*O* is also for other), *R* is for rubella, *C* is for cytomegalovirus, and *H* is for herpes. Herpes is actually rarely transmitted transplacentally. Most herpes infections occur transcervically or during the process of birth. Other organisms *(O)* with transplacental routes of infection include parvovirus, some but not all human immunodeficiency viruses (HIV), some hepatitis viruses, Coxsackie viruses, ECHO viruses, and many other organisms. Most perinatal infections with HIV and hepatitis viruses, especially hepatitis B, infect the baby during birth since the baby is exposed to large amounts of infected maternal blood. Villitis may be subtle with only a mild proliferative response of villus connective tissue cells and Hofbauer cells. On the other hand, a distinct lymphocytic and even plasmacytic infiltrate may ensue, especially with syphilis and with cytomegalovirus infections. *Listeria monocytogenes* is a bacterium that is transmitted transplacentally. It induces an acute suppurative villitis with multiple small microabscesses of villi.

Circulatory Problems

The umbilical cord, especially if excessively long (> 80 cm) may tangle about the fetal limbs or wrap around the fetal neck or trunk. Long cords are also

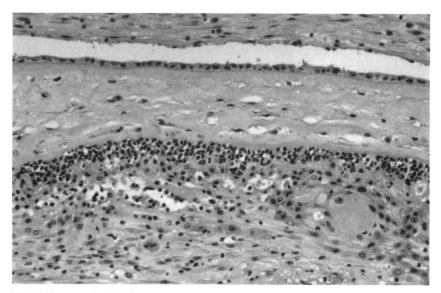

Fig. 4-12. Amnionitis due to transcervical bacterial infection. Maternal leukocytes migrate through the membranes to reach the infected contents of the sac.

prone to true knots due to fetal tumbling movements. These events rarely produce problems unless the umbilical vessels become excessively stretched and compressed. Wharton's jelly in the umbilical cord provides a cushion that protects against vascular compression. The umbilical cord may prolapse into the birth canal before the head descends. In such cases the oncoming head can compress the cord against bony prominences in the mother's pelvis and the umbilical vessels may become occluded. Disturbances in the fetal circulation produce few untoward effects in the placenta. In fact, complete cessation of fetal blood flow and fetal demise are associated with few lesions in the placenta until several days have passed.

The most common of all placental lesions, infarcts and intervillus thrombi, are due to maternal circulatory problems. Both lesions are prominent in *pregnancy-induced hypertension*, also known as *eclampsia, preeclampsia,* or *toxemia of pregnancy.* (In Europe, this condition is called *gestosis.*) This disease may start in the second trimester but usually is manifest toward the end of pregnancy. Few lesions are found in the decidua but the second invasion of vessels by trophoblast has apparently failed. Spiral or coiled arterioles remain intact. This results in continued spasm of vessels, placental ischemia, infarcts, and intervillus thrombi due to stagnant circulation. In some cases, decidual arterioles may have thickened walls with lipid deposits.

Another placental circulatory problem is associated with maternal antiphospholipid or anticardiolipin antibodies, and lupus anticoagulant. Multiple placental infarcts and intervillous thrombi develop, often in midgestation. Fetal death is common. Low doses of aspirin are often effective in preventing placental lesions and fetal death. Cortisone analogs are also used in treatment of this condition.

Abruptio Placenta

If the decidua and the associated anchoring villi become necrotic, bleeding into the area can cleave the placenta away from its attachment to the maternal tissues. This bleeding may dissect along the plane between the chorion and the decidua and emerge as vaginal bleeding. The hematoma forming between the placenta and the uterus produces irritation to the uterine muscle. Contractions may be mild or they may produce considerable pain. The triad of pain, vaginal bleeding, and fetal compromise suggests the diagnosis of a subplacental hematoma, also known as *abruptio placenta*. Even though the bleeding may cease, the portion of the placenta overlying the hematoma will undergo necrosis. On rare occasions, the hematoma leaves a depression in the placental tissue that can be detected by examining the maternal surface.

Meconium Staining

Meconium staining occurs in about 15 to 20 percent of all deliveries. The results are usually benign but in about 2 or 3 percent this finding is pre-

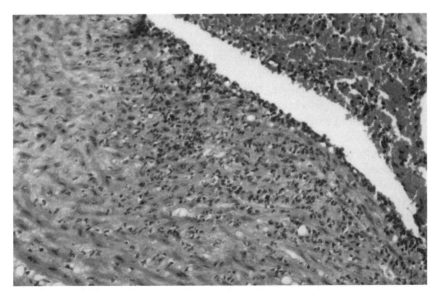

Fig. 4-13. Umbilical vessel with fetal leukocytes responding to an amnionic sac infection.

ceded by significant fetal asphyxia. *Asphyxia* is defined as hypoxia and hypercarbia with the corollary association of acidosis (see Chap. 5). Meconium is laden with bile pigments and other chemical constituents that alter the amnion. The pigment seeps into the amnionic connective tissue where, in a matter of minutes, it is picked up by macrophages and is then carried deep into the chorion. It is estimated to take about 3 hours for the meconium-laden macrophages to migrate from the superficial to the deep chorion and superficial decidua. By examining placental membranes, one can estimate the duration of time from passage of meconium to birth and delivery of the placenta.

Miscellaneous Placental Lesions

Another pathologic condition of the placenta is *placenta previa.* Here the placenta is implanted low in the uterus and grows over the internal cervical os. This area bleeds, sometimes profusely and dangerously, especially when the cervix dilates and effaces at the onset of labor or when the area is probed.

Placental edema, or hydrops, may develop when there is fetal infection, heart failure, vascular anomalies, or severe fetal anemia. In past times, the most common cause was erythroblastosis fetalis due to fetal-maternal Rh incompatibility. Now that Rh-negative women receive anti-Rh immune globulin during pregnancy, destruction of their fetuses' red blood cells is avoided. Other causes of placental hydrops are alpha-thalassemia, other heritable metabolic or red blood cell disorders, and infections with parvovirus, cytomegalovirus, and syphilis.

Tumors of the Placenta

Chorangiomas are hemangiomas of fetal villous vessels. They are usually small (less than 2 cm in diameter) but may occupy up to a third or more of the placental mass, in which case fetal heart failure develops due to shunting of circulation through the tumor.

Trophoblastic tumors include *partial hydatidiform mole, complete hydatidiform mole, placental implantation site tumors,* and *choriocarcinomas.* The partial mole is associated with an embryo or a fetus and usually has a portion of normal placental tissue. Within the abnormal tissue, the trophoblast layer is hyperplastic and the villi become severely swollen and hydropic, forming 0.5- to 1.5-cm masses in clusters like bunches of grapes. Individual cells in the trophoblast may be normal or hyperchromatic and anaplastic. Triploidy (three haploid sets of chromosomes, i.e., 69 chromosomes) is common in partial moles. The extra set of chromosomes is of paternal derivation. Partial moles are almost never malignant but careful follow up with serial measurements of hCG in the mother's serum are warranted. The values should fall to zero in a matter of a few weeks or 2 or 3 months.

Complete moles have no associated fetus or embryo. Grossly, they may appear similar to partial moles but normal-appearing placental tissue is absent. The uterus is filled with grape-like masses of hydropic villi. This produces a uterus much larger than expected for the duration of gestation. Trophoblast cells are usually enlarged, hyperchromatic, and may appear anaplastic. The chromosome complement is usually diploid (46 chromosomes) but both haploid sets may be derived from the father. Complete moles are usually benign but require careful follow up with serial measurements of hCG. Like the partial mole, values should fall to zero in a few weeks or 2 or 3 months.

Placental site tumors are composed of intermediate trophoblast that persist after the end of a pregnancy. Human placental lactogen is the predominant hormone secreted by these tumors, although some hCG may also be secreted. These tumors are commonly benign, but several cases have ended with metastatic disease and fatality.

Choriocarcinoma is a frankly malignant tumor of trophoblast with marked anaplasia of cells and distinct invasion of maternal uterine tissues. These are solid tumors and show no grape-like clusters as are seen in partial and complete moles. Choriocarcinomas are rapidly progressive tumors. Fortunately, most choriocarcinomas are exquisitely sensitive to chemotherapeutic agents such as methotrexate.

Recommended Reading

Baldwin, V. Multiple Births. In J. S. Wigglesworth, and D. B. Singer (eds.), *Textbook of Fetal and Perinatal Pathology.* Boston: Blackwell, 1991.

Benirschke, K., and Kaufman, H. *The Human Placenta.* New York: Springer, 1991.

Fox, H. *Pathology of the Placenta.* Philadelphia: Saunders, 1978.

Naeye, R. L. *Disorders of the Placenta, Fetus and Neonate. Diagnosis and Clinical Significance.* St. Louis: Mosby-Year Book, 1992.

Robertson, E. G., and Neer, K. J. Placental injection studies in twin gestation. *Am. J. Obstet. Gynecol.* 147:170–174, 1983.

Rushton, I. Placental Pathology. In J. S. Wigglesworth and D. B. Singer (eds.), *Textbook of Fetal and Perinatal Pathology.* Boston: Blackwell, 1991.

Sibai, B. M., et al. Maternal and perinatal outcome associated with the syndrome of hemolysis, elevated liver enzymes and low platelets in severe eclampsia. *Am. J. Obstet. Gynecol.* 155:501–509, 1986.

Fetal and Neonatal Pathology

Don B. Singer and Patricia A. O'Shea

Abnormal Growth

In embryonic and early fetal life, cellular proliferation accounts for most of the body's growth. From midgestation (approximately 18–20 weeks) onward, proliferation slows and is combined with enlargement of individual cells. If disease occurs in the first half of gestation, proliferation is retarded and fewer cells develop. A generalized smallness is the result. This is *symmetric growth retardation*. If cell enlargement is retarded, the brain tends to be spared and continues to grow normally while somatic tissues, particularly the bones, muscles, subcutaneous tissues, heart, lung, liver, and kidney will all have smaller cells. The result is a relatively large head and small body, i.e., *asymmetric growth retardation*.

Infants who are within two standard deviations of their expected average weight at a given gestation are called *appropriate for gestational age* (AGA); those less than two standard deviations are *small for gestational age* (SGA); and those greater than two standard deviations are *large for gestational age* (LGA). The approximate birth weights at various stages of gestation are listed in Table 5-1. These data are for infants born at sea level. Those born in cities such as Denver will be slightly smaller. Infants with congenital defects or those born to mothers with severe hypertension tend to be SGA. Most LGA babies are born to mothers who are themselves large or who were large at birth. Infants with Beckwith-Wiedemann syndrome, infantile giantism, or those born to mothers with poorly controlled diabetes mellitus tend to be LGA. The size of the father has little to do with the size of the fetus or newborn baby in most instances.

Table 5-1. Approximate birth weights at various stages of gestation

Gestational age (weeks)	Approximate birth weight (g)
20	200
23	500
28	1060
32	1500
36	2500
40	3400
42	3600

Pathologic Processes in Fetuses and Neonates

A few pathologic processes account for virtually all morbidity and mortality in fetuses and neonates. These processes are asphyxia, aspiration of meconium, infection, neonatal jaundice, congenital diseases (metabolic conditions and malformations), trauma, iatrogenic diseases, and tumors.

Asphyxia

Asphyxia is defined as hypoxia, hypercarbia, and as a corollary to both of these, respiratory or metabolic acidosis, or both. Severe perinatal asphyxia may cause neurologic deficits. Recently defined criteria for severe asphyxia include: (1) profound metabolic or mixed acidemia (pH < 7.00) on an umbilical arterial sample of blood; (2) Apgar score of 0 to 3 at 5 minutes; (3) clinical neurologic signs including neonatal seizures, hypotonia, coma, or hypoxic-ischemic encephalopathy; and (4) multiorgan system dysfunction.

Respiration in utero is conducted not by the lungs but by the placenta. Any process that interferes with placental exchange of oxygen and carbon dioxide results in asphyxia. Maternal pregnancy-induced hypertension, cord accidents that impede the flow of blood in the umbilical vessels, retroplacental hematomas (also called abruptio placentae, or placental abruptions), and placental infarcts are possible causes of fetal asphyxia. Up to 10 percent of the placenta may be infarcted without ill effect to the fetus. At least 30 percent must be infarcted, and acutely so, to produce fetal death. In placental abruption, bleeding cleaves the placenta from the uterus and forms hematomas that compress the overlying placental villous tissue. When hematomas have been present for a few days or weeks, the overlying placental tissue will become necrotic and eventually fibrotic.

Postnatal asphyxia may result from pulmonary hypoplasia, respiratory distress syndrome, pneumonia, aspiration of foreign material (amniotic fluid or meconium), or malformations of the respiratory tract such as choanal atresia, laryngeal stenosis or webs, tracheomalacia, congenital cystic adenomatoid malformation, diaphragmatic hernia or other intrathoracic masses, agenesis of the lungs, and certain forms of congenital heart disease.

In the pathophysiology of fetal asphyxia, the fetal heart rate is decreased, usually markedly, below 100 beats per minute. Umbilical arterial acidosis (pH 7.0) is another of the critical markers for fetal asphyxia. The umbilical blood PO_2 may be in the 12 to 15 mm Hg range. Because of hypoxia, hypercarbia, and acidosis, the fetus responds with deep respiratory movements. Fetal respiratory movements normally are shallow and aspiration of amniotic fluid into the acinar (alveolar) lung tissues does not occur. With asphyxia, deep inspiratory movements pull amniotic fluid and the cellular material to the periphery of the lung. The increased negative pressure in the thorax, associated with hypoxia, produces petechiae in the visceral pleura, the visceral pericardium, and on the surface of the thymus. In either fetal or neonatal asphyxia, myocardial infarcts, liver necrosis, and necrosis and hemorrhage of the adrenals and kidneys may develop (Figs. 5-1, 5-2). The gastrointestinal tract may show necrosis of mucosa, particularly in the terminal ileum and cecal region, i.e., necrotizing enterocolitis (NEC) (Fig. 5-3). The pathogenesis of NEC may include other factors such as infection and ischemia.

In premature babies the periventricular germinal matrix in the brain is vulnerable to asphyxic damage. Venules and capillaries rupture, and small subependymal hemorrhages form and coalesce, breaching the ependymal

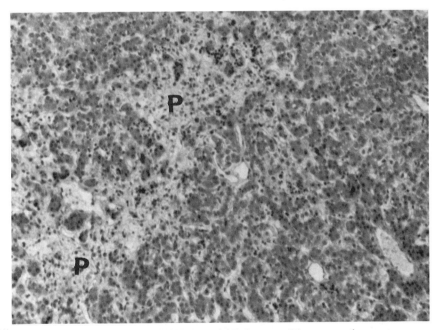

Fig. 5-1. Liver from neonate with asphyxia. Pale areas *(P)* are necrotic zones irregularly distributed in the lobules. Hematoxylin and eosin stain, original magnification x100.

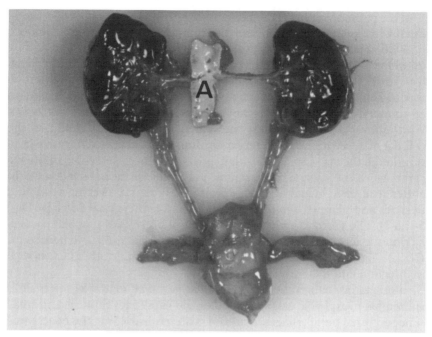

Fig. 5-2. Genitourinary tract from an asphyxiated neonate. The kidneys have hemorrhagic medullae. The aorta *(A)* and renal arteries are free of thrombi, which indicates that the process is a generalized one with the kidney representing a particularly vulnerable organ.

lining and leading to intraventricular hemorrhage (Fig. 5-4). If the ventricles become dilated with blood or clots or if blood dissects into surrounding brain parenchyma, the prognosis for normal function is poor. If the bleeding is confined to the subependymal zone or to the lumens of undilated ventricles, nearly normal function in infancy and later life can be predicted.

Small infarcts of white matter in the centrum semiovale region (periventricular leukomalacia) may result from asphyxia or ischemia. When the lesions are large, liquifactive necrosis will produce cavities in the brain. The pathogenesis of either germinal matrix hemorrhage or periventricular leukomalacia is not completely understood. Hypoxia and ischemia are both implicated as is poor autoregulation of circulatory hemodynamics in the premature fetus or infant. Neonatal sepsis is an associated and possibly predisposing factor in some cases.

In the living infant, damage to the surfactant-producing cells will result in atelectasis with congestion of the collapsed parenchyma. After about 3 hours of air breathing, *hyaline membranes* may form along the larger air spaces such as the terminal bronchioles and alveolar antra. Continued efforts at ventilation, usually with respirators and high-pressure settings, will

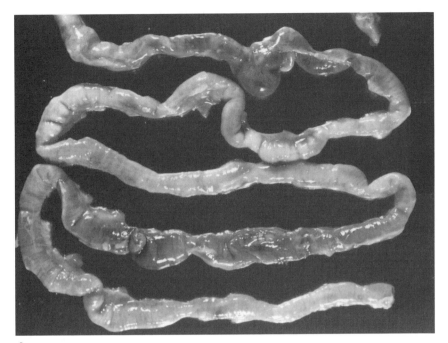

A

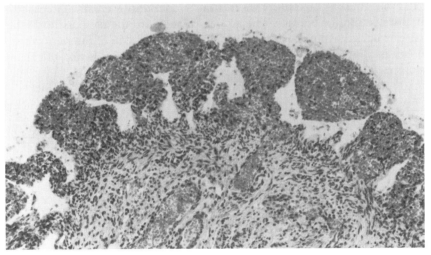

B

Fig. 5-3. (A) Portion of small intestine. The dark areas are bowel with full-thickness hypoxic-ischemic necrosis (i.e., necrotizing enterocolitis). (B) Microscopic view of necrotizing enterocolitis with the process of necrosis most severe at the lumenal surface. The villi are swollen and have lost the lining epithelium. Hematoxylin and eosin stain, original magnification X20.

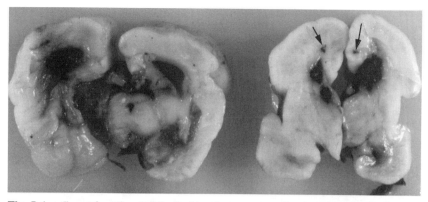

Fig. 5-4. Coronal sections of the brains of premature twins, both of whom were asphyxiated. The one on the left has severe intraventricular hemorrhage. The one on the right has less severe intraventricular hemorrhage but areas of necrosis in the centrum semiovale *(arrows)*. These processes are more characteristic of ischemia than asphyxia, but both processes are often present in premature neonates.

result in rupture of air sacs and the production of interstitial air around vessels, along the interlobular septae, and around bronchi. If the air dissects to the pleura, subpleural air blebs form and if these rupture, pneumothorax will result. This is a fairly common event in babies who require respirator therapy. The air can dissect into the mediastinum, the pericardial sac, or upwards into the soft tissues and skin of the neck where it can be detected by palpating crepitance. For a tabular listing of the lesions of fetal or neonatal asphyxia, see Table 5-2.

Table 5-2.   Effects of fetal or neonatal asphyxia

Acidosis (lactic acid)
Myocardial necrosis
Pulmonary pneumocyte necrosis
Hyaline membrane disease
Necrotizing enterocolitis
Hepatic midzonal necrosis
Adrenal hemorrhage
Renal lesions
    Cortical necrosis
    Medullary hemorrhage
    Acute tubular necrosis
Hypoxic-ischemic encephalopathy
    Germinal matrix hemorrhage
    Periventricular leukomalacia
Microvascular thrombi (disseminated intravascular coagulation)

Aspiration of Meconium

The literature contains numerous descriptions of meconium "pneumonitis" or chemical pneumonitis from aspirated meconium. This is a medical myth passed from one textbook to the next without critical evaluation. Pneumonitis, when it is associated with meconium, is virtually always due to bacteria mixed with the meconium in the amniotic fluid. When the aspirated meconium is sterile, it induces no inflammation (Fig. 5-5). However, the meconium itself is extremely dangerous since it occupies lung spaces intended for air and it is eliminated from the lung with great difficulty. It may cause severe or fatal asphyxia. If the meconium remains in the distal air space for a week or more, the bile salts and enzymes can damage the alveolar epithelium and result in a mild inflammatory response.

Infection

Fetuses and neonates are more vulnerable to infections than are older infants, children, and adults. The humoral and cellular immune mechanisms are not fully developed. Phagocytes respond more slowly and less effectively to invading organisms. The response of the complement system is also less effective than in more mature individuals. Interleukins are

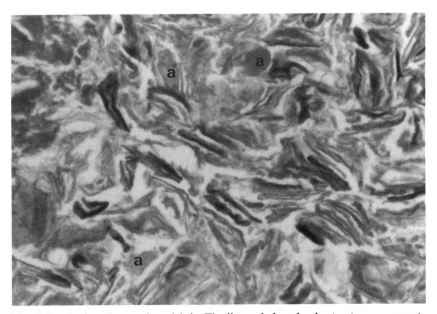

Fig. 5-5.   Aspirated meconium debris. The linear dark and pale structures represent squamous epithelial cells swallowed and digested in the fetal intestinal tract. The rounded and granular amorphous deposits *(a)* are other elements of the meconium that are expelled from the rectum into the amniotic fluid and then aspirated into the lungs. Hematoxylin and eosin stain, original magnification X100.

similarly less effective in the perinatal period than in infants, children, or adults.

Amniotic Sac Infection Syndrome

The most common type of bacterial infection of fetuses and neonates is that which ascends from the maternal cervix to the amniotic sac and then by aspiration to the fetal respiratory and gastrointestinal tracts. This is the amniotic sac infection syndrome. Even with a competent cervix, certain virulent bacteria can breach the barriers of cervical mucus, the amnion membrane, and the bactericidal activity of the amniotic fluid. The most common organisms responsible for amniotic sac infection syndrome in the United States are the group B *Streptococci* and *Escherichia coli.* Other organisms that have been implicated include coagulase-negative *Staphylococci, Streptococcus viridans,* group A *Streptococcus, Haemophilus influenzae, Fusobacterium,* other enteric organisms, and rarely, *Pseudomonas* and *Proteus* organisms (I. M. Gladstone, et al., 1990).

The diagnosis of amniotic sac infection is not readily made before birth. The mother may have low-grade fever, pelvic pain or tenderness, purulent vaginal discharge or purulent cervicitis, but often she has no symptoms. The neonate may have either an early-onset syndrome (0–6 days of age) or a late-onset syndrome (≥ 7 days of age). Early-onset sepsis is characterized clinically by rapid onset of severe symptoms with pneumonia, septicemia, septic shock, and a relatively high mortality rate of about 20 percent. Late-onset sepsis develops more gradually, is less severe, is more apt to have associated meningitis, joint or skin infections, and has a low mortality rate.

The pathologic features of the amniotic sac infection syndrome include acute chorioamnionitis, funisitis (inflammation of the umbilical cord), and vasculitis involving the fetal umbilical vessels and the fetal chorionic plate vessels. Aspirated bacteria induce a diffuse pneumonia in the fetus that can persist after birth. Pneumonia of intrauterine origin has a characteristic pathologic feature that is neither lobar nor bronchial in distribution. The distribution is diffuse and, less commonly, in a patchy aspiration pattern. Polymorphonuclear leukocytes predominate in the inflammatory response, and fibrin is rarely found (Fig. 5-6). In babies who survive, respiratory distress is common and hyaline membranes may form that are indistinguishable from those of the idiopathic respiratory distress syndrome. With appropriate studies, colonies of bacteria may be identified within the hyaline membranes. Tracheitis may accompany the pneumonia but usually the trachea and bronchi are free of inflammation. The aspirated infected amniotic fluid may also extend through the eustachian tubes to the middle ears, so fetuses and newborns may have otitis media.

Inflammatory foci are not usually found in organs other than the placenta, membranes, or lung. In a minority of cases of early-onset disease, meningitis or cerebral ventriculitis may be found. Swallowed infected and inflamed amniotic fluid containing polymorphonuclear leukocytes may be

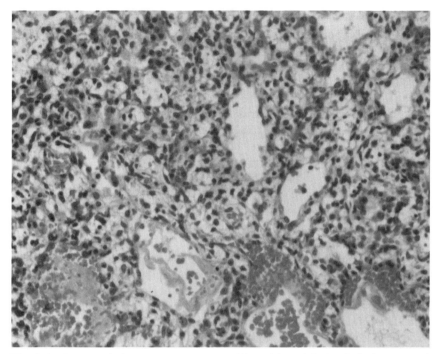

Fig. 5-6. Pneumonia in a premature neonate's lung. The acini contain leukocytes and amorphous exudate. Hematoxylin and eosin stain, original magnification X400.

detected in the gastrointestinal tract, particularly in the mucus of the stomach. Occasionally, polymorphonuclear leukocytes and bacteria are identified in the small bowel, colon, or rectum. Such findings may be observed in stillborn fetuses. These do not represent inflammation of the gastrointestinal tissues but rather swallowed exudate.

In many cases, the infection invades the bloodstream and, if the organisms are sufficiently virulent, septicemia results. The features of septicemia clinically include either hypo- or hyperthermia, neutrophilia or neutropenia, lethargy, poor feeding, and cyanosis. Many of the signs and symptoms of neonatal septicemia are nonspecific. Shock and disseminated intravascular coagulation with attendant lesions of necrosis and microvascular thrombi may be found in the skin, brain, lungs, liver, kidneys, and other tissues and organs. Disseminated abscesses are uncommon except when the infections are due to *Staphylococcus aureus, Pseudomonas aeruginosa,* or *Candida albicans.* These organisms are more often encountered as superinfections when intensive care is prolonged, i.e., with antibiotics, invasive procedures, indwelling catheters, or feeding tubes.

Early recognition of the infection in neonates is important since the process can move very quickly from total lack of symptoms to a fulminant course leading to death within a few hours. Antibiotic treatment may be curative if it is appropriate to the organism and if it is instituted quickly.

Transplacental Infection Syndromes
Fetuses may be infected by organisms coming from the mother's blood-stream through the placenta. The organisms responsible for most of these transplacental infections are viruses, but many bacteria and some protozoa may also reach the fetus across the placenta. The acronym TORCH has been applied to this group of conditions (toxoplasmosis, rubella, cytomegalovirus, and herpes) but these only partially tell the story. The acronym can be stretched to read TORCHSHPHL and even beyond. The additional microbes are syphilis, hepatitis B virus, parovirus, human immunodeficiency virus (HIV), and *Listeria monocytogenes.*

Most transplacental infections occur early in gestation or in midgestation. The effects are reduction in the number of cells or reduction in the size of cells, or both. Inflammatory foci are chronic (i.e., lymphocytes, plasma cells, and macrophages predominate) and many are fibrotic. Generalized interstitial fibrosis is characteristic of congenital syphilis.

Stimulation of the fetal immune system is evident in chronic fetal infections. The lymphoid tissues are hyperplastic and germinal centers may form. Ordinarily, follicles and germinal centers do not form in human lymph nodes or spleens until 2 or 3 months of postnatal life.

Toxoplasmosis is due to a large protozoan that crosses the placenta and invades many fetal tissues. Periventricular calcifications in the brain and chorioretinitis are characteristic lesions.

Cytomegalovirus can cause devastating disease in fetuses. The ballooned infected cells have large intranuclear inclusions (Fig. 5-7). Growth retardation is prominent. Almost every tissue in the body can be infected, but the periventricular region of the brain and the retina are special targets.

Parvovirus is another devastating prenatal transplacental infection. The fetal nucleated red blood cell precursors are the targets of human parvovirus. Intranuclear viral inclusions are small, lavender to purple in routine hematoxylin and eosin–stained tissues, and most readily detected in the liver, where hematopoiesis is prominent (Fig. 5-8). A severe fetal anemia results in hydrops fetalis and placental hydrops. The placenta may be massively enlarged due to edema.

Of the transplacental infections represented by the acronym TORCH, the initial *H*, for herpes simplex infections, is erroneously included. These infections are almost always acquired in the same fashion as the amniotic sac infections, namely, at the end of pregnancy when membranes have ruptured or when the baby passes through the birth canal. The inoculation takes place from the infected maternal genitalia. Some cases of hepatitis B are contracted early but most are contracted at the time of delivery when exposure to maternal blood is extensive. The same may be true for some cases of HIV infection.

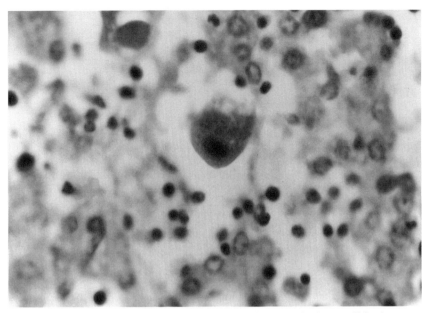

Fig. 5-7. Lung from fetus infected with cytomegalovirus. The large cell in the center has a smudged enlarged nucleus that represents an inclusion composed of the viral colony. Hematoxylin and eosin stain, original magnification X1000.

Neonatal Jaundice

Causes of neonatal hyperbilirubinemia fall into three main categories:

1. Overproduction of bilirubin. This is always the result of excessive red cell destruction, either because of hemolysis or from mobilization of hemoglobin from a hematoma.
2. Failure of the hepatocyte to conjugate or to excrete bilirubin.
3. Mechanical or functional obstruction to the excretion of the bile from the liver.

In overproduction hyperbilirubinemia and in failure to conjugate, the unconjugated bilirubin is elevated, whereas in obstructive jaundice, the conjugated fraction is high. Unconjugated bilirubin is fat-soluble and capable of entering the brain across the blood-brain barrier. It is toxic to the developing nervous system, especially in acidotic states, and causes irreversible neuronal necrosis and pigment deposition, especially in the basal ganglia (kernicterus). Long-term sequelae are motor disturbances, deafness, mental retardation, and seizures.

Historically, the most common cause of neonatal hyperbilirubinemia has been Rh incompatibility leading to hemolytic disease of the newborn, but widespread use of Rh immune globulin has made that condition a

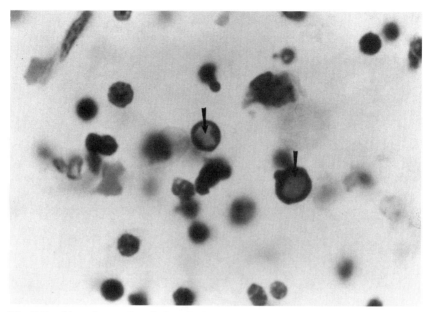

Fig. 5-8. Liver from a fetus infected with parvovirus, B19. The two larger cells in the center each have cleared chromatin in the center of the nucleus. These lighter areas are colonies of parvovirus *(arrows)*. Hematoxylin and eosin stain, original magnification X1000.

rarity. Problems with other blood groups, especially ABO incompatibilities, are frequently associated with neonatal jaundice. In certain populations red-cell membrane defects and hemoglobinopathies such as alpha-thalassemia constitute important causes of neonatal anemia and jaundice. Mobilization of excess bilirubin from extravasated red cells is a complication of neonatal hemorrhage, for example from intracerebral hemorrhage or trauma.

The normal neonatal liver does not conjugate bilirubin effectively during the first few days of life, and consequently some otherwise normal neonates become jaundiced in the first days of life, until the conjugation pathway "matures." This maturation delay is referred to as physiologic jaundice, and resolves spontaneously or may be treated with minimal phototherapy. The problem may be prolonged by breast milk feedings and is exacerbated by prematurity. Inborn errors of bilirubin conjugation (for example, Crigler-Najjar syndrome) are extremely rare.

Two main groups of diseases cause conjugated or direct hyperbilirubinemia: anatomic or mechanical lesions that physically obstruct the flow of bile, and functional or metabolic deficits in bile excretion. Bile plugs, atresia of the extrahepatic biliary tree, and choledochal cysts are the most common mechanical obstructions. Extrahepatic biliary atresia is thought to result from intrauterine or perinatal inflammatory sclerosis of the bile ducts and is considered a disruption rather than a malformation. The etiology is at present unknown. Until recently, biliary atresia has been a uniformly fatal condition, but advances in surgical treatment (porto-enterostomy and orthotopic liver transplantation) now permit survival of many infants (Fig. 5-9).

So-called intrahepatic biliary atresia is a feature of many different conditions. The preferred name is *paucity of intrahepatic ducts*. In some cases the condition is inherited as part of an autosomal-dominant syndrome with pulmonary stenosis or atresia; this constellation is called *Alagille syndrome*.

Cholestasis without a demonstrable anatomic obstruction is a feature of many inflammatory, infectious, and metabolic conditions (Fig. 5-10). The excretory defect may be intracellular, in the hepatocyte, or at the level of the bile canaliculi. Some of the metabolic conditions associated with cholestasis are familial and are inherited in Mendelian fashion. Galactosemia and alpha-1-antitrypsin deficiency are the most common metabolic disorders that cause neonatal jaundice. Neonatal bacterial sepsis, many of the congenital viral infections, and toxoplasmosis may also cause hepatitis and cholestasis. The most common iatrogenic cause is parenteral nutrition.

Neonatal giant cell transformation is a peculiar morphologic reaction of the neonatal liver to many different stimuli, including most of the above conditions. When all known infectious, metabolic, or anatomic causes have been excluded, the diagnosis of idiopathic neonatal giant cell hepatitis is appropriate.

The differential diagnosis of neonatal jaundice is difficult and the list of causes is lengthy. Hemolysis and hemorrhage are relatively easy to detect with routinely available imaging and laboratory testing, but differentiation of the myriad infectious, metabolic, and obstructive conditions may ultimately require sophisticated imaging techniques, liver biopsy, or exploratory surgery. An outline of the differential diagnosis of neonatal jaundice is given in Table 5-3.

Metabolic Diseases

Neonatal metabolic disorders can lead to irreversible damage to the brain and other organs, and can cause death. For some of these disorders, dietary or endocrine treatment is available and may ameliorate or even completely prevent long-term sequelae.

Newborn screening for certain metabolic disorders is mandated in most states. The test menu varies, but screening for phenylketonuria, galactosemia, and hypothyroidism is almost universal. These diseases illustrate and fulfill the basic criteria for effective neonatal screening, namely:

1. That the disease be detectable in the neonate with the test used.
2. That effective treatment is available that prevents many or all of the ill effects of the disease.

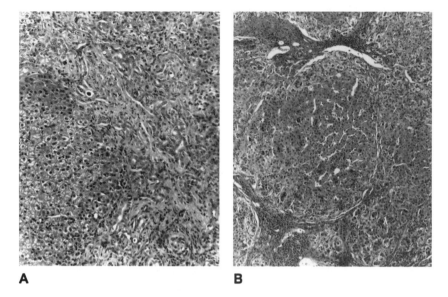

A   B

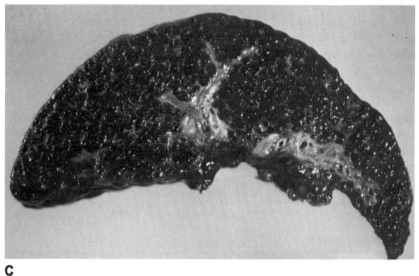

C

Fig. 5-9.   The evolution of cirrhosis in extrahepatic biliary atresia. The early (A) and
the late (B) stages of the disease. Obstruction causes proliferation of bile ducts and
fibrosis in the portal areas. This proliferation evolves over months to years into dense
fibrosis, marked cholestasis, and gradual disappearance of interlobular bile ducts.
Hematoxylin and eosin stain, original magnification x100. (C) The shrunken and
nodular appearance of a cirrhotic liver removed at the time of orthotopic liver
transplantation.

Table 5-3.   Differential diagnosis of neonatal jaundice

Obstruction
  Biliary atresia
  Choledochal cyst
  Paucity of intrahepatic bile ducts
Infection
  Neonatal sepsis
  Congenital or perinatally acquired bacterial or viral infection
  Toxoplasmosis
Increased red cell destruction
  Hemolytic anemias
  Isoimmunization
  Thalassemia
  Sickle-cell disease
  Hemorrhage
Metabolic disorders
  Galactosemia
  Alpha-1-antitrypsin deficiency
  Tyrosinemia
  Neonatal hemachromatosis
  Niemann-Pick disease, type C
Chromosomal disorders
  Trisomy 18, 22
  Monosomy X
Iatrogenic disorders
  Parenteral nutrition
  Drug toxicity
"Physiologic jaundice"
Idiopathic neonatal hepatitis

---

3. That the prevalence in the screened population and the severity
    of the condition warrant the costs of the screening program.

Screening programs may reflect geographic and ethnic variations in prevalence of some diseases. It makes sense for example to screen black persons
for sickle-cell disease and Asian persons for alpha-thalassemia. Screening
tests are more sensitive than they are specific and always require confirmation by definitive testing. Screening programs, however effective, can detect only a portion of newborn metabolic diseases. Accurate and timely
diagnosis of most metabolic disorders still relies on recognition of clinical
and laboratory findings that raise the suspicion of metabolic disease. These
features are summarized in Tables 5-4 and 5-5.

The list of metabolic diseases that may be manifested in the newborn
period is very long; Table 5-6 lists some of the more important ones. All
are rare and may require definitive diagnostic tests that are performed in

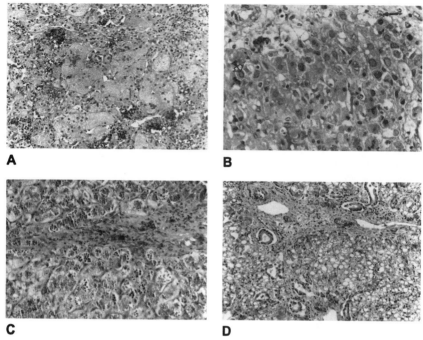

Fig. 5-10. Some of the conditions that cause neonatal jaundice have highly characteristic or even diagnostic morphologic features. (A) Idiopathic neonatal giant cell hepatitis. Many different diseases cause this peculiar appearance of the hepatocytes. Hematoxylin and eosin stain, original magnification x200. (B) Neonatal disseminated herpes infection. The diagnostic intranuclear inclusions are of two types: glassy inclusion *(clear arrow)* filling the entire nucleus and smaller haloed forms *(solid arrow)*. Hematoxylin and eosin stain, original magnification x400. (C) In alpha-1-antitrypsin deficiency liver cells contain cytoplasmic inclusions that consist of alpha-1-antitrypsin trapped in the endoplasmic reticulum (dark granular deposits). Hematoxylin and eosin stain, original magnification x200. (D) Extensive hepatocyte fatty change with fibrosis is a hallmark of metabolic derangement, in this case galactosemia. Hematoxylin and eosin stain, original magnification x100.

a few highly specialized laboratories. In many cases, readily available laboratory tests may serve to narrow the list of possibilities once suspicion is raised. Some of these useful and widely available laboratory methods are listed in Table 5-7 and may point the way to specific enzyme or DNA studies.

Disorders Associated with Multiple Births

The natural incidence of twinning in the United States is once in 90 live births. Triplets occur naturally once in $(90)^2$, or 8100 live births; quadruplets once in $(90)^3$, or 729,000 live births, and so on. Multiple gestations occur with higher frequencies but many if not most of these are spontaneously reduced in early gestation to singletons or are completely aborted. Drugs used to increase fertility may induce polyovulation so that multiple

Table 5-4. Signs and symptoms of metabolic disease in the newborn

Disorders of growth (intrauterine growth retardation, macrosomia)
Skeletal abnormalities (dwarfism, fractures, growth delay, abnormal bone density)
Dysmorphic features
Altered neurologic states (lethargy, coma, seizures)
Abnormal muscle tone (floppiness, jitteriness)
Feeding difficulties (vomiting, diarrhea)
Edema or hydrops
Hepatomegaly or cardiomegaly, or both
Jaundice
Abnormalities of skin and hair color or texture
Peculiar odors (maple syrup, sweaty feet)
Ocular abnormalities (cataract, corneal clouding, cherry red spots)

Table 5-5. Laboratory data suggestive of metabolic disease in the newborn

Anemia or leukopenia (especially with abnormal morphology)
Hyperbilirubinemia
Hypo- or hyperglycemia
Acidosis or alkalosis
Hyperammonemia
Ketosis
Electrolyte abnormalities

births have recently become iatrogenically increased. Monozygous (identical) twins are born in similar proportionate numbers to mothers of all races and ethnic groups, whereas dizygous twins are much more frequent among some ethnic groups, e.g., central African women, than among other ethnic groups, e.g., central European women.

Intrauterine growth of each twin, triplet, or quadruplet progresses at the same rate as that of a singleton until the sum of fetal weights is about 3000 g. Growth rates then slow as gestation continues. In the case of twins, when each is about 1500 g, or at about 33 to 34 weeks' gestation, growth rates diminish; in the case of triplets, growth rates diminish when each weighs about 1000 g, or at about 27 to 28 weeks' gestation.

Monozygous (identical) twins have up to a three-fold increase in congenital malformations compared with dizygous (fraternal) twins or singletons. A single umbilical artery is commonly observed in the umbilical cord of monozygous twins. More serious malformations, e.g., congenital heart disease and genitourinary and gastrointestinal anomalies are also observed.

The first-born of twins or triplets is more apt to be infected than her or his second- or third-born siblings. This is because of proximity to the birth canal from which ascending amniotic sac infections originate. The second-born of twins or the third-born of triplets is more apt to be asphyxi-

Table 5-6. Metabolic diseases in newborns

Disorders of carbohydrate metabolism
  Galactosemia
  Some glycogen storage diseases
  Hereditary fructose intolerance
  Mucopolysaccharidoses
Disorders of amino- and organic-acid metabolism
  Tyrosinemia
  Maple syrup urine disease
  Methylmalonic acidemia
  Disorders of pyruvate metabolism
  Nonketotic hyperglycinemia
Disorders of urea metabolism
  Ornithine transcarbamylase deficiency
  Carbamyl phosphate synthetase deficiency
Cystic fibrosis
Disorders of mitochondrial oxidation
Peroxisomal disorders
Alpha-1-antitrypsin deficiency
Endocrine disorders
  Congenital adrenal hyperplasia
  Congenital hypothyroidism
  Congenital hypoparathyroidism (DiGeorge syndrome)

ated than her or his earlier-born siblings. The reason is not entirely clear although parturition of the first-born results in reduced utero-placental blood flow and this is repeated with parturition of the second (and third) fetus.

The twin-to-twin transfusion (T^4) syndrome occurs only between monozygotic twins (or monozygotic siblings in triplets, quadruplets, etc.) through anastamoses between the siblings' circulations in a common placenta. In chronic T^4 syndrome, marked disparities occur in the sizes of the fetuses and their viscera. The recipient's heart, spleen, liver, and kidneys are much larger than the donor's organs. The hematocrit of the recipient is often 20 percent higher than that of the donor, so plethora is common in the recipient, and pallor is common in the donor. The recipients have more morbidity and higher rates of death than the donors because of circulatory overload, heart failure, or hyperviscosity with tissue hypoxia. In acute T^4 syndrome, the donor may have profound anemia that is sometimes fatal.

The dead twin syndrome occurs only in monozygotic twins (or between monozygotic siblings in triplets, quadruplets, etc.). In such cases, one of the siblings dies in utero while the other survives. In a small proportion of such cases, probably fewer than 25 percent, the surviving twin has necrotic lesions of the skin, extremities, brain, or viscera. Portions of the skin may

Table 5-7. Laboratory aids to diagnosis of metabolic diseases

Placental examination for storage diseases, hydrops, and erythroblastosis
Urinary metabolites
  Reducing substances
  Mucopolysaccharides
  Organic acids
  Amino acids
Peripheral blood smear for vacuolated leukocytes
Biopsy of skin, conjunctiva, bone marrow, or liver for light and electron microscopy
Muscle biopsy for electron microscopy, enzyme histochemistry
Protein and hemoglobin electrophoresis

be absent. The kidneys, spleen, and brain are particularly prone to necrosis. In babies who do not succumb to these lesions, fibrosis and atrophy are noted. The pathogenesis is unclear. One explanation is that the dead twin releases necrosis-promoting substances (perhaps cytokines) into the circulation of the surviving twin. A second explanation is that a single critical event occurs, lethal to one twin and sublethal but devastating to the surviving twin.

Congenital Malformations

Central Nervous System
Because development of the CNS occurs over the entire gestational period and well into postnatal life, the nervous system is subject to a wide variety of types and severity of defects. Structural malformations of the brain and spinal cord may be classified in three broad categories with considerable overlap.

    1. Disorders of induction of neurulation and closure of the neural tube. These are examples of true developmental malformation and occur very early in gestation, within the first month.

    2. Disorders of neural proliferation and migration. These are for the most part disorders arising in the third to fifth months of gestation; they may be either malformations or disruptions.

    3. Encephaloclastic defects are caused by destruction or disruption of a normal developmental process and may occur at any time. It is important, though often difficult, to distinguish these lesions from malformations so that appropriate genetic counseling may be done.

    Disturbances of induction of the neural plate are relatively rare and usually are anterior. The one most frequently encountered in clinical practice is holoprosencephaly, which is the result of failure of the forebrain to divide sagittally into two halves. Because the anterior neural tube induces development of the eyes, olfactory apparatus, and face, this anomaly is frequently associated with facial defects that may range from barely perceptible hypotelorism (closely set eyes) to cyclopia. Holoprosencephaly is sometimes a part of chromosomal syndromes, especially trisomy 13 (Fig. 5-11).

Disorders of closure of the neural tube, or dysraphism, are thought to be multifactorial. The geographic incidence varies widely. They are amenable to prenatal diagnosis with ultrasound and maternal serum alpha-fetoprotein and recent data indicate that some may be prevented with maternal preconceptional folic acid supplementation. The spectrum of closure defects ranges from small defects within the cord, invisible externally (diastematomyelia, or split cord, and hydromyelia, a cyst in the cord), to absence of the brain (anencephaly) and completely open spinal cord (rachischisis or craniorachischisis). Intermediate lesions are cystic herniations of meninges (meningocele) or of meninges and nervous tissue (encephalocele, meningomyelocele). A minority of these deficits occur as part of malformation syndromes, with recognized Mendelian inheritance, and others may be mimicked by acquired destructive or deforming conditions, particularly premature amniotic rupture or "amniotic band" sequence.

Hydrocephalus consists of enlargement of the ventricular system at the expense of the brain; it is frequently a component of dysraphic conditions such as meningomyelocele in the Arnold-Chiari malformation.

Hydrocephalus may result from stenosis of the aqueduct (either developmental or acquired), obstruction of reabsorption of CSF by arachnoidal fibrosis, and "hydrocephalus ex vacuo" resulting from loss of brain parenchyma and its replacement by CSF. During fetal and infant life, the cranial sutures are not fused; the cranial vault can expand in response to increased CSF pressure. For this reason hydrocephalus frequently leads to a large head.

Disorders of neuronal proliferation, migration, and maturation give rise to defects characterized by disorganization of the cerebrum and cerebellum. Serious disturbances result in abnormal gyration patterns: lissencephaly (smooth brain, or lack of normal gyri), pachygyria (fat gyri), polymicrogyria (excessive tiny convolutions), or heterotopic gray matter masses.

Once neurons achieve their correct location, disorders of arborization, synaptic connection, and myelination may interrupt the normal developmental progression. Some disorders of migration and maturation are obvious, and others require extremely intricate procedures for their demonstration at the microscopic level. It appears that these subtle abnormalities may be responsible for some forms of retardation, epilepsy, and other neuronal dysfunctions.

Encephaloclastic lesions also take many forms, depending on the timing, nature, and severity of the insult. These defects are caused by destruction of the developing nervous system by toxic or metabolic insult,

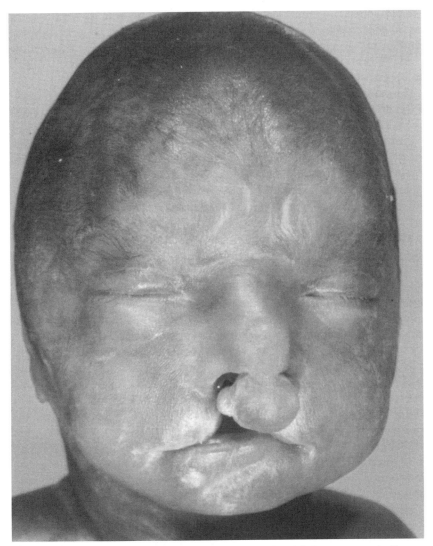

Fig. 5-11.   Cleft lip and cleft palate may occur as isolated defects or as part of a malformation complex as in this infant with trisomy 13.

infection, vascular accidents, or anoxia. An example is the microcephaly and hydrocephalus resulting from intrauterine necrosis of brain, as in congenital toxoplasmosis.

Cardiovascular System
Congenital heart defects may occur as part of a genetically determined syndrome in which recurrence risk is high and prenatal diagnosis is

feasible. Most congenital heart diseases occur as sporadic isolated defects with multifactorial causes and are of two physiologic types: abnormal shunts between pulmonary and systemic circuits and obstructions to blood flow in one or both circuits. Frequently these occur in combinations of considerable complexity.

The most common shunts are persistent patency of the foramen ovale or the ductus arteriosus. Patent foramen ovale or other atrial septal defects are rarely symptomatic in newborns. Patent ductus arteriosus is a frequent finding in premature infants, and in the setting of elevated pulmonary artery pressure may significantly contribute to morbidity by further decreasing pulmonary blood flow. Ventricular septal defects (VSD) are less common but more serious. The severity depends on the size of the hole and on associated defects. Some VSDs close spontaneously. About one-fifth of VSD patients have other serious defects that contribute to morbidity and mortality. Large combined atrial and ventricular septal defects are called atrioventricular canal defects and result from failure of or defective endocardial cushion development. This defect is frequently associated with Down syndrome. Because both mitral and tricuspid valves are defective, atrioventricular canal defects cause heart failure at an early age.

Persistent truncus arteriosus (or common aortopulmonary trunk) is a rare left-to-right shunt usually leading to early heart failure.

Transposition of the great arteries (i.e., aorta arising from the right ventricle and pulmonary artery from the left ventricle) is a fairly common form of congenital heart defect (Fig. 5-12). The pulmonary and systemic circuits operate in parallel instead of in series, and survival is dependent on the coexistence of a shunt, usually patent foramen ovale, patent ductus arteriosus, or ventricular septal defect.

Obstruction to flow is almost invariably associated with an intracardiac shunt at some level. Obstruction to pulmonary blood flow acts to decrease oxygenation and these babies are cyanotic. Systemic circuit obstructions produce heart failure, tissue hypoxia, and acidosis.

Babies with severe pulmonary arterial obstruction and an intact ventricular septum are critically ill in the neonatal period. Pulmonic stenosis or atresia with VSD usually occurs as tetralogy of Fallot (VSD, aorta displaced to the right overriding the VSD, pulmonary valvar or infundibular stenosis or atresia, and right ventricular hypertrophy). The condition is ameliorated by surgically creating systemic-to-pulmonary shunts.

Mitral and aortic stenosis accompanied by hypoplasia of the left ventricle and aorta is referred to as hypoplastic left heart syndrome. It usually causes death in the neonatal period. Operative repair is rarely successful but neonatal heart transplantation may offer some a chance of survival. Of concern are the associated congenital and acquired CNS defects in some babies with hypoplastic left heart syndromes.

Coarctation of the aorta and interrupted aortic arch may occur as isolated lesions or as part of complicated malformation.

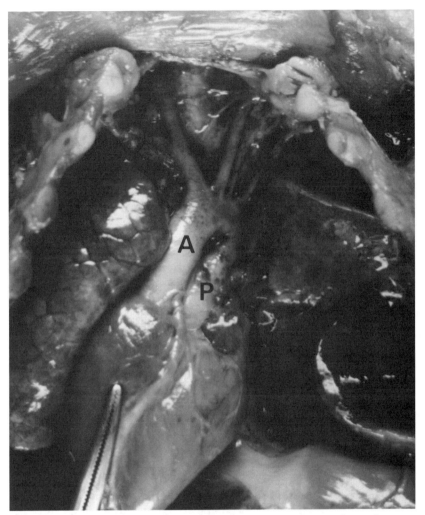

Fig. 5-12. Transposition of the great arteries. This is an infrequent form of congenital heart disease but is one of the more common cardiac anomalies seen at autopsy in neonates because of the severity of the disease. The aorta *(A)* arises from the right ventricle and the pulmonary artery *(P)* arises from the left ventricle. Surgical repair is feasible but difficult because of the need to switch the coronary arteries.

Anomalies of pulmonary venous return are uncommon but diagnostically challenging forms of left-to-right shunt. Anomalous pulmonary venous return may involve all or only part of the pulmonary veins, and the anomalous connections to the systemic veins occur in several anatomic varieties both above and below the diaphragm. Anomalies of systemic venous return usually do not cause clinical problems for the neonate.

Patients with asplenia or polysplenia have defective regulation of sidedness during embryologic development that leads to anomalies of visceral and atrial situs and of cardiac looping. The resulting cardiac lesions are varied and extremely complex.

Progress in surgical repair of congenital defects and in cardiac transplantation permits increasing duration and quality of survival for many infants with congenital heart diseases, but they remain an important cause of morbidity and mortality in neonates.

Respiratory System

Defects in the upper airway include choanal and laryngeal atresia and tracheoesophageal fistula. Cystic lung lesions are uncommon causes of neonatal respiratory distress. Bronchogenic cysts are probably related to aberrant rests of bronchial tissue. Segments of lung without connection to the bronchial tree are called *sequestrations*. Intralobar sequestrations are enveloped within the pleura of the ipsilateral lung; extralobar sequestrations have a separate pleural covering. Either may have a blood supply from the aorta. Other conditions that may present as cystic lung lesions are congenital cystic adenomatoid malformation of lung, a hamartomatous change that may be localized or involve an entire lobe, and congenital lobar emphysema (which is actually hyperinflation).

Hypoplastic lungs have a decreased number of bronchial generations or decreased acini (alveoli) and are usually less than half of the expected weight. Unilateral hypoplasia almost always results from a space-occupying mass in the hemithorax. Diaphragmatic hernia with displacement of intestine and liver into the chest is a common cause. Bilateral hypoplasia results from oligohydramnios; neuromuscular disease that limits intrauterine motion; and cartilaginous or bony disorders that limit thoracic size.

Gastrointestinal Tract

Anomalies of the intestinal tract include stenosis, atresia, and duplications. Esophageal atresia is usually associated with tracheoesophageal fistula and is the most frequent esophageal abnormality. These babies develop respiratory distress early because of aspiration of saliva or feedings. Tracheoesophageal fistula without atresia may go undetected until the infant or child develops recurrent aspiration pneumonia.

Gastric duplication is extremely rare, but gastric outlet obstruction due to hypertrophic pyloric stenosis is common. It is usually discovered after the first few weeks of life because of repeated vomiting, visible peristaltic waves, and a palpable epigastric mass.

Small intestinal duplications are uncommon and tend to become clinically evident only after they have amassed enough secretions to cause intestinal obstruction. This rarely occurs in the newborn period. Intestinal atresia, on the other hand, is discovered as soon as feeding begins, when signs of obstruction appear. Atresias may be single or multiple. Many are the result of intrauterine volvulus or other vascular catastrophes and are therefore disruptions rather than malformations. Meconium ileus associated with cystic fibrosis is an important cause of intestinal atresia.

Large intestinal duplication and atresia are very unusual. The most important congenital lesion of large bowel is Hirschsprung's disease, or congenital megacolon. Defective migration of autonomic ganglion cells results in an aganglionic segment of distal colon. The aganglionic segment does not contract in normal peristaltic waves, resulting in functional obstruction. Hirschsprung's disease does not often present in the neonatal period. Short aganglionic segments are relatively easily corrected surgically, but removal of long segments results in severe nutritional deficiency. Anorectal atresia (imperforate anus) may be associated with anomalies of the lower genitourinary tract. A constellation of vertebral, anal, tracheoesophageal, and renal anomalies (of undetermined etiology) is given the acronym VATER association. Sometimes congenital heart defects are a feature as well.

Genitourinary Tract
Renal agenesis is quite rare and may be either unilateral or bilateral; the bilateral condition is one of the many causes of the oligohydramnios sequence and is incompatible with life. True renal hypoplasia (i.e., a small but otherwise normal kidney with reduced number of calyces) is also quite rare. Most small kidneys in infants are dysplastic or atrophic.

Renal cysts are of several types, and it is important to distinguish them. Polycystic renal disease in childhood may be either autosomal recessive or dominant. These genetically determined bilateral diseases must be distinguished from cystic renal dysplasia, also known as multicystic kidney. The latter is a sporadic lesion with a very low recurrence rate. The differences are shown in Table 5-8. Many other rare forms of cystic disease are associated with a wide variety of inherited conditions like chondrodysplasia, Meckel's syndrome, and tuberous sclerosis.

Important malformations of the bladder include bladder exstrophy, in which the bladder opens directly in the defective anterior abdominal wall, and massive bladder dilatation associated with urethral obstruction. The latter is called *prune belly syndrome* because the anterior abdominal musculature is stretched over the huge bladder and fails to develop properly during intrauterine life. When the bladder is decompressed, the abdominal wall is lax and redundant with folds of skin resembling the surface of a prune (Fig. 5-13).

Duplications, ectopias, and fusions of all or part of the upper urinary tract usually become clinically apparent when complicated by urinary tract infections in older children (Fig. 5-14).

Ambiguous genitalia comprise a serious problem in the newborn and warrant prompt genetic, endocrine, and anatomic evaluation to determine appropriate gender assignment. Apart from important psychosocial

Table 5-8. Cystic diseases of neonatal kidneys

	Inheritance	Laterality	Liver cysts	Size/ Shape	Pathogenesis	Cysts
Infantile polycystic disease	Autosomal recessive	Bilateral	Always	Large reniform	Unknown	Collecting ducts, small radial cysts
Adult polycystic kidney	Autosomal dominant	Bilateral	Sometimes	Large, huge, irregular	Unknown	All parts of nephron, irregular, variable size
Renal dysplasia with cysts	Sporadic	Unilateral or bilateral	No	Small or large, irregular	Intrauterine obstruction of urethra, ureter, calyx, or tubule	Very irregular, all parts of nephron; may have cartilage

considerations, children with dysgenetic gonads are at risk for development of gonadal neoplasms, and some children with congenital adrenal hyperplasia have life-threatening salt loss.

Musculoskeletal System
Skeletal abnormalities and dwarfism in the newborn are frequently the result of inborn errors of metabolism affecting the growth and remodeling of bone and cartilage and disordered enchondral ossification. Dozens of skeletal dysplasias are recognized at present; genetically they are dominant, recessive, X-linked, and sporadic. Differentiating one from another is difficult. Some, like autosomal-dominant achondroplasia, are compatible with long life. Others, particularly those in which thoracic underdevelopment causes pulmonary hypoplasia, are lethal in the neonatal period (Fig. 5-15). Some are associated with renal disease.

  Osteogenesis imperfecta is a family of collagen disorders, of which many different types exist, characterized by fragile bones and multiple fractures. AD and AR inheritance are reported and new dominant mutations account for some sporadic cases. Congenital forms are usually lethal.

  Deformities of the skeleton also result from limited intrauterine space, as in oligohydramnios, and from a variety of neuromuscular diseases. Extreme positional deformities resulting in multiple contractures are termed arthrogryposis congenita. Arthrogryposis is not a disease entity but a phenotype that results from many different primary neuromuscular conditions.

Trauma and Iatrogenic Diseases
Throughout history, obstetric practices have been continuously monitored and modified in an effort to reduce maternal, fetal, and neonatal morbidity and mortality. This effort has been particularly successful in reducing

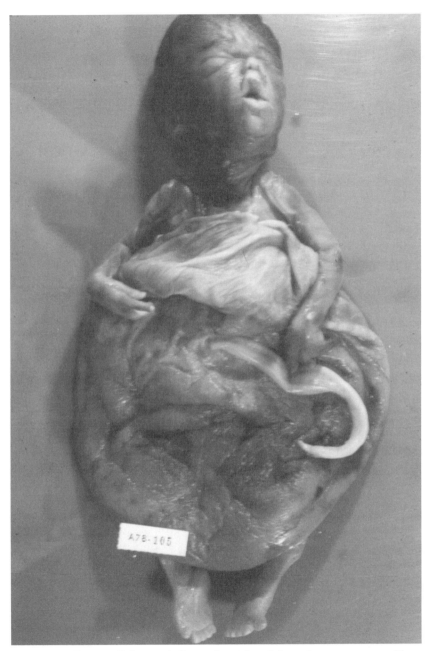

Fig. 5-13. The so-called prune belly syndrome is a deformation sequence resulting from massive bladder and abdominal distention due to lower urinary tract obstruction. Patients less severely affected than this infant may survive, though most have severe impairment of renal function.

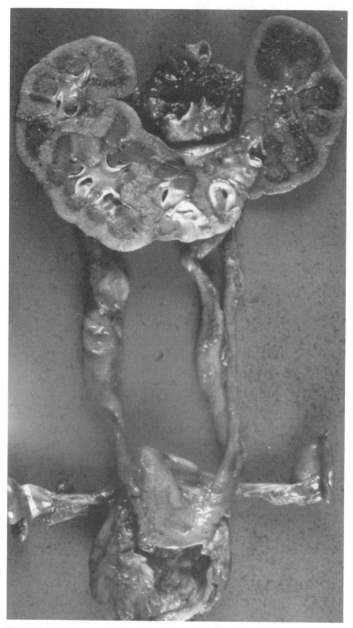

Fig. 5-14. The most common urinary tract malformations are
ectopias and duplications; this horseshoe kidney represents both.
Such defects are usually discovered only when altered anatomic
configuration leads to urinary tract obstruction and infection.

traumatic lesions of the fetus and neonate. Erb's palsy is paralysis and atrophy of an upper limb due to avulsion of the brachial plexus. Erb's palsy and spinal injuries most often occur in difficult breech deliveries or in cases of shoulder dystocia. Bell's palsy (facial nerve paralysis) is usually transient and results from trauma to the nerve. Fractures of the clavicle, humerus, and femur occur with difficult fetal presentations and deliveries. Skull fractures may be due to difficult presentations. Torticollis (wry neck) is believed, in some instances, to result from trauma to the sternocleidomastoid muscle in which a small benign fibrous tumor develops at the clavicular insertion. Skin abrasions are common and cause serious disease only rarely. Scalpel wounds occasionally result from cesarean section deliveries. (Few reports of such lesions have appeared in the literature. Most such wounds are small and easily repaired with practically no visual residual.) Needle punctures have been reported as complications of amniocentesis, percutaneous umbilical blood sampling (PUBS), and other invasive

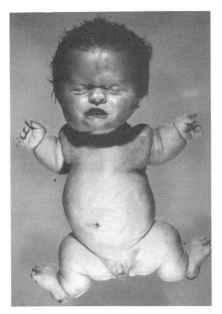
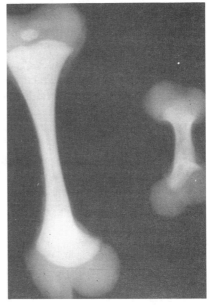

A   **B**

Fig. 5-15.   The chondrodysplasias are a large group of inborn disorders of bone and cartilage development. (A) Child with thanatophoric dysplasia, with short limbs and small thoracic cavity. Because of pulmonary hypoplasia, the condition is uniformly fatal. Most cases are thought to represent new dominant mutation, and recurrence risk is negligible. Thanatophoric dysplasia is easily confused with other mainly autosomal-recessive dysplasias. (B) Radiograph of a normal femur *(left)* and an affected femur *(right)*.

procedures. These are rarely serious lesions. Chorionic villus sampling (CVS) is associated with a minimal increased risk for spontaneous abortion. Recent studies associate CVS with defective growth of one or more limbs but the mechanism for this is unclear.

Trauma to visceral organs is rare. Ruptures of the liver or the adrenals were often mentioned in the past; however, it appears now that capsular rupture of the liver with hematoma or hemorrhage is a disease of premature infants with very low birth weights and is most often associated with infection and asphyxia, not trauma. Adrenal hemorrhage is now recognized as a lesion associated with severe asphyxia.

The advent of neonatal intensive care has produced a remarkable improvement in the outcome of babies born prematurely or with difficulties preceding or during labor. On the other hand, artificial respiration has been associated with such lesions as bronchopulmonary dysplasia (BPD), the neonatal form of oxygen toxicity. This condition is considered a part of the sequence of unrelenting respiratory distress syndrome of the premature neonate. The changes of BPD are different from those in adults in whom the lung has long since ceased to develop. BPD includes vascular proliferation and fibrous proliferation in an irregular pattern throughout the lobules of the lung. Areas of atelectasis, congestion, fibrosis, and destruction of the pulmonary parenchymal tissue alternate with areas that are normally formed but often hyperdistended. This imparts a coarse bubbly appearance to the lung on x-ray.

Other common iatrogenic conditions result from indwelling catheters and tubes. Insertion of an endotracheal tube for respirator therapy may result in necrosis of the laryngeal, tracheal, and bronchial mucosa. Mechanical trauma is not entirely the cause. The more distal lesions are attributed to a combination of oxygen and barotrauma. In a noncompliant lung, mechanically assisted respiration can result in pneumothorax. The treatment may require a chest tube. If inserted carefully, this is usually without untoward incident but in some instances, pulmonary tissue may be pierced by the chest tube. If more than one chest tube is required in the same area of the same lung, the first one probably pierced the lung and created another source for pneumothorax.

Indwelling catheters in vessels may result in thrombi if left for more than a few days. The intravascular thrombi can break away and embolize to smaller radicals in the vascular tree. Gangrene of the toes or feet is sometimes a result. Infarcts of the kidneys and adrenals and gastrointestinal tract may also result. For some reason, pulmonary infarcts are rare in neonates, even when a catheter has been placed in the venous system for long periods of time.

Another iatrogenic syndrome is also an infectious syndrome, namely, sepsis in intensively treated neonates. The organisms responsible for this type of sepsis are coagulase-positive and coagulase-negative *Staphylococci*, *Pseudomonas,* and fungal and yeast organisms, especially *Candida albicans.*

Disseminated lesions including abscesses are found throughout the organs of the entire body.

Neonatal Neoplasms

Congenital and neonatal tumors are rare, occurring only at a rate of 1 to 4 per 100,000 live births. Because they are frequently very large, even grotesque, they are alarming to both parents and physicians. The majority are benign, and even in cases in which the morphology is unmistakably malignant, the clinical behavior in the newborn is frequently (and paradoxically) that of a benign neoplasm.

Most types of neoplasia have been reported in the neonate, but only four groups account for the majority of congenital and neonatal tumors: neuroblastoma, soft-tissue tumors, teratoma, and congenital leukemia.

Neuroblastoma is the most common truly malignant congenital neoplasm. Morphologically, neonatal neuroblastomas are indistinguishable from those of older children, but it is clear that neonatal and young infants have neuroblastomas that frequently behave in a clinically benign fashion even when widely disseminated. Spontaneous regression is more common in neuroblastoma than any other human malignancy, and differentiation and maturation to benign neural tumors are well documented. A minority behave as fully malignant neoplasms. It has so far been difficult to predict malignant behavior, but lytic skeletal lesions and large numbers of copies of N-*myc* oncogene are poor prognostic signs. Because of this unpredictability and also because of the enhanced risks of cytotoxic therapy in the very young, treatment for newborns and young infants with neuroblastoma is very conservative. Up to one-third of neonates with neuroblastoma have other growth disturbances or developmental defects, often involving the autonomic nervous system, such as Beckwith-Wiedemann syndrome, von Recklinghausen's neurofibromatosis, or Hirschsprung's disease. These and other associations of congenital neoplasms with genetic and developmental defects strongly suggest that the development of neoplasia is related to dysembryogenesis and genomic alterations.

Soft-tissue tumors are overall the most common neoplasms in the neonate. The overwhelming majority are benign. Vascular neoplasms (hemangiomas and lymphomas) constitute the majority, and virtually all behave in a benign fashion, though the clinical and microscopic appearance may be alarming. Many hemangiomas undergo spontaneous regression. Tumors of adipose tissue and fibrous tissue also may be large and histologically very active but these usually do not metastasize and are controlled by surgery. Some biologically nonmetastasizing lesions may be fatal because of local invasiveness and compromise of vital unresectable structures.

An exception to the generally innocuous behavior of soft-tissue neoplasms is embryonal rhabdomyosarcoma. Benign skeletal muscle tumors are extremely rare; most of the skeletal muscle tumors are truly malignant.

Peripheral nerve sheath tumors and bone neoplasms are rarely encountered in neonates but may be malignant. Wilms' tumor is also very rare in newborns. Most newborn renal masses are either dysplastic kidneys or mesoblastic nephroma, a benign connective tissue tumor unique to the young infant's kidney.

Germ cell tumors in the neonatal period are mainly represented by benign cystic teratomas. The most frequent site is the sacrococcygeal area. Teratomas frequently contain immature elements that are histologically alarming but not necessarily indicative of malignancy. Rare examples exist of neonatal malignant germ cell tumors, mainly endodermal sinus tumors.

Congenital leukemias are rare and congenital dysmyelopoietic syndromes are unusual. In contrast to the situation in older children, most newborn leukemias are myeloid, not lymphoid. Congenital leukemia has a very high mortality rate, and so must be distinguished, often with difficulty, from leukemoid reactions accompanying other conditions. Congenital leukemia is associated with genetic or chromosomal disorders including trisomies 13, 15, and 21; Bloom syndrome; Turner's syndrome; and Fanconi's anemia.

Recommended Reading

Carter, B. S., Haverkamp, A. D., and Merenstein, G. B. The definition of acute perinatal asphyxia. In S. Shankaran (ed.), *Clin. Perinatol.* 20:287–305, 1993.

Coffin, C., and Dehner, L. P. Congenital tumors. In J. T. Stocker and L. P. Dehner (eds.), *Pediatric Pathology.* Philadelphia: Lippincott, 1992. Pp. 325–354.

Galdstone, I. M., et al. A 10-year review of neonatal sepsis and comparison with the previous 50 years experience. *Pediatr. Infect. Dis. J.* 9:819–825, 1990.

Gilbert-Barness, E., and Opitz, J. *Congenital Anomalies and Pediatric Pathology.* Philadelphia: Lippincott, 1992. Pp. 73–116.

Nelson, K. B., and Ellenberg, J. H. Antecedents of cerebral palsy. *N. Engl. J. Med.* 315:81–86, 1986.

Wigglesworth, J. S., and Singer, D. B. *Textbook of Fetal and Prenatal Pathology.* Boston: Blackwell, 1991.

Neonatal Adaptation

William Cashore

After delivery, the newborn infant must independently assume all functions performed or regulated by the placenta during fetal life. These include oxygen and carbon dioxide exchange and transport, temperature stabilization, nutrition, maintenance and development of body composition, and excretion. Major functional changes must occur immediately after birth, followed by gradual adaptation and maturation in many body systems.

Respiration

During the later stages of labor, fetal PO_2 decreases and PCO_2 increases slightly. These physiologic changes in blood gas tension may contribute to the biochemical stimuli for the onset of breathing at birth. In fact, term infants undergoing more severe hypoxemic stress may begin gasping respirations while still in utero, with some risk of aspirating amniotic fluid and its contents. At delivery, the onset of breathing is also stimulated by cold stress and tactile sensation, as well as the physiologic perinatal increase in PCO_2 and decrease in PO_2 just before birth. The physiologic forces of labor may also elaborate secretion of stored surfactant in the terminal airways, preparing the lung for mechanical stabilization with the onset of breathing. This apparent increase in the availability of pulmonary surfactant is most notable in term infants and may be mediated by an increase in circulating cortisol and thyroxin levels during labor.

Vaginal delivery may expel some amniotic fluid from the trachea and other airways by chest compression during passage through the birth canal. Immediately after delivery, elastic recoil of the compressed thorax may then add to the mechanical forces that help to initiate the first breath. The physiologic onset of regular breathing occurs within the first 1 to 2 minutes after birth in normal infants. Breathing usually starts with one or two gasps, which create a large gradient in transthoracic pressure, to open first the proximal and then the distal airways. Transthoracic pressure and airway patency are then maintained by expansion of the distal airways and forced expiration against a closed glottis, often noted by those attending at birth as a series of grunts, whimpers, or lusty cries. The cry effectively stabilizes the airways and creates a functional residual capacity, as the elaborated surfactant forms a monolayer to coat the distal airways. Within the first few minutes, the normal lung stabilizes, a functional residual capacity develops, and the work of breathing changes from the initial strong gasps that first open the lung, to more shallow and stable respirations, usually at a rate of 30 to 50 breaths per minute.

Even though thoracic compression expels some amniotic fluid from the upper airway, for some time after birth the newborn lung contains small residual amounts of amniotic fluid. Over the first several hours of normal respiration, the fluid in the more distal airways is absorbed across the epithelium and carried away by the lymphatics. In the first few hours, many newborns, while making a satisfactory adjustment, have somewhat "wet" breath sounds on auscultation with a stethoscope. A few infants fail to reabsorb the amniotic fluid promptly; these infants may show signs of a mild aspiration pneumonia, or retained water in the interstitial spaces of the lung. Such infants may persist for some hours or even a few days with rapid, nondistressed respirations and occasionally a low-level requirement for supplemental oxygen. The condition of tachypnea with failure to clear the amniotic fluid promptly is known clinically as *transient tachypnea of the newborn*, or "retained lung fluid." This condition is occasionally seen in otherwise normal infants, and usually takes 1 to 3 days for spontaneous resolution.

Several more pathological conditions are worth mentioning here. *Respiratory distress syndrome* of the newborn is caused by deficiency of pulmonary surfactant and is seen predominantly in premature infants, although occasionally it is seen in term infants. It is characterized by progressive atelectasis and oxygen need over the first several postnatal days, as the surfactant-deficient lung cannot maintain stable expansion. Respiratory distress syndrome due to surfactant deficiency is the most common pulmonary disorder of newborn infants. *Neonatal pneumonia* may result from antenatal or perinatal aspiration of bacterially contaminated amniotic fluid. Although group B *Streptococcus* is the most common cause of neonatal bacterial pneumonia, a number of other bacterial pathogens can also cause this condition, which clinically resembles respiratory distress syndrome and which requires prompt recognition and antibiotic treatment. On physical and radiologic examination, respiratory distress syndrome and neonatal pneumonia may appear similar in their initial stages.

Postnatal Circulatory Adaptation

Following delivery, the neonatal circulation undergoes a complex set of adjustments, some of them immediately postnatal and others more gradual. With the first few breaths, both arterial and venous oxygen tension (PO_2) markedly increase in the neonatal circulation. In response to increasing PO_2, and perhaps in response to the mechanical forces of delivery and cord clamping as well, the umbilical arteries and vein constrict. This constriction is mainly an effect of endothelial exposure to increased oxygen concentration. The pulmonary capillary bed rapidly expands. With stabilization of the lung, and an abrupt local increase in PO_2, the pulmonary end arteries and capillaries dilate, while the circumferential smooth muscle of the ductus arteriosus constricts. Dilation of the pulmonary vascular bed and constriction of the ductus arteriosus both appear to be mediated by prostaglandin released on exposure of the vessel walls to increased oxygen.

As the lungs expand, pulmonary vascular resistance decreases and pulmonary blood flow increases. With constriction of the ductus arteriosus, which previously shunted blood from the right ventricle to the descending aorta, the right ventricular output is now directed to the pulmonary arteries and the lungs. The right and left ventricular outputs, which in fetal life existed "in parallel" through intracardiac and extracardiac shunts, now become functionally separate and take place "in series" starting with venous return to the right atrium and pulmonary circulation via the right ventricle (Fig. 6-1). The pulmonary circulation therefore becomes right-sided, and the systemic circulation left-sided, with return of oxygenated blood to the left atrium via the pulmonary veins. As pulmonary vascular and right ventricular pressures fall, systemic or left-sided pressures rise as the left ventricle now becomes the chamber perfusing the rest of the body. This change also elevates left atrial pressure to slightly above right atrial pressure. The foramen ovale, which shunted right to left before birth as a result of high right-sided pressures, now reverses flow as left atrial pressure rises in response to the systemic load. A membranous flap that permitted a right-to-left shunt through the foramen ovale now closes over the foramen, functionally separating the atria from each other. Gradually, this flap is molded to the atrial wall, forming a permanent atrial septum.

In summary, the closure of antenatal shunts with the onset of neonatal breathing and circulation is mediated by both biochemical and mechanical forces. Oxygen and prostaglandin $F_{2\text{-alpha}}$ constrict the ductus venosus, the ductus arteriosus, and the umbilical vessels. The change in pressure gradient between the left and the right atria closes the foramen ovale. Gradually, the endothelium of these closed shunts grows together, making the closures permanent.

Shunts may persist at the level of the foramen ovale or the ductus arteriosus during the initial period of neonatal circulatory adaptation (12–24 hours, or slightly longer in some infants). These shunts may be left-to-right, right-to-left, or bidirectional (alternating in flow direction with

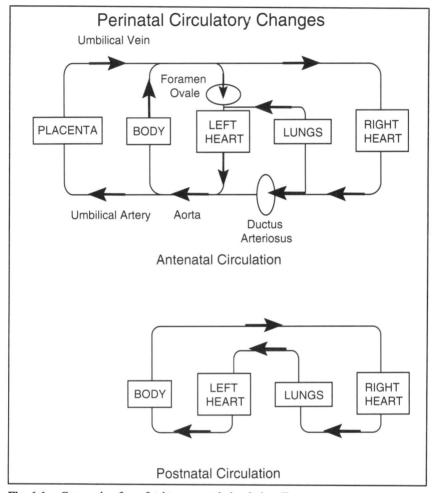

Fig. 6-1. Conversion from fetal to neonatal circulation. Exposure to oxygen constricts the ductus arteriosus. As the placenta, a low-resistance circuit, is removed, left ventricular and left atrial pressures rise, and a membranous portion of the left atrial wall closes over the foramen ovale. Right- and left-sided circulations, which were partially in parallel during fetal life, are now fully in series.

systole and diastole), depending on metabolic demands and the time course of pressure changes between pulmonic and systemic circulations. Occasionally, increased intrathoracic pressure, e.g., with crying, may briefly produce right-to-left shunting associated with transient cyanosis. Clinically, the persistence of shunts means that up to one-third of newborns without anatomic heart disease may have heart murmurs at some time during the neonatal period. These "functional" murmurs without signs of obstructive or cyanotic heart disease are usually evanescent incidental findings in asymptomatic healthy-appearing infants. These murmurs become less frequent and less audible as shunts close permanently.

Thermal Regulation and Energy Requirements

Regulation of body temperature is another important physiologic function in neonatal adaptation. Most infants accomplish this without difficulty, but the ability of a newborn to respond to extremes in environmental temperature is somewhat limited, compared to that of an adult. Newborns do not generate heat by shivering or dissipate heat by perspiration. Newborns dissipate excess heat by radiant and convective heat loss, and by tachypnea, which produces some evaporation and heat loss from the airways.

In response to a marked lowering of environmental temperature, newborns produce heat by recycling subcutaneous brown fat, which is found in several body regions, but chiefly in the posterior neck and subscapular areas. Because the production of heat by lipolysis of brown fat is a less efficient and more energy-consuming process than shivering, neonatal energy and oxygen consumption to regulate temperature is greater than in adults.

For maintenance of normal body temperature, the newborn does best in a *thermal-neutral zone* of environmental temperature. The thermal-neutral zone is the environmental temperature at which thermal regulation is optimal, and temperature is maintained by normal physiologic processes with minimum oxygen consumption. Although no specific single environmental temperature is optimal for every newborn, certain ranges of temperature and humidity are appropriate for newborns of different weights, gestational ages, skin thickness, fat content, and body composition. For term babies, environmental temperatures of 24 to 28°C are generally suitable. For premature infants of 2000 to 2500 g, environmental temperatures of 28 to 30°C may be needed. For infants of 1000 to 1500 g, the initial incubator temperatures may need to be in the range of 32 to 36°C. Finally, for premature infants of less than 1000 g, the thermal-neutral environmental temperature may need to be nearly as high as body temperature.

Ambient humidity also contributes to thermal neutrality by reducing transcutaneous insensible water loss, an energy-consuming process in the newborn. In general, increased atmospheric humidity or increased humidity by warm mist administered to an incubator will somewhat reduce the thermal-neutral environmental temperature for a particular infant.

The thermal-neutral temperature zone for a particular infant is that at which oxygen consumption to maintain body temperature is least (Fig. 6-2). In temperate or warm climates, most healthy infants will quickly adjust to a thermal-neutral temperature next to the skin if they are dressed in layers, wrapped, or held skin-to-skin by their mothers. Distressed infants and infants subjected to temperature extremes have greater difficulty

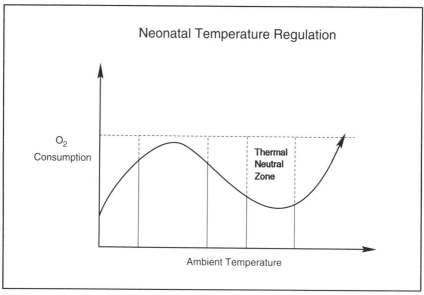

Fig. 6-2. The relationship of ambient temperature to control of body temperature in the newborn. Because infants do not efficiently produce heat by shivering or dissipate it by sweating, chemical heat production by lipolysis and insensible heat loss from the skin and airways become important processes in neonatal temperature regulation.

achieving optimal thermal regulation. Departure of environmental temperature from the thermal-neutral zone in either direction markedly increases oxygen consumption. Because the infant's temperature-regulating mechanisms are less mature and less flexible than those of adults, subjection to extreme environmental heat may produce hyperthermia at a marked energy cost and the occasional development of irreversible hyperthermia, whereas cold exposure with hypothermia rapidly increases oxygen consumption and may result in extreme hypothermia with death from cold stress.

Unfed infants principally consume endogenous glucose as their main energy source for metabolic regulation. In response to the normal metabolic stress of labor and birth and a change in thermal environment from amniotic fluid at body temperature to ambient air at a lower temperature, most unfed infants just after birth undergo a fall of approximately 40 percent in plasma glucose compared to the umbilical cord glucose concentration. Although there is a slight developmental delay in the maturation of hormonal pathways for glycogenolysis and gluconeogenesis, most infants will respond to the initial thermal stress and meet their energy requirements by consumption of glucose and lipolysis. There is an approximately 40 percent fall in blood glucose. In response to thermal stress and a decrease in plasma glucose, circulating catecholamines increase and free fatty acids, glycerol, and ketone bodies increase two- to threefold in an inverse relationship to plasma glucose. As plasma glucose decreases in the first several hours after birth, ketone bodies, free fatty acids, and glycerol show a corresponding and proportionate increase (Fig. 6-3). After reaching a nadir several hours after birth, plasma glucose begins to correct itself spontaneously and also increases in response to feeding. As the infant achieves self-regulation of plasma glucose, lipolysis decreases, and the circulating concentrations of lipolytic products also decline toward baseline levels and become more finely regulated. These metabolic regulatory responses may be exaggerated in response to thermal stress (i.e., ambient temperatures outside the thermal-neutral zone). Also, infants of diabetic mothers and infants without adequate fat stores (e.g., extremely premature infants) may have a more precipitous and persistent fall in plasma glucose with a diminished ability to compensate by lipolytic processes or gluconeogenesis. These infants are metabolically more at risk and may at times become acidotic in response to hypoglycemia or thermal stress. Normal newborns regulate temperature and energy requirements more efficiently than premature infants or infants of diabetic mothers, despite the larger size of the latter infants.

Oxygen Transport

Until term, fetuses and newborn infants have predominantly fetal hemoglobin. This form of hemoglobin is well suited to intrauterine oxygen transport and exchange, because of its high affinity for oxygen in a low-oxygen environment. Compared to adult hemoglobin, fetal hemoglobin is more

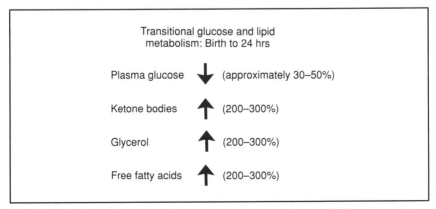

Fig. 6-3. Postnatal changes in plasma glucose concentration and lipid components during the first 6 to 12 hours after birth.

highly saturated at lower blood-oxygen tension. The p50 of fetal hemoglobin, i.e., the oxygen tension at which hemoglobin is 50 percent saturated, is 18 mm Hg for typical fetal hemoglobin and 27 to 28 mm Hg for adult hemoglobin. At a PO_2 of 40 mm hg, fetal hemoglobin is approximately 85 percent saturated, whereas the saturation of adult hemoglobin at the same PO_2 is less than 80 percent.

High circulating oxygen tensions that follow birth and the onset of breathing suppress new hemoglobin production for several months. Postnatal hemoglobin production is predominantly of hemoglobin A. In the postnatal oxygen environment, hemoglobin A is adequately saturated and has the additional physiologic benefit of releasing oxygen more readily into the tissues. The binding of 2,3,diphosphoglycerate to adult hemoglobin slightly decreases hemoglobin oxygen affinity, but increases the availability of transported oxygen to the tissues. In a postnatal milieu of adequate oxygen and rapid growth, this shift from fetal to adult hemoglobin is in general physiologically beneficial.

Fetal hemoglobin persists somewhat longer in the premature infant. Oxygen saturation of hemoglobin may be adequate at somewhat lower PO_2, but with a slightly decreased availability of hemoglobin-bound oxygen to the tissues. The conversion from fetal to adult hemoglobin and the "shift to the right" of the oxygen dissociation curve proceeds gradually throughout the first year of postnatal life.

Nutritional Requirements

The basal caloric expenditure of a newborn infant is approximately 50 to 60 kcal/kg/day. Sustained growth approximating the third-trimester intrauterine rate requires approximately 100 kcal/kg/day in normal term infants. Basal water requirements increase from approximately 65 to 70 ml/kg/day on day 1, to 90 to 100 ml/kg/day by days 3 and 4 as the infant becomes more active and solute intake increases with the ingestion of breast milk or formula. The newborn infant's water requirement includes 30 to 50 ml/kg/day for urine formation, approximately 15 ml/kg/day in stool, and 20 to 25 ml/kg/day for insensible water loss. Water requirement increases with the intake and excretion of dietary solute during the first week. Specific dynamic absorption, i.e., the water and energy needed for the digestive and regulatory functions in the GI tract, is about 10 percent of the water and calories ingested.

A protein intake of 2.5 to 3.5 g/kg/day is required for sustained normal postnatal growth. The intake of other nutrients in breast milk or formula is approximately 15 to 16 g/kg/day of carbohydrate (as lactose in human milk) and 3 to 4 g/kg/day of fat. The caloric concentration of human milk and most formulas is approximately 20 calories per 30 ml, so that a total milk intake of 150 ml/kg or more provides the calories needed for growth.

Changes in Body Composition

Total body water and extracellular body water decrease throughout gestation and also postnatally; after birth there is a postnatal adjustment of extracellular water that generally appears as a water diuresis and weight loss between days 1 and 3 in many babies. Muscle mass, fat stores, and brain growth increase with gestational and postnatal development at the expense of the extracellular water compartment. Fat storage is particularly evident in the third trimester and during early postnatal growth, and the triglyceride and cholesterol concentrations of human milk are correspondingly high to meet these requirements for the development of fat stores and brain growth. Late in the first year, rates of fat accumulation, head growth, and overall somatic growth slow down, and the caloric intake and the rate of weight gain decline noticeably after the first year of postnatal life. It is a rule of thumb that the fetus will double in weight from approximately 1000 to 2000 g between 28 and 34 weeks' gestation, and then increase from 2000 to approximately 3000 g or more between 34 and 40 weeks' gestation. Birth weight usually doubles within the first 5 to 6 months, from 3 kg to approximately 6 kg, and triples within the first year from 3000 g at birth to approximately 9 to 10 kg at 1 year of age. The further increase in growth between 1 and 2 years of age is only about 50 percent of the first year's weight gain, or from 10 kg at 1 year to 15 kg at age 2.

Maturation of Renal Function

In the newborn period, both glomerular filtration and tubular reabsorption are balanced but are reduced compared to later ages. The renal concentrating capacity of the newborn kidney is reduced to approximately 400 to 600 mOsm/L, compared to a maximum concentrating capacity of about 1400 mOsm/L in the adult. Consequently, the volume of urine required to excrete a given solute load is greater in the newborn infant than it is for the older child or adult. Newborn infants are particularly vulnerable to dehydration as a consequence of gastroenteritis or hypertonic feedings, because of their inability to concentrate their urine. One of the advantages of human milk for human newborns is the smaller solute load of human milk compared to formula, so that for a given caloric intake with breast milk, a smaller solute load is presented to the kidney.

Gradual renal maturation occurs postnatally (Table 6-1). Maturation of renal plasma flow and concentrating ability occur in approximately 3 to 6 months. Maximum rates for glomerular filtration and urea clearance are achieved by approximately 12 months of age. Premature infants show somewhat accelerated maturation of the kidney. For example, a 1-month-old 28-week premature infant (postconceptional age, 32 weeks) will have already developed renal function comparable to that of a term infant. Postnatal renal maturation in premature infants is an important physiologic adjustment contributing to their eventual survival.

Table 6-1. Renal maturation in newborn infants

	Term newborn	Adult	Time to mature (mo)
Glomerular filtration ($ml/min/1.73$ m^2)	40–60	120	12–24
Urea clearance ($ml/min/1.73$ m^2)	20–50	75	12–24
Maximum concentration of urine (mOsm/L)	400–600	1400	3
Extreme dilution of urine (mOsm/L)	50	50	
Hydrogen ion excretion	Somewhat decreased		1–3

The consequences of some failures of neonatal adaptation should be recognized. Asphyxia interferes with neonatal cardiorespiratory adaptation and may also damage other organ systems. The short-term consequences of asphyxia are hypoxemia, acidosis, and sometimes persistence of fetal circulatory patterns, as persistent acidosis sustains high pulmonary vascular pressures and right-to-left shunts. Hypothermia markedly increases energy consumption, and is also associated with acidosis and failure of the transitional circulation to convert to normal postnatal pathways. Hypoglycemia in the face of cardiorespiratory or metabolic instability produces a pathophysiologic condition in which the newborn fails to provide enough energy for physiologic adaptation and brain metabolism. Hypoglycemia is sometimes associated with central nervous system irritability and profound hypoglycemia, with cortical damage.

In summary, during the transition from the fetal to the newborn period, the newborn infant must maintain temperature and oxygen transport, must ingest and independently metabolize all nutrients, and must excrete all wastes. Failure of a smooth transition in any of these functions may lead to significant perinatal and postnatal morbidity.

Recommended Readings

Cornblath, M., and Schwartz, R. *Disorders of Carbohydrate Metabolism in Infancy* (3rd ed.). Philadelphia: Saunders, 1991. Chaps. 1 and 2, 1–86.

Holliday, M. A. (ed.). *Pediatric Nephrology* (2nd ed.). Baltimore: Williams & Wilkins, 1987. Section 12: "The Perinatal Period." Pp. 901–961.

Serwer, G. A. Postnatal Circulatory Adjustments. In R. A. Polin and W. W. Fox (eds.), *Fetal and Neonatal Physiology.* Philadelphia: Saunders, 1992. Chap. 70, 710–721.

Swyer, P. R. Thermoregulation in the Newborn. In L. Stern and P. Vert (eds.), *Neonatal Medicine.* New York: Masson, 1987. Chap. 35, 773–790.

7

Genetics

David L. Meryash

The physician caring for the pregnant woman has a unique opportunity to obtain information that can have a positive impact on the health of the entire family. Today there are numerous ways of determining the presence within a family of deleterious genes. In addition, the prospects for treatment of genetic diseases or disabilities continue to improve rapidly. A careful family history during early pregnancy with special attention to genetic disorders could result in the prevention or amelioration of medical or developmental problems in the infant. It could also result in uncovering information that will be useful for counseling members of the extended family. The first prenatal visit is the opportune time to explore the possibility that the unborn child is at risk for having a birth defect or genetic disorder.

Frequency of Genetic Disorders
Collectively genetic disorders are not rare (Table 7-1). Approximately 5 percent of children are born with a genetic disease or birth defect. Congenital heart disease, the most frequently occurring major defect, occurs 9 times in every 1000 births. Cystic fibrosis has an incidence of 1 in 2000 live births among whites and has a carrier frequency of 1 in 22 individuals. Many conditions occur more often among people of particular ethnic backgrounds. One of every 10 black Americans is a carrier of the gene for sickle cell anemia. Among American Jews of Ashkenazi ancestry, 1 of every 27 is a carrier for Tay-Sachs disease and there is a similarly high carrier frequency among French Canadians. The thalassemias together are the most common single-gene disorders worldwide. They are more likely to be found among individuals of Mediterranean or Southeast Asian descent. It is

Table 7-1. Incidences of some birth defects and chronic illnesses with a genetic basis

Birth defects and chronic illnesses	General incidence
Cleft lip with or without cleft palate	1.6/1000 children
Congenital heart disease	9/1000 children
Neural tube defect	
Spina bifida	0.7/1000 children
Encephalocele	0.15/1000 children
Neurofibromatosis	0.4/1000 children
Cystic fibrosis	0.5/1000 children
Phenylketonuria	0.1/1000 children
Duchenne's muscular dystrophy	0.2/1000 males
Fragile X syndrome	1/1000 males
	1/2000 females
Sickle cell anemia	10–20/1000 blacks
Tay-Sachs disease	0.17–0.4/1000 Ashkenazi Jews, French Canadians
Thalassemia	10–20/1000 Mediterraneans, Asians

nearly impossible to estimate the number of children affected by genetic disorders since many such conditions are mild or often remain undetected, whereas others are manifested late in life. Some of the most common human afflictions (alcoholism, epilepsy, diabetes mellitus, hypercholesterolemia, and cancer) have a significant genetic component but, unfortunately, little intervention is available for them prenatally or in infancy. Many genetic conditions in which the genetic mechanisms are better defined, however, are detectable during pregnancy or at the time of birth, when critical management decisions can be made.

Definitions

Genetic

A condition is *genetic* if there is an abnormality in the quantity of DNA, its structure, or its function. The aberration may be missing material, extra material, an alteration of the sequence of nucleotides, or the failure of a gene to be turned on or suppressed at the appropriate time.

Inherited

A genetic disorder is *inherited* if one or both parents have contributed the deleterious genes. Many genetic disorders, however, present as a sporadic event or as the result of a new mutation in either the egg or sperm. Trisomy 21, the chromosomal cause of Down syndrome, occurs 95 percent of the time as a result of nondisjunction during gamete production. In these instances, both parents have a normal chromosome complement and the condition was not inherited. The risk of nondisjunction increases with maternal age.

Many dominantly inherited disorders have a high rate of new mutation. For example, in about one-half of the individuals with neurofibromatosis (NF-1 and NF-2), neither parent is affected. In achondroplasia, another common dominantly inherited condition, new mutations are associated with advancing paternal age.

Congenital

A *congenital* condition is one in which the adverse influence has been exerted by the time of birth. Thus, diseases or conditions caused by environmental factors during pregnancy in addition to genetic disorders are congenital.

Gene and Chromosome Structure

The normal human has 22 pairs of autosomes and one pair of sex chromosomes for a total of 46. Each pair consists of one paternally derived and one maternally derived chromosome. A chromosome contains a single continuous strand of DNA with instructions for the development and growth of the organism. The DNA is embedded in protein that renders it visible when prepared and stained for cytogenetic analysis. Modern methods of molecular analysis can detect variations in DNA that can signal disease or distinguish the maternal and paternal chromosomes.

DNA is composed of sequences of four nucleotides, or bases—adenine (A), cytosine (C), guanine (G), and thymine (T)—joined together by phosphate-sugar links. Along the string of DNA there are stretches of nucleotides, called genes, that code for the synthesis of a particular protein. The human genome is estimated to contain about 100,000 genes. The sequence of nucleotides within a gene determines which amino acids form its product. The entire sequence of nucleotides is *transcribed* into a messenger RNA molecule. The messenger RNA (mRNA) then serves as the template for protein synthesis. Individual amino acids are then brought together with transfer RNA (tRNA) as the mediator in the process called *translation*. Only some segments of the gene, however, are translated into protein. These segments are called *exons*. Along the gene there are also intervening sequences of DNA, called *introns,* which are not translated. A gene also contains sequences that regulate its synthesis.

Nature of Genetic Abnormalities

Until recently genetic defects could be divided neatly into two types: single gene disorders and chromosome abnormalities. Advances in methods of chromosome analysis and the emergence of DNA analysis have resulted in a blurring of this distinction. We now recognize a continuum of possible genetic mutations in which the stretch of DNA involved varies in size (Table 7-2). At one end of the spectrum lies a single base substitution, insertion, or deletion within a single gene and, at the other extreme, the addition or lack of an entire chromosome. In between lie partial gene duplications, disorders due to unstable DNA sequences, and contiguous gene syndromes.

Single-Gene Disorders

Single-gene disorders are localized either to autosomes or to the X chromosome and are transmitted in a dominant or recessive fashion. While the male-determining locus is on the Y, as of this writing no significant disorders have been assigned to the Y chromosome. A condition is dominant or recessive depending on whether one or both genes of a pair must be in the aberrant form in order for it to be expressed clinically. The distinction is actually arbitrary, especially for X-linked conditions, since quite often heterozygotes express some characteristics of the disease. For example, although only males are affected by severe muscle weakness and loss of

Table 7-2. Classification of common genetic conditions according to the nature of the underlying defect[a]

Single-gene disorders	Multifactorial
Autosomal-dominant	Anencephaly
Achondroplasia	Cleft palate
Neurofibromatosis NF-1 (17), NF-2 (22)	Meningomyelocele
Huntington's chorea (4)	Congenital heart disease
Marfan syndrome (15)	Pyloric stenosis
Myotonic dystrophy[b]	
Polycystic kidney disease	Contiguous gene syndromes
Cleft lip with or without cleft palate	Angelman syndrome (15)
Autosomal-recessive	Aniridia-Wilms' tumor (11)
Cystic fibrosis (7)	Prader-Willi syndrome (15)
Phenylketonuria (12)	Retinoblastoma–Mental
Sickle cell anemia (11)	retardation (13)
Tay-Sachs disease	
Thalassemia-alpha (16), -beta (11)	Chromosome disorders
	Cri du chat syndrome (5
X-linked	Down syndrome (21)
Duchenne's and Becker's muscular	Klinefelter's syndrome (X)
dystrophy (X)	Trisomy 13 (13)
Hemophilia A and B (X)	Trisomy 18 (18)
Fragile X syndrome (X)[b]	Turner's syndrome (X)
Rett syndrome (X)	

[a]Where known, the chromosome involved is indicated in parentheses.
[b]The genetic mutation consists of a several-fold amplification or lengthening of an unstable region of DNA. In fragile X syndrome, this often results in a visible chromosomal change.

function, some female carriers of Duchenne's muscular dystrophy have muscle weakness, and many demonstrate elevated creatine phosphokinase levels that reflect subclinical muscle destruction. The mode of inheritance of single-gene disorders is often apparent from the family history (Fig. 7-1). When a specific diagnosis cannot be made in a proband (the individual under consideration), simply determining the mode of inheritance from historical information and examination of relatives can sometimes provide useful information for counseling the family.

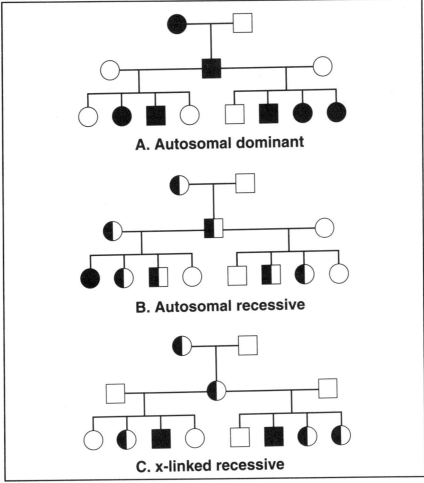

A. Autosomal dominant

B. Autosomal recessive

C. x-linked recessive

Fig. 7-1. In all three pedigrees, squares represent males and circles represent females. A symbol that is completely filled in represents an affected individual. Half-filled symbols represent asymptomatic carriers. Individuals represented by empty symbols are neither affected nor carriers of the disease-producing gene. In the autosomal-dominant pedigree, all affected individuals carry a single copy of the abnormal gene.

Autosomal-dominant Inheritance

Each child of a person with an autosomal-dominant disorder (Fig. 7-1A) has a 50 percent chance of inheriting the abnormal gene. If a child is affected by an autosomal-dominant condition often he or she has inherited the gene from one or the other parent. However, there is a high frequency of new mutation among autosomal-dominant conditions, in which case neither parent is affected. Therefore, to determine the risk for recurrence for a couple with an affected child, it is essential to establish whether or not a parent is affected. This is complicated further by the fact that autosomal-dominant conditions frequently vary considerably in their expression, with some individuals being minimally affected. If it can be established with reasonable certainty that neither parent is a carrier, the couple does not have a significantly increased risk for bearing another affected child.

Autosomal-recessive Inheritance

A child affected by an autosomal-recessive disorder (Fig. 7-1B) inherited one abnormal gene from each parent. Both parents are heterozygotes and, with each pregnancy, they have a 1 in 4 chance of bearing an affected child. The risk that a person affected by an autosomal-recessive disorder will have an affected child depends first on whether the condition results in diminished fertility, and secondly, the chance that his or her spouse is heterozygous for the condition, i.e., the frequency of the carrier state in the population. A person who is a known carrier of the cystic fibrosis gene, for example, has a 1 in 22 chance of marrying someone who is unknowingly a carrier. If both have the gene, each has a 1 in 2 chance of transmitting it. Therefore their chance of bearing an affected child with a given pregnancy is approximately $1 : 22 \times 1 : 2 \times 1 : 2$ or $1 : 88$. This risk will be considerably higher if the couple shares a common ancestor. Biologic relatedness between mates is called *consanguinity* and a mating between relatives is referred to as *consanguineous*. In the example given, in which one member of a couple is known to be a carrier of the cystic fibrosis gene, the other member should also be examined, by DNA analysis, for abnormalities of the CF gene (see below). Based on the results, the couple's risk for bearing an affected child can be redetermined.

X-linked Inheritance

A woman who is a carrier of an X-linked disorder (Fig. 7-1C) has, with each pregnancy, a 50 percent chance of passing on the affected gene. In general, if the child receiving the gene is a male, he will have signs of the disorder. A female child will be unaffected. There are, however, important exceptions to this rule. So that female individuals do not receive a double dose of the effects of genes lying on the X chromosome, one of the Xs in each cell of the developing embryo becomes inactivated (the Lyon hypothesis). The process is random so that on a cell-by-cell basis it is either the paternally derived or maternally derived X chromosome that is inactivated. If by chance the X containing a disease-producing gene is more often active than the X containing the normal gene, a female may be affected by the disease (unfavorable Lyonization). A female who carries the gene for an X-linked disorder and who, through a chromosomal rearrangement, is missing a portion of her normal X might also be affected by an X-linked condition.

A man who carries the gene for an X-linked disorder will pass the gene to each of his daughters, all of whom will be carriers. He cannot pass the gene to a son. Thus in X-linked inheritance there is never father-to-son transmission.

As is the case for autosomal-dominant conditions, in X-linked conditions there is a high frequency of new mutation. This is particularly true of Duchenne's muscular dystrophy, in which 1 out of 3 affected males and 1 out of 2 carriers have the gene as a result of a fresh mutation.

The Variable Nature of Single-Gene Mutations

We now recognize that many different types of alterations within a gene can result in a reduction, absence, or the abnormal function of a protein product. An alteration in one nucleotide can change the amino acid occurring at a particular position (missense mutation) or stop protein synthesis before it is complete (nonsense mutation). Sickle cell anemia arises from a single base substitution in the β-globin gene. The base change results in a product that differs from the normal protein by one amino acid. All individuals with sickle-cell hemoglobin possess the same mutation. Other disorders arise from the deletion, insertion, or inversion of a small group of nucleotides.

In contrast to sickle-cell disease, some disorders can arise from one of many different mutations within the responsible gene. Cystic fibrosis (CF) can be caused by as many as 100 distinct mutations within the CF gene, which is located on chromosome 7. One of these, a deletion of three base pairs that results in the omission of a single amino acid (phenylalanine) in the CF transmembrane conductance regulator protein, however, accounts for 70 percent of the abnormal genes in the white population.

Neurofibromatosis type 1 (NF-1) is characterized by variable and diverse abnormalities that appear in tissues derived from the neural crest. The gene for NF-1, which has been genetically mapped to the long arm of chromosome 17, is a relatively large one, which makes it vulnerable to many different mutations. In fact deletions of variable length of several different regions of the NF-1 gene have been found in separate families. In other families chromosome translocations, each disrupting the gene at a different location, have been identified.

At least 60 mutations of different types and locations have been found in the phenylalanine hydroxylase gene, which helps explain the considerable phenotypic heterogeneity of phenylketonuria (PKU).

Recently, partial duplications of a gene have also been recognized as a cause of human disease. In these mutations, segments of a gene are repeated from one to several times and arranged in tandem. About 6 to 7 percent of the mutations responsible for Duchenne's and Becker's muscular dystrophy are partial gene duplications.

Inherited Unstable DNA Sequences

Several disorders are now known to be due to a newly discovered form of genetic mutation. In these disorders there is amplification, or repetition, of short strings of nucleotides. The number of copies seems to change during meiosis or mitosis, producing phenotypic variation. A very important example is the fragile X syndrome, the most common inherited form of mental retardation. The condition owes its name to a characteristic appearance of the affected X chromosome, in which the tip appears to be breaking off. The fragile X syndrome presents an interesting variation on X-linked inheritance. As in more typical X-linked disorders, there is no father-to-son transmission. However, in contrast to other X-linked conditions, heterozygotes are frequently affected, and show intellectual impairment or typical physical characteristics. Furthermore, approximately 1 out of 5 males who have transmitted the gene are *unaffected*. The mutation responsible for the full-blown syndrome is a several-fold increase in the length of a normally occurring string of cytosine and guanine nucleotides near the end of the long arm of the X chromosome. The normal function of this string of nucleotides appears to be regulation of transcription of an adjacent gene called FMR-1. In the presence of the mutation, transcription is blocked. The fragile X syndrome is transmitted by individuals of normal intellectual ability who carry a gene of a length intermediate between that of the normal gene and that of a mentally retarded individual. The intermediate-length gene, known as a *premutation*, is converted to a full-length gene or *full mutation* during passage through oogenesis of a carrier female. Diagnosis of the carrier state and the full mutation is possible by direct DNA analysis.

This kind of mutation is also responsible for Huntington's chorea and for myotonic dystrophy, an autosomal-dominant disorder that results in weakness of facial and distal limb muscle and delay of relaxation of contracted muscles. The congenital form is one cause of neonatal hypotonia. Within the myotonic dystrophy gene, the number of copies of the repeated sequence and the severity of the disorder increases with each generation.

Chromosome Disorders

In many disorders there is a visible alteration of one or more chromosomes. The so-called chromosome disorders are the result of the deletion or addition of a relatively large segment of DNA. In some conditions there is an extra or missing copy of an entire chromosome. In others there are deletions or additions of small parts of a chromosome. The manifestations of chromosomal disorders relate both to the number and specificity of the genes present in the extra or missing portion of the genome. If a chromosome or a portion of it is missing, the individual is *monosomic* for that part of the genome. If there is extra genetic material attached to an otherwise normal chromosome it can usually be identified as a misplaced part of a different chromosome. The individual would be *trisomic,* or have three copies of a portion of his or her genome. In order for there to be a visible change on chromosomal analysis, the span of DNA involved almost always will contain a large number of genes. Consequently chromosome disorders as a rule produce a wide range of effects. Multiple congenital anomalies or patterns of malformation are nearly always present and often can be recognized in the delivery room (Table 7-3). Developmental delay and mental retardation are a usual feature of chromosome disorders.

Table 7-3. Incidence and features of the three most common autosomal trisomies recognizable in newborns

Autosomal trisomy	Incidence	Features
Trisomy 21 (Down syndrome)	1/800	Hypotonia Short stature Brachycephaly, flat occiput Upslanting palpebral fissures Epicanthal folds Congenital heart disease Single palmar crease Moderate mental retardation
Trisomy 18	1/8000	Hypertonia, clenched fists Severe congenital heart disease Prominent occiput Receding jaw Low-set ears Short sternum Rocker-bottom feet, prominent calcanei Severe mental retardation Failure to thrive
Trisomy 13	1/8,000	Central nervous system malformations Growth retardation Ocular hypertelorism, microphthalmia Cleft lip, cleft palate Overlapping digits, polydactyly Rocker-bottom feet Congenital heart disease

Down syndrome is the most common example of a chromosome disorder that presents with a recognizable pattern of malformation and developmental disability. About 95 percent of the time the child with Down syndrome has in each cell 47 chromosomes with an extra number 21. This situation arises from nondisjunction of the pair of 21s during meiosis in the production of either the father's sperm or the mother's ovum. Nondisjunction can also occur during mitosis during embryogenesis; this will lead to a mixture of cells, some with 46 chromosomes and some with 47. The result is *mosaicism*, which accounts for a few instances of Down syndrome. In both of these situations, the parents' genotypes are normal and the Down syndrome was not inherited.

In about 3 to 5 percent of children with Down syndrome, the extra 21 is attached to another chromosome (either a 13, 14, 15, 21, or 22). Such a rearrangement of chromosomal material is called a *translocation*. About half of the time these translocations occur during gametogenesis. The rest of the time, however, one or the other parent is discovered to be a translocation carrier. This parent, who is phenotypically normal, will have only 45 chromosomes and two number 21s. One of the 21s, instead of being freestanding, will be attached to another chromosome. If the parent transmits this translocation chromosome along with his or her other 21, the infant will inherit Down syndrome. Translocations can involve virtually any of the 46 chromosomes and result in monosomy or trisomy of genetic material.

Trisomy 13 and trisomy 18 can also be suspected in the newborn period by a characteristic appearance. Although they are less common than Down syndrome, the clinical picture for these conditions is more severe, with expectation for survival typically ranging from a few days to 1 or 2 years.

Altered number, or *aneuploidy*, of the sex chromosomes results in more subtle phenotypic alteration than aneuploidy of the autosomes. Individuals with Klinefelter's (XXY) syndrome, or XXY and XXX karyotypes, cannot be detected by physical features in utero or in the newborn period. Infants born with 45,X karyotypes and Turner's syndrome, however, often have edema of the dorsum of the feet or coarctation of the aorta that can lead to early diagnosis. A fetus with 45,X may be identified through ultrasound by the presence of a cystic hygroma, a swelling of the neck caused by lymphedema.

Contiguous Gene Syndromes

A few conditions have been identified in which several deleterious adjacent genes appear together. Depending on the number of genes involved, affected individuals may demonstrate varying combinations of features. These resultant recognizable patterns of characteristics, in association with their altered genetic substrate, are known as *contiguous gene syndromes*. In a proportion of these patients cytogenetic analysis demonstrates a small but visible deletion of chromosomal material. Examples include the Prader-Willi syndrome and Angelman syndrome, due to a missing sequence of genes on the long arm of chromosome 15 (15q-); the aniridia Wilms' tumor association, in which the abnormalities lie on 11p; and retino-blastoma–mental retardation, due to defects on 13q. Prader-Willi syndrome and Angelman syndrome, two distinct conditions with few features in common, are both due to a deletion of the same region of chromosome 15. However, although the parents' chromosomes are normal, the deletion in the affected individual is found on the 15 inherited from the father in the case of Prader-Willi, and on the maternally derived 15 in the case of Angelman. Such differences in chromosomal function that depend on parental origin are known as *imprinting;* this is a relatively recently discovered phenomenon.

Multifactorial Conditions

A group of isolated congenital defects appear to recur within sibships with a frequency of about 2 to 5 percent. These conditions include neural tube defects (anencephaly and meningomyelocele), congenital heart disease, pyloric stenosis, congenital hip dysplasia, and some forms of cleft lip and cleft palate. This recurrence risk is considerably lower than that expected for autosomal-recessive disorders, but significantly higher than the background occurrence rate for these disorders in the general population. The predisposition for these defects to occur within certain families implies a strong genetic influence but the number of genes involved and their locations are unknown. It is thought that both parents contribute some of the predisposing genes. Studies in animals suggest that an environmental factor might trigger the occurrence of these defects in genetically susceptible individuals. Because of the combined genetic and environmental contribution, these conditions are referred to as having *multifactorial* etiologies. Specific environmental factors—elevated maternal temperature, nutritional deficits, and consumption of large amounts of alcohol—have induced neural tube defects in laboratory animals. One large survey in humans showed a reduction in the recurrence of neural tube defects among families in which the mother began vitamin supplements around the time of conception. This result suggested a possible role of vitamin deficiency. It is generally thought that which particular adverse environmental influence is present is not as important as the fact that it is present during a critical stage of embryonic development (see Chap. 3).

Genetic Diagnosis

There are a variety of ways of determining whether an individual carries an abnormal gene.

Phenotypic Evidence

Some conditions present with a cluster of typical clinical features, fit a recognizable pattern of human malformation, and are diagnosable largely by physical examination. Examples are meningomyelocele, Williams syndrome, achondroplasia, and Apert syndrome. Some conditions, such as Down syndrome, trisomy 13, and trisomy 18, although recognizable by examination, are confirmed by chromosome analysis. Chronic illnesses are most often diagnosed by their clinical manifestations. The inborn errors of metabolism—PKU, galactosemia, the mucopolysaccharidoses, and the glycogen storage diseases, for example—are identified by biochemical means through measurement of the deficient or aberrant gene product.

Pedigree Analysis
Often, by examining the pedigree, even in situations in which the basic metabolic defect or the nature of the genetic mutation is not known, it is possible to determine the carrier status of unaffected individuals (Fig. 7-2).

Chromosome Analysis (Cytogenetics)
A chromosome analysis is usually performed on lymphocytes acquired by venipuncture that have been stimulated to divide in a nutrient-rich culture using phytohemagglutinin, a potent mitogen. After 48 to 96 hours, mitosis is arrested by the addition of colchicine to the culture. Then the cells are stained and viewed under a microscope. A more rapid diagnosis (4–6 hours) is possible if the examination is performed on bone marrow cells that are already rapidly dividing, but the chromosome preparation is often less clear, and the added discomfort that bone marrow aspiration presents to the patient is usually not justified. A quick count of unbanded chromosomes can be performed if a trisomy is suspected. However, definitive identification of chromosome rearrangements, deletions, or additions requires banding, a special staining method that allows identification of specific portions of each chromosome. If a baby is recognized in the delivery room to have multiple congenital anomalies or is suspected of having a specific chromosomal syndrome, a cord blood specimen can be heparinized and sent to the laboratory.

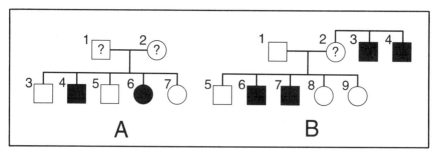

Fig. 7-2. In A two of the children (4,6) have a disorder known to be autosomal-recessive. Both parents (1,2) must be heterozygous for the condition. In B individual 2 is an obligate carrier of the X-linked disorder affecting 2 of her sons and her 2 brothers, all of whom share similar clinical features.

In order to demonstrate the very small deletions associated with the contiguous gene syndromes, special techniques must be employed in the laboratory to arrest cell division while the chromosomes are relatively long. To study chromosomes for these abnormalities, one must request *prometaphase*, or high-resolution, banding. This technique results in a several-fold increase in the number of light and dark bands that can be seen on each chromosome and enables the recognition of relatively small deletions.

Direct Detection by DNA Analysis

Until recently one could determine that a person carried a deleterious gene only if that gene expressed itself either by causing disease in that person or his or her descendents or if it produced minor biochemical alterations that could be detected. Now, using DNA analysis, it is possible to determine carrier status for the genes of many conditions long before the disease is manifest. Unlike chromosome analysis, which must be performed on rapidly dividing cells, DNA can be isolated from any available tissue.

When a genetic disorder can be attributed to a known alteration or deletion of a base sequence, it is possible to detect the abnormality directly using molecular means. The DNA obtained from the patient is fractionated using special enzymes, called *restriction endonucleases*. The segment of DNA containing the gene is then isolated using a radioactively labelled gene probe that will bind specifically to it. Restriction enzymes recognize specific nucleotide sequences and cut DNA wherever these sequences occur. Wherever there is an alteration in the base sequence from the one recognized by a particular restriction enzyme, a cut is not made. Depending on where and how often the restriction site is recognized along a given strand of DNA, there will be variability in the length of the fragments that will result. The lengths of these fragments then can be determined by electrophoresis. The effect of the presence of the genetic mutation is to alter the length of the DNA segment isolated by the gene-specific probe. For example, sickle cell anemia arises as a result of a single base substitution in the beta-globin gene (Fig. 7-3) and can be detected by direct DNA analysis.

Indirect Detection by DNA Analysis

For many disorders, although the gene itself may not have been isolated, its approximate location on a particular chromosome has been determined by chromosomal and molecular analysis of blood samples from families in which the disorder is present. When one or both parents in a family unit are known to carry the deleterious form of the gene, it is often possible, through molecular means, to determine with reasonable accuracy whether a child (or fetus) has inherited their affected or unaffected chromosomes. To understand how this works, it is necessary to know what it means for two genetic loci to be "linked."

During the first stage of meiosis there is always a certain amount of crossing over that takes place between the homologous chromosomes of each

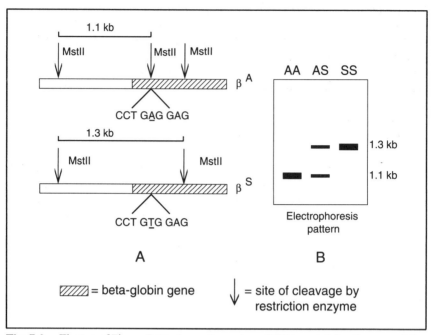

Fig. 7-3. The top of Figure 7-3A shows the region of DNA containing the normal β-globin gene. The bottom shows the same region indicating the substitution of a T for A, representing the sickle cell mutation, within a segment (CCT GTG GAG) of the gene. This substitution removes a restriction site recognized by the restriction eyzyme Mst II. Figure 7-3B shows the pattern of distribution of the segments of DNA on an electrophoresis gel that results when Mst II is used to cleave the DNA of individuals with the 3 possible genotypes. Where the normal β-globin gene is present, a fragment 1.1 kilobases (kb) in length results. The absence of the restriction site in the sickle cell gene produces a longer 1.3 kb fragment. A heterozygote, or carrier of the sickle cell gene (AS), will demonstrate both fragments. An individual with sickle cell (SS) disease will demonstrate only 1.3 kb fragments and an individual homozygous for the normal gene (AA) will show only 1.1 kb fragments.

pair. It is this crossing over or recombination of the genetic material between maternally and paternally derived chromosomes that contributes to the heterogeneity of the genetic material contained in sperm and ova. The further apart two genetic loci on a given chromosome are from each other, the more likely a crossover (recombinant) can take place between them. If two loci are close to each other, they are said to be tightly linked and are likely to be inherited together. In such a case, a closely linked genetic locus, if it is more readily detected, then can serve as a marker for the disease locus (Fig. 7-4).

In actuality the genes for such measurable traits rarely lie close enough to the genetic loci one wishes to study. However, restriction fragment–

length polymorphisms allow analysis using extremely close markers. Throughout the genome there are numerous regions in which there are differences in base sequences among individuals, which are harmless from a functional point of view, but which provide a valuable method for examining genetic diversity. In effect this is what constitutes an individual's genetic fingerprint. These variations, or polymorphisms, are inherited as if they were single genes. Their presence can be detected indirectly using restriction endonucleases. It is the resulting lengths of the "restriction fragments" that serve as markers for the presence or absence of the deleterious gene (Fig. 7-5).

The likelihood that a recombinant event will interfere with the predictive accuracy of linkage analysis decreases with the distance between the restriction site and the disease locus. The predictive accuracy of the analysis can be increased greatly if several linked polymorphic loci are used, particularly if they flank, or lie on opposite sides of, the gene locus.

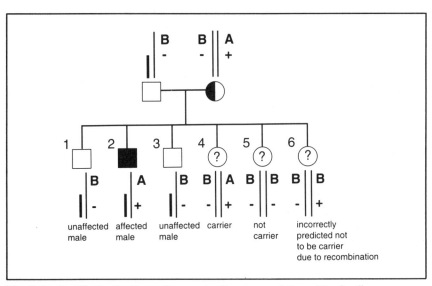

Fig. 7-4. In this family, the mother carries the abnormal form (+) of a disease-producing gene on one of her two X chromosomes. This gene is not detectable in a silent carrier. There is, however, another gene lying close to it that exists in two harmless, but different, forms (A and B) that can be distinguished in the laboratory. Perhaps they might produce two forms of a protein, both of which are fully functional. The father carries form B of the protein and the mother carries a mixture of the two forms (i.e., is heterozygous). Individual 2 is affected by the (+) gene. He also has form A of the enzyme. Thus, it can be assumed that whichever offspring has form A of the enzyme, or a mixture of form A and B, also inherited the disease-bearing gene (+) from the mother. Thus, daughter 4 will be predicted to be a carrier and daughter 5 will be predicted not to be a carrier. However, if a recombinant event takes place, thus separating the A and (+) alleles, the prediction will be inaccurate (individual 6).

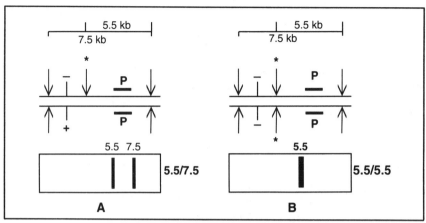

Fig. 7-5. In this example, (+) is the abnormal and (–) is the normal form of a disease-causing gene. There is a closely linked polymorphism (*) that in one form yields a fragment 5.5 kilobases (kb) in length and the other yields a 7.5kb fragment that can be isolated by a genetic probe *(P)* and identified by electrophoresis. In a particular family the longer fragment is associated with (+) and the shorter fragment with (–). (A) Individual A shows two bands on electrophoresis representing both fragment lengths. She is then heterozygous for the restriction fragment–length polymorphism and therefore heterozygous for the disease-producing gene. (B) Individual B shows one wider band representing a double dose of 5.5-kb fragments and is therefore homozygous for the shorter fragment and therefore not a carrier of the disease-producing gene.

The Polymerase Chain Reaction

Use of the polymerase chain reaction (PCR) can greatly facilitate diagnosis by DNA analysis. This technique allows one to make millions of copies in vitro of a short region of a gene so that the amplified DNA can be analyzed directly. PCR is initiated by oligonucleotide primers (short strtetches of synthesized DNA that recognize complementary DNA in a sample from a patient), and is propagated by a DNA polymerase. The PCR enables genetic diagnosis to be performed within hours instead of weeks, thus making it quite suitable for large-scale and relatively inexpensive screening. With computer-assisted automated technology some medical centers now have the ability to read and print out the actual base sequence of a DNA segment that has been amplified through the PCR.

Genetic Screening Tests

A variety of screening tests for genetic diseases is now available during pregnancy (prenatal screening) and in the newborn period (neonatal or newborn screening). Some of these tests are performed on the future parents to determine their carrier status, the risk for fetal disease, or to prevent abnormalities in the newborn. Others allow for determination of the presence of a genetic disorder in a fetus.

Carrier detection testing is now commonly offered to prospective parents early in pregnancy for Tay-Sachs disease, sickle cell anemia, alpha- and beta-thalassemia, and CF.

Obstetricians and prenatal clinics now routinely perform glucose tolerance tests on pregnant women to screen for diabetes. If maternal diabetes is poorly controlled during the first trimester it can produce congenital malformations. Inadequate control of blood sugar during the later stages of pregnancy can cause macrosomia in the infant, leading to possible difficulties with labor and delivery or hypoglycemia in the first hours of life (see Chap. 6).

Open neural tube defects (meningomyelocele and anencephaly) can be detected on the basis of elevated alpha fetoprotein (AFP) in the mother's serum at 16 to 19 weeks. AFP, a normal product of the fetal liver, is excreted into amniotic fluid. If the fetus has a neural tube defect, abnormally large amounts are present in the amniotic fluid. Some of the AFP finds its way into the maternal bloodstream. Elevated levels in amniotic fluid will be reflected in similar elevations in maternal serum. Because AFP levels normally rise during pregnancy, it is important to compare the level with the length of gestation. The most common reason for an "elevated" AFP is a pregnancy that is further along than it was thought to be. The AFP will also be elevated in the case of a multiple gestation. Fetal ultrasound can be used to determine the gestational age or the presence of twins. If the AFP is still abnormal after confirmation of the gestational age and multiple pregnancy is ruled out, the amniotic AFP level can be determined by amniocentesis and the spine can be explored using directed ultrasound in order to make a definitive diagnosis. Omphalocele, congenital nephrosis, and duodenal atresia are other congenital anomalies that can produce abnormally high levels of AFP.

The measurement of maternal serum AFP (MSAFP) is quick, easy, and sufficiently inexpensive to examine all pregnant women, and fulfills the requirements of a good screening test. Consequently it is now widely offered. After several years of experience with MSAFP measurement, it was discovered that abnormally *low* levels of the protein are associated with the presence of fetuses with Down syndrome (trisomy 21). Thus MSAFP became, in addition to maternal age, another mechanism of screening for Down syndrome. Using the MSAFP results and maternal age, a combined risk for Down syndrome can be calculated. If the combined risk is high, amniocentesis for chromosome analysis should be offered. In an effort to increase the accuracy of prenatal screening for Down syndrome, researchers found additional useful biochemical markers. Now, in addition to MSAFP, some laboratories measure maternal serum human chorionic gonadotropin (hCG), which is increased, and unconjugated estriol, which is decreased in the presence of a fetus with Down syndrome. Though it is less common than Down syndrome, trisomy 18 can also be detected through measurement of these same markers.

Like other screening tests, maternal serum analysis yields both false-positive and false-negative results. It is important, therefore, to stress to patients that an abnormal screening test is not diagnostic but rather signals the need for further examination.

In most states newborn screening for certain inborn errors of metabolism is now mandatory. Screening began in 1963 for PKU, a disorder of amino acid metabolism which, if untreated, leads to mental retardation. Early detection and treatment with a low phenylalanine diet can prevent serious developmental consequences. Many state laboratories now include screening for galactosemia, tyrosinemia, maple syrup urine disease, and homocystinuria. Though not known to be genetic, congenital hypothyroidism is also included in the screen. All of these disorders can be screened for using a dried drop of blood obtained by heelstick on a piece of filter paper during the first few days of life. Some states now screen for sickle cell anemia and related hemoglobinopathies by testing blood specimens obtained from newborns.

Early Identification and Intervention

Genetic conditions vary in the severity of their clinical expression. Some genetically determined traits have little or no impact on an individual's growth, health, or development. Others present cosmetic concerns, and others still can significantly impair an individual's well-being. Many of the most severe genetic disorders frequently result in intrauterine demise. However, the vast majority of genetic disorders are compatible with full-term gestation and require special management during life, frequently at the time of birth.

For those conditions that are detectable prenatally and would result in serious malformations, intellectual impairment, or drastically foreshortened lives, elective termination of pregnancy can be an option. If, in a given instance, abortion is not an acceptable option, prenatal diagnosis allows preparation for the management of the affected newborn and his or her family. If, for example, it is known ahead of time that a child with spina bifida will be delivered, all the consultants who will care for the infant can be alerted and be ready to intervene. The opening in the back will need to be closed surgically within hours of delivery. Children with spina bifida are also at increased risk for developing hydrocephalus, which will require a ventriculoperitoneal shunt insertion within the first few days to weeks. Equally important, the parents can be counseled ahead of time regarding what they will see at delivery and the type of treatment that will be necessary.

If the birth of a child with Down syndrome is anticipated, a developmental pediatrician with expertise in the long-term management and expectations for children with the condition can be available to answer the family's questions. The existence of special educational services and other supports should be discussed with parents of any newborn having a genetic disorder associated with developmental disability. The family can also benefit tremendously by being put in touch with a support group of parents of children with the same or similar disabilities. Because there is a high incidence of congenital heart disease among children with Down syndrome, they must be evaluated in the neonatal period for any evidence of it. If Down syndrome is diagnosed prenatally, directed ultrasound of the fetus can reveal a heart defect.

Knowledge that a newborn has sickle cell anemia will allow surveillance from day one for life-threatening infection and the earliest signs of other related crises. Newborns with sickle cell anemia are placed on prophylactic antibiotics.

Early recognition of CF will also lead to a more favorable course. Provision of supplemental pancreatic enzymes improves the nutritional status of children with CF. Vigorous, early prevention and treatment of pulmonary infections with antibiotics and chest physiotherapy are credited with prolonging the life span of children with this disease.

Diagnosis of biochemical disorders in the neonatal period can result in the prevention of symptoms by dietary manipulation. Now that PKU is normally diagnosed via newborn screening, individuals who have it usually grow up to have normal lives. Paradoxically a new issue arose as a consequence. As adults, women with PKU may no longer be on a phenylalanine-restricted diet. We now know that the high levels of phenylalanine that these women may have can be teratogenic during pregnancy. Although their children may not be at high risk for having the genetic disorder, they are at risk for disability produced by exposure to an environmental toxin, i.e., high levels of phenylalanine. Problems can be averted if the woman with PKU returns to her diet prior to conception. It is therefore essential that women with PKU and their mates be carefully counseled.

We are at the dawn of gene therapy for various diseases and the future holds promise for the primary prevention and cure of many genetic conditions. The chance to profit from these developments depends on timely diagnosis.

Early identification of a genetic disorder in a fetus or newborn also yields information that may be helpful to relatives who may be pregnant or considering pregnancy. Such information can be invaluable to their reproductive decisions.

Obtaining a Family History

The first step to early diagnosis is obtaining a family history designed to uncover any genetic condition for which the couple is at risk. The first prenatal visit should include a careful history of both the prospective mother and father's families. The ages of both parents and their ethnic backgrounds should be noted. Ethnic background alone or parental age may be an indication for specific carrier testing or genetic screening. The physician should ask whether the parents are related to each other in any way other than marriage. Then, starting with both prospective parents, followed by their previous children, and then their own parents and siblings, the physician should inquire for each individual the presence of:

- Mental retardation, a learning disability, speech problems, or considerably lower achievement than his or her siblings
- A nerve or muscle problem
- Early nonaccidental death
- A chronic illness or known genetic disorder or known carrier status for specific conditions (e.g., Tay-Sachs or sickle-cell disease)
- A birth defect
- History of frequent miscarriages, stillbirths, or neonatal deaths

A systematic review performed in this manner will increase the chances that a genetic disorder can be diagnosed sufficiently early to provide helpful intervention.

How Family History can be Negative in Genetic Diseases

The absence of a positive family history does not rule out the possibility that an isolated instance of an abnormality in a family is due to genetic causes. Situations in which the family history may be negative include (1) an incomplete history or missing information, (2) nonpaternity, (3) new mutation, (4) variable expression or penetrance, (5) initial appearance in a family of an autosomal-recessive or multifactorial disorder, or (6) an X-linked condition with relatively small sibships. Furthermore, a family history that is apparently negative for any genetic disorder does not indicate that a couple is not at increased risk for some condition.

Genetic Consultation

Whether a particular couple should be referred to a medical geneticist or genetic counselor should depend on the knowledge, expertise, and time constraints of the referring obstetrician. Consultation with a geneticist may be helpful for (1) confirmation or assistance in establishing an etiologic diagnosis for a disorder that has previously appeared within the family; (2) assurance of obtaining a comprehensive fully informative family history; (3) assistance in the interpretation of a family tree; (4) determination of the persons at risk for having affected children and the magnitude of risk; (5) discussion with the family concerning the mode of transmission of a disorder and other genetic factors; (6) assistance in setting up carrier testing and prenatal diagnosis procedures; and (7) discussion of reproductive options for couples determined to be at risk. The referring physician should explain that a geneticist is a source of information and will not dictate a course of action when important reproductive decisions must be made. The American Society of Human Genetics defines genetic counseling as

> ... a communication process which deals with the human problems associated with the occurrence, or the risk of occurrence, of a genetic disorder in a family. This process involves an attempt by one or more appropriately trained persons to help the individual or family (1) to comprehend the medical facts, including the diagnosis, the probable course of the disorder, and the available management; (2) to appreciate the way heredity contributes to the disorder, and the risk of recurrence in specified relatives; (3) to understand the options for dealing with the risk of recurrence; (4) to choose the course of action which seems appropriate to them in view of their risk, their family goals, and their ethical and religious standards, and to act in accordance with that decision; and (5) to make the best possible adjustment to the disorder in an affected family member and/or to the risk of recurrence of that disorder.

Summary

The rapid advances taking place in genetic diagnosis and the treatment of genetic disease can overwhelm the most diligent practitioner. Discoveries now being made are setting the stage for repairing genetic errors at the molecular level. However, various forms of early intervention are already available to ameliorate or repair the effects of many genetic conditions. The treatment of genetic diseases often transcends the boundaries of any single medical discipline. Identifying a couple as being at risk for bearing a child with a genetic condition opens up the possibility that other relatives are also at risk. From the genetic perspective, therefore, the family is the patient. For these reasons the prudent physician should adopt a team approach and feel free to collaborate with other specialists, including a geneticist, in the care of the family with a pregnancy.

Recommended Reading

American Society of Human Genetics Ad Hoc Committee on Genetic Counseling. Genetic counseling. *Am. J. Hum. Genet.* 27:240, 1975.

Emery, A. E. H., and Rimoin, D. L. *Principles and Practice of Medical Genetics.* London: Churchill-Livingstone, 1991.

Schmickel, R. Contiguous gene syndromes: A component of recognizable syndromes. *J. Pediatr.* 109:231–241, 1986.

Smith, D. W. *Recognizable Patterns of Human Malformation* (4th ed.). Philadelphia: Saunders, 1988.

Thompson, M. W., McInnes, R. R., and Willard, H. F. *Thompson and Thompson Genetics in Medicine* (5th ed.). Philadelphia: Saunders, 1991.

8

Congenital Defects and Their Causes

Patricia A. O'Shea

The study of human birth defects, in many respects a frustrating undertaking, is nonetheless a stunning illustration of acceleration in the rate of change in scientific understanding in our time. The earliest known record of a human birth defect is a small statuette of laterally conjoined twins that dates from 6500 B.C. and that is believed to have represented a goddess. For the next 8000 years, written and pictorial images of congenital malformation abound, testifying to man's fascination with these phenomena.

Malformed individuals have been regarded with both awe and horror, sometimes deified, more often shunned or castigated as symbols of the gods' curse or as retribution for some maternal or societal wrongdoing. Witchcraft was a leading etiologic theory, but species cross-fertilization, or "hybridization," and psychic influences, or "maternal impressions," were occasionally invoked as well. There were early attempts to demystify the process of human development; Aristotle and Galen both studied embryos and human fetuses, but their scientific approach was buried in the superstition and mysticism of the Dark Ages.

The roots of modern teratology may be found in the anatomic studies of the great painters and sculptors of the Renaissance. Leonardo da Vinci in his *Quaderni d' Anatomia* counselled study of the sequential development of the fetus, and Fabricius published a remarkably accurate account of embryology, *De Formatu Foetu.* To the great English physician William Harvey goes credit for the realization that defective embryogenesis leads to malformation. In 1651, Harvey proposed in *De Generatione Animale* that arrest of embryonic development might explain many common malformations. It took another 200 hundred years for his work to be accepted. In 1851,

Wardenburg proposed that Down syndrome might be a chromosomal disorder. Confirmation came a century later, in the work of LeJeune, but from then on progress was rapid indeed. Watson and Crick described the structure of DNA in 1962, and the discovery in 1978 by Smith and Nathans of restriction endonucleases provided the tools for detecting minute alternations of DNA. The development in rapid sequence of technologies for synthesis, sequencing, and amplification of DNA has created an explosive growth in our understanding of genetic defects.

In contrast, understanding of environmental influences on human development has been painfully slow and in many cases has been the result of a tragic therapeutic or environmental disaster. Thus, the first recognition of a virus teratogenic in humans followed the rubella epidemic of 1939 to 1940; in 1941 Sir Norman Gregg described the major clinical features of the congenital rubella syndrome: congenital cataract, hearing defects, and congenital heart disease. Thalidomide embryopathy was recognized by Lenz and McBride in 1961 following an epidemic of limb reduction defects in Europe. Awareness of the teratogenic effects of irradiation owes much to Hiroshima.

The real incidence of human birth defects is not easily determined; much depends on the definition of birth defect, on the population under study, on the diligence of the search, and on the level of technology brought to

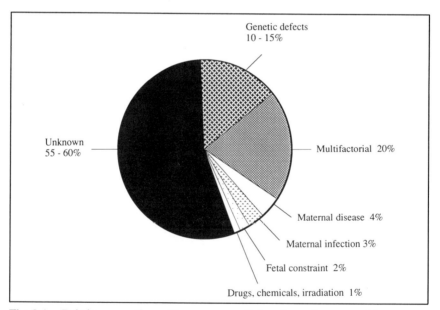

Fig. 8-1. Relative proportions of human congenital malformations caused by recognized teratogenic agents. In a majority of cases, no etiology can be determined.

bear on the question. For the present purpose, we will define a congenital malformation as a structural (as opposed to physiologic) defect of prenatal origin, present at birth, which seriously interferes with function, health, or viability. Approximately 2 to 3 percent of live born individuals have defects of this type. If one surveys infants who have died in the perinatal period, almost one-fourth have malformations. Recent advances in cytogenetics and molecular genetics have resulted in significant progress in determining the cause of many birth defects, but at present one is able to ascribe a definite etiology only in a minority of cases (Fig. 8-1). This does not mean, however, that useful information may not be available in every case. Utilizing detailed family histories, empirically derived recurrence risks, and increasingly sophisticated prenatal diagnostic testing, it is possible to provide a reasonably accurate estimate of the possibility of recurrence of a given defect and to initiate appropriate diagnostic or therapeutic measures. In a recent Belgian study of congenital anomalies, three-fourths of the conditions identified were associated with a known increased recurrence risk; in half of these, prenatal diagnosis was feasible. Understanding of the mechanisms of normal and abnormal development is an essential step toward accurate and complete diagnosis, detection, and treatment or prevention of congenital defects.

Terminology: Categories of Congenital Defects

Normal human development is a series of complicated and precisely orchestrated molecular, cellular, and physiologic events. Cell division, differentiation, migration, and growth occur as interrelated components of a developmental process in which each new step depends on preceding events. The program is completely contained in the genetic material in each fertilized zygote, but the execution of that program is subject to influence by the particular intrauterine environment in which the zygote develops. To understand how birth defects arise, it is necessary to understand the mechanisms by which normal development is perturbed. In 1980, an international working group established a terminology that is widely used to describe human anomalies in terms of their pathogenesis. For single defects, the terminology is straightforward. The term *malformation* is reserved for primary and fundamental aberration in the zygote by which it is irretrievably programmed to abnormal development, regardless of environmental influences. The vast majority of malformations are newly acquired or inherited defects in the genetic material. For most defects caused by abnormalities of the intrauterine environment, we use the terms disruption or deformation. *Disruption* refers to destruction of normally developing tissue by some outside influence; examples are most of the infectious and drug-related defects. *Deformation* describes aberrations of development in which the tissues and organs develop normally but are constrained by physical forces into odd shapes, sizes, or positions; a good example is the flat face and equinovarus (club foot) deformity that results from fetal compression by uterine muscle in the absence of adequate amniotic fluid cushioning. If the mechanism is unknown, a defect is categorized as a malformation. Abnormal differentiation or organization of tissues is termed *dysplasia.*

Every step in development depends on what has gone before; one defect may affect subsequent events. We use the term *sequence* to describe a pathophysiologically interrelated set of defects following from a single defect, which may be a malformation, disruption, or deformation, or some combination thereof (Fig. 8-2). There are malformation sequences, disruption sequences, and deformation sequences. If there are multiple structural defects that cannot be explained on the basis of a single primary defect, the term *syndrome* is employed. Most syndromes are malformation syndromes; these generally constitute a predictable set of anomalies that occur in concert, and are thought to be due to a single cause, which may or may not be known. The major chromosomal disorders (Turner's syndrome, Down syndrome, and trisomies 13 and 18) fall into this group.

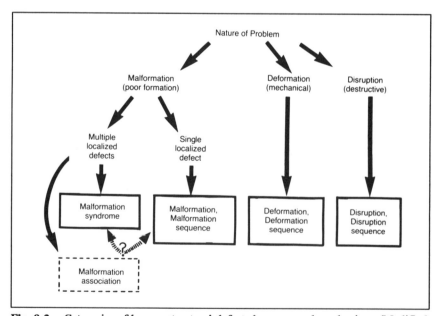

Fig. 8-2. Categories of human structural defects by presumed mechanism. (Modified from Jones, K. L. *Smith's Recognizable Patterns of Human Malformation.* Philadelphia: Saunders, 1988, with permission.)

A Developmental Anatomic Approach to Congenital Defects

In order to provide optimal treatment for the patient with a birth defect, and appropriate genetic counselling to his or her parents, the diagnosis must be as complete and accurate as possible. The aim is to determine the basic developmental defect that led to the observed pattern of malformation. One asks the question "Which anomaly represents the earliest morphogenetic defect?" This permits timing of the in utero onset of the developmental error, and is useful in excluding certain factors as causes of the defect. As an example, closure of the neural tube occurs at the end of the first month of embryonic development. The occurrence of a neural tube defect (spina bifida, meningomyelocele, encephalocele) could not, therefore, be the result of a maternal infection or drug exposure in the second trimester.

The next step is to try to determine whether all of the anomalies observed can be explained as the result of a single problem; i.e., is there an identifiable sequence? Knowledge of normal human development is an obvious necessity for this step. If there is an apparent sequence, what is the likely mechanism? Can the defects be explained by tissue necrosis, inflammation and scarring, mechanical obstruction of a hollow viscus, or compression of the fetus? Once the anomalies are accurately defined anatomically, and their relationship (if any) to one another established, an attempt is made to arrive at a diagnosis of some recognized pattern of malformation.

The necessity for this developmental approach arises from the nonspecificity of individual defects. Hydrocephalus, for example, is a common congenital defect that can result from at least 30 to 50 different genetic, infectious, and toxic conditions ranging from trisomy to retinoic acid embryopathy (Fig. 8-3). In addition, hydrocephalus commonly results from postnatal aqueductal scarring following neonatal intraventricular hemorrhage or neonatal meningitis. Thus, a common phenotype can result from a large number of pre- or postnatal causes with very different implications for treatment, recurrence risk, and prevention.

Conversely, there is wide variability in the spectrum of phenotypic changes resulting from a given developmental error. That is, the severity of a defect among individuals with the same basic problem may vary. A tiny umbilical hernia and a large and life-threatening omphalocele represent different degrees of the same basic defect, namely failure of retraction of the bowel into the abdominal cavity. The wide variation in expression of Down syndrome is another example. Mental deficiency is really the only ubiquitous clinical feature; not all patients with trisomy 21 have epicanthal folds, short necks, or a simian crease, yet all have an extra chromosome.

The approach to diagnosis, prevention, and treatment of birth defects therefore requires that adequate anatomic and clinical data be collected, and that it be interpreted by persons who are knowledgeable and qualified to deal with developmental problems.

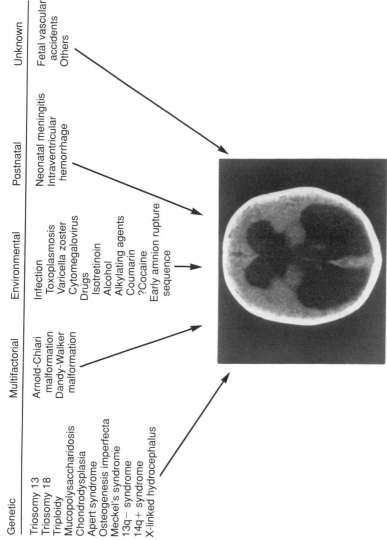

Genetic	Multifactorial	Environmental	Postnatal	Unknown
Triosomy 13	Arnold-Chiari malformation	Infection	Neonatal meningitis	Fetal vascular accidents
Triosomy 18	Dandy-Walker malformation	Toxoplasmosis	Intraventricular hemorrhage	Others
Triploidy		Varicella zoster		
Mucopolysaccharidosis		Cytomegalovirus		
Chondrodysplasia		Drugs		
Apert syndrome		Isotretinoin		
Osteogenesis imperfecta		Alcohol		
Meckel's syndrome		Alkylating agents		
13q− syndrome		Coumarin		
14q+ syndrome		?Cocaine		
X-linked hydrocephalus		Early amnion rupture sequence		

Fig. 8-3. Hydrocephalus is an example of the nonspecificity of individual defects. Many different disease entities produce a similar phenotype. Correct diagnosis depends on accurate and complete history, assessment of associated anomalies, and appropriate imaging and laboratory testing.

Thorough and accurate history-taking is essential. The family history must be ascertained in detail to look for similar or related problems, unexplained infant or childhood death, unexplained spontaneous abortion, and consanguinity. The pregnancy history must be examined with reference to previous pregnancy loss, infectious disease, and drug or toxic exposure. Preconceptional history may be important in the genesis of many birth defects, and may account for mutation in germ line cells or abnormalities of the intrauterine environment. The major organ systems are formed by the end of 6 weeks after conception; this means that major anomalies are likely to have developed before pregnancy is even recognized. Indeed, it is apparent that many pregnancies are lost before they are recognized, many of them with major chromosomal abnormalities. Prevention of the birth defects associated with maternal diabetes mellitus, for example, requires careful prepregnancy planning to optimize metabolic control prior to conception and particularly during the period of embryogenesis. One cannot prevent a thing after it has happened.

Etiology of Congenital Defects

Much is known about etiology and pathogenesis of birth defects in experimental animals; less is known about humans. This is so in part because ascertainment of etiology in humans is complicated by many confounding conditions for which it is difficult or impossible to control. The timing of an insult may be critical. Some teratogens are operative only during a very short period of time, whereas others may act any time during pregnancy, to effect variable manifestations depending on the stage of development of the embryo or fetus. Thalidomide produces the characteristic limb reduction anomalies only when exposure occurs 35 to 50 days after the last menstrual period. Rubella virus can cause trouble at any time during pregnancy, but the incidence and type of defect vary with gestational age. Exposure dose is frequently undeterminable in human pregnancy; size of viral inoculum, doses of over-the-counter medications or drugs of abuse, alcohol intake, and exposure to environmental irradiation can at best only be estimated. Extrapolation of data from animal experiments is risky because of the many problems of species specificity. To use thalidomide again as an example, extensive testing in mice and rats had not uncovered the drug's teratogenic effects, which became apparent only after the fact, when thalidomide was tested in rabbits. Even in situations in which exposure and dose can be precisely determined, as with therapeutic agents, it may be difficult to determine whether it is the drug itself, a metabolite, or the condition for which it is prescribed (or some combination thereof) that is really the teratogen. The lay press, juries, and judges have sometimes failed to realize that coexistence does not necessarily equal cause and effect; this has given rise to a whole new class of drugs known as "litogens," drugs that do not cause birth defects but do cause lawsuits.

A Brief Survey of Known and Putative Human Teratogens

Known causes of human birth defects fall into four main categories: genetic and chromosomal abnormalities; environmental influences of intrauterine or extrauterine origin; multifactorial processes that represent a synergy between genetic and environmental causes; and unidentified or idiopathic causes, the latter shrinking but still the largest group.

Single-gene defects and chromosomal abnormalities together account for 10 to 15 percent of anomalies in live born infants. The true incidence of chromosomal defects is much greater; studies of fetuses aborted spontaneously in the first trimester show that over 50 percent of these conceptuses have major structural chromosomal abnormalities, mainly trisomy, monosomy, and triploidy. Most conceptuses with monosomy X (45X, or Turner's syndrome) are aborted spontaneously in the first trimester; autosomal monosomy is almost always lethal. In general, the major structural chromosomal defects are malformation syndromes; there are anomalies of many different organ systems that cannot be explained by a single developmental sequence gone awry. Common examples include Down syndrome, Turner's syndrome, and the major trisomies 13 and 18. For purposes of genetic counselling and prevention, it is important to distinguish trisomy due to nondisjunction from trisomy due to parental balanced translocation. The former is associated with advanced maternal age and is not inherited. Trisomy resulting from balanced translocation is independent of maternal age and is inherited.

As the ability to detect short segments of the chromosome improves, many disorders not previously known to be chromosomal have been found to result from structural chromosomal changes: translocation, deletions, isochromosomes, and ring chromosomes. Examples of disorders attributed to deletions include the heritable form of retinoblastoma (del 13q), the aniridia-Wilms' tumor syndrome (del 11p), diGeorge syndrome (del 22q), and Duchenne's muscular dystrophy (del Xp). Triploidy may result from a variety of mechanisms; the most common is dispermy, which is a sporadic event and is unlikely to recur in future pregnancies.

Most individuals with chromosomal abnormalities will have multiple defects in many organ systems; hence the importance of genetic (karyotypic) analysis of patients with multiple defects.

Single-gene defects inherited according to mendelian principles account for about one-twelfth of congenital defects. This is an interesting group; most of these are point mutations that produce metabolically defective molecules that then cause disordered embryogenesis. In a sense, then, the fetus is programmed to produce its own teratogenic metabolites. Examples include Zellweger syndrome (a disorder of peroxisomal biosynthesis) and some of the chondrodystrophies that produce short-limbed dwarfism. The term *metabolic dysplasia* has been used to describe morphologic abnormalities that result from inborn errors of metabolism.

Approximately one-fifth of congenital defects are thought to be multi-factorial in cause; there appears to be some genetic predisposition to the defect, but certain environmental factors are also necessary. Examples of defects thought to be multifactorial include neural tube defects and congenital heart disease. This group of disorders is not well understood and it is possible that some will prove on further study to be genetic.

Alterations of the intrauterine environment usually produce disruptions, deformations, or dysplasia. These conditions include three groups of defects: those due to maternal disease, those due to fetal disease, and those due to physical disturbances in the intrauterine environment.

Chief among teratogenic maternal diseases is diabetes mellitus. Infants of diabetic mothers are three times as likely to have birth defects as infants of nondiabetic mothers. Common malformations in these infants include congenital heart disease and defects in the axial skeleton and limbs (Fig. 8-4). The spectrum of severity of skeletal change is wide, and ranges from mild shortening of the legs to a severe mermaid-like deformity known (inaccurately) as *caudal regression*. The exact mechanisms by which diabetes

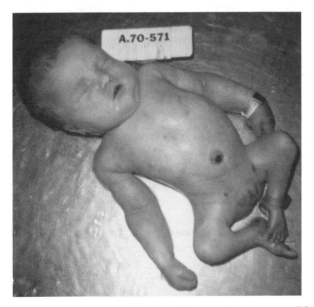

Fig. 8-4. Infant of a diabetic mother with caudal regression sequence. Maternal diabetes mellitus is a potent teratogen that produces a wide spectrum of anomalies. This infant has shortening and deformity of the lower extremities, a small pelvis with absent sacrum and coccyx, defective lumbar vertebrae, and multiple lower urinary tract anomalies including horseshoe kidney and bilateral hydronephrosis. Anal and lower genital tract anomalies are often present. The mechanism is not known but presumably the primary defect is a very early insult to the caudal end of the developing embryo. When renal disease is severe, these infants also have oligohydramnios and its sequelae.

influences embryologic development are incompletely understood. It is clear, however, that good metabolic control of maternal diabetes prior to and during pregnancy can dramatically reduce the rate of malformation. That the teratogenic factor is environmental rather than genetic is confirmed by the absence of increased malformations in infants of diabetic fathers.

Maternal phenylketonuria (PKU) is a new teratogen resulting from medical progress. As women with PKU survive into the childbearing years with normal intelligence, an increased rate of low birth weight, microcephaly, mental retardation, and congenital heart disease has been noted in their offspring. The teratogenic effect appears to be the result of hyperphenylalaninemia, and, like maternal diabetes, maternal PKU-related defects can be largely averted by meticulous dietary control before and during pregnancy. (The offspring, of course, are still obligate carriers of PKU.)

Unusual physical or mechanical conditions in the intrauterine environment give rise to deformations or disruptions. The consequences of oligohydramnios illustrate a deformation sequence (Fig. 8-5). Deprived of a normal cushion of amniotic fluid, the fetus is compressed by uterine muscle, fetal movement is constrained, and the normal movement of fluid into the developing respiratory tree is lacking. This condition results in a relatively flattened fetal face with canthal folds, low-set and maldeveloped ears, fixed positional defects of the legs, flattened hands, and underdevelopment of the lungs. The example also illustrates how many different underlying conditions may result in the same phenotype. Oligohydramnios is responsible for the external dysmorphisms and lung hypoplasia, but known causes of oligohydramnios are many. These include chronic leaks of amniotic fluid, abdominal and tubal pregnancy, inherited renal cystic disease (of many types), fetal urinary tract obstruction, and renal agenesis. The terms *oligohydramnios sequence,* or *fetal compression syndrome,* describe a phenotype that may have any of a large number of underlying defects; unless the primary defect is known, appropriate treatment and counselling are seriously compromised.

The early amniotic rupture sequence exemplifies a disruptive and deforming sequence. Premature amniotic rupture leads to oligohydramnios and also to the formation of band-like scars bridging the amniotic cavity. The fetus becomes entrapped in the scar tissue or adherent to the amnion,

Fig. 8-5. Two different infants with a common phenotype, the oligohydramnios sequence, or Potter's sequence, but with very different underlying diseases. Both infants have Potter's facies, low-set abnormal ears, limb deformities, and marked pulmonary hypoplasia. The one on top (A–D) has autosomal-recessive infantile polycystic kidney disease; there is a 1 in 4 chance of recurrence in each subsequent pregnancy. The infant in E–H has bilateral cystic renal dysplasia resulting from bilateral ureteral obstruction. This is a sporadic occurrence, unlikely to recur in subsequent pregnancies. Many different etiologies may work by a common mechanism to produce similar defects.

OLIGOHYDRAMNIOS SEQUENCE

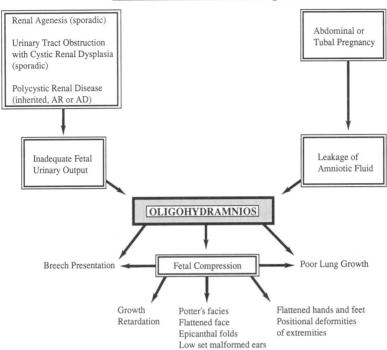

```
┌─────────────────────────────┐                    ┌─────────────────┐
│ Renal Agenesis (sporadic)   │                    │ Abdominal or    │
│                             │                    │ Tubal Pregnancy │
│ Urinary Tract Obstruction   │                    └─────────────────┘
│ with Cystic Renal Dysplasia │                            │
│ (sporadic)                  │                            │
│                             │                            ▼
│ Polycystic Renal Disease    │                    ┌─────────────────┐
│ (inherited, AR or AD)       │                    │ Leakage of      │
└─────────────────────────────┘                    │ Amniotic Fluid  │
         │                                          └─────────────────┘
         ▼
┌─────────────────┐
│ Inadequate Fetal│
│ Urinary Output  │
└─────────────────┘
```

OLIGOHYDRAMNIOS

Breech Presentation ← Fetal Compression → Poor Lung Growth

Growth Retardation

Potter's facies
Flattened face
Epicanthal folds
Low set malformed ears

Flattened hands and feet
Positional deformities
of extremities

A B C D

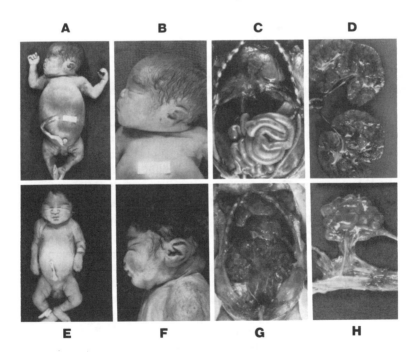

E F G H

and the result is a bizarre and completely unpredictable pattern of limb amputations, body clefts, and adhesions that on occasion mimic conditions of genetic or multifactorial cause that have a high recurrence rate. The importance of recognizing this so-called amniotic band syndrome is that it is sporadic and the chance of recurrence in subsequent pregnancies is very low.

The fetus may exert a teratogenic effect on himself or herself, as for example in so-called prune belly syndrome and the fetal hypokinesia or akinesia effect. In the former, massive bladder dilatation, usually due to lower urinary tract obstruction, leads to massive abdominal distention, which in turn leads to failure of the anterior abdominal wall muscles to develop properly. When the bladder is emptied, either via rupture or cystostomy, the abdomen deflates and the thin, noncontractile abdominal wall indeed looks like a prune. Secondary elevation of the diaphragm and oligohydramnios resulting from fetal oliguria or anuria may lead to lung hypoplasia and the oligohydramnios sequence. This is one of the few defects currently amenable to intrauterine surgery. If the bladder can be decompressed before renal and lung development are seriously impaired, there is potential for good prognosis.

Limitation of fetal movement (hypokinesia or akinesia) may result in fixed positional deformities of the limbs and contractures of the joints; the most severe end of this spectrum is arthrogryposis. Conditions that limit fetal movement include fetal crowding and a wide variety of neurologic, muscular, and connective-tissue disorders, each with its own implications for recurrence. Examples of different causes of fetal movement limitation include maternal myasthenia gravis, meningomyelocele (multifactorial), and anterior horn-cell disease (autosomal-recessive).

Table 8-1 lists the important teratogens in the extrauterine environment. Of these extrinsic teratogenic influences, infectious diseases constitute a most important group, accounting for a small (2–3%) but clearly preventable proportion of birth defects. Many microorganisms are capable of fetal infection, but only four are established teratogens. Rubella virus, cytomegalovirus, varicella zoster, and *Toxoplasma gondii* all produce consistent patterns of abnormality. Human immunodeficiency virus (HIV) infection has been postulated as a teratogen, but the frequent presence of confounding variables (substance abuse and concurrent infection with other agents) would appear to warrant caution in ascribing a teratogenic role for this virus at present.

All of these agents are capable of crossing the placenta early or late in gestation. They produce tissue necrosis, inflammation and scarring, and inhibition of cell growth and differentiation, and they are all systemic (i.e., widespread) illnesses. The pattern of the resulting disruption depends on the timing and severity of the insult, and therefore the dysmorphogenetic syndromes caused by infectious agents are variable in type and severity, although the main features remain relatively consistent. The congenital

Table 8-1. Known and suspected environmental human teratogens

Infectious agents	Rubella virus
	Cytomegalovirus
	Toxoplasma gondii
	Varicella zoster virus
	(?) Human immunodeficiency virus
	Treponema pallidum
Drugs	Alcohol
	Cocaine
	Thalidomide
	Isotretinoin
	Coumarin
	Androgens
	Diethylstilbesterol
	Phenytoin
	Trimethadione
	Valproic acid
	Tetracycline
Pollutants	Organic mercury
	Lead
	PCBs
Physical agents	Ionizing radiation
	Hyperthermia

rubella syndrome is perhaps the best studied of the group. Rubella virus reaches the fetus in the course of maternal viremia at any time during pregnancy. The earlier the infection, the more numerous and severe the resulting defects. Congenital cardiac defects result from first-trimester infections, deafness and neurologic deficits are seen through the fourth month, and retinopathy through the fifth month of gestation. Infections later in gestation, after all major organs have developed, cause mainly inflammatory and destructive lesions; in the central nervous system, these may produce serious deficits. A recently recognized example of fetal disruption is intrauterine varicella zoster infection. Though apparently rare, this infection can be devastating to the fetus, causing extensive necrosis of the central nervous system and severe scarring of skin in dermatome distribution (Fig. 8-6); this results in hydrocephalus and limb deformities.

Of the infectious teratogens, rubella embryopathy is clearly preventable with current immunization programs. Cytomegalovirus, varicella zoster, and HIV embryopathy are at least theoretically treatable in utero with antiviral agents. Recent attempts to treat fetal toxoplasmosis by treating the mother have appeared to lessen the severity of the fetal effects.

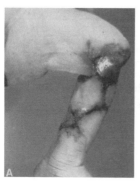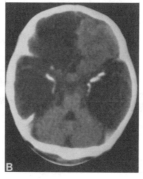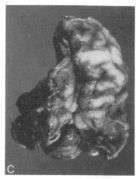

Fig. 8-6. Fetal varicella zoster, a disruptive sequence contracted from the mother. The route of infection is not yet known, but the fetus develops a severe herpes zoster–like pattern of skin and nerve involvement that leads to (A) dermal and epidermal scarring in a dermatome distribution and (B) cavitary necrosis of the central nervous system, shown in CT scan and (C) photo of the brain at autopsy.

Studies of fetuses exposed in utero to high doses of radiation present convincing evidence of increased rates of microcephaly, microphthalmia, and skeletal defects involving the skull, vertebrae, and limbs. Fetal x-ray exposure may occur during the course of therapeutic maternal radiation or as a result of nuclear accident or explosion. Studies relating the incidence of fetal anomalies to proximity to the hypocenter of thermonuclear explosion demonstrate a dose effect for microcephaly and mental retardation. Diagnostic x-ray in low (<5 rad) dose is not usually considered a danger to the fetus, but no safe lower threshold has been established, and unnecessary exposure of the embryo or fetus should be avoided. Improvements in ultrasound and magnetic resonance imaging have obviated the need for extensive use of pelvic radiation in pregnancy. Radio-iodine administration after the fetal thyroid begins to concentrate iodide at 10 to 12 weeks of gestation ablates fetal as well as maternal thyroid and may lead to congenital hypothyroidism (cretinism). Exposure to video display terminals has not been associated with increased risk of congenital defects.

Environmental contamination by a wide variety of additives, chemical contaminants, and pollutants is of serious concern. An enormous group of metals, coloring agents, dyes, propellants, solvents, and industrial and agricultural chemicals has been investigated for embryotoxic and teratogenic effects. Applicability of experimental and animal data to human risk is particularly difficult to assess in this group for reasons already cited. Environmental contaminants are ubiquitous, difficult to detect, and rarely occur as isolated single-agent contamination. Nowhere is the uncontrolled nature of human exposure more frustratingly apparent, or the need for careful study and cautious interpretation of data more compelling.

Attempts to solve by litigation questions that have not been answered by scientific inquiry would not appear to represent a positive or rational approach.

Although not attempting to minimize the real or potential dangers of environmental contamination, it is fair to say that as of this writing investigations have turned up large numbers of litogens but only a single confirmed teratogen, organic mercury. In Japan and Iraq, methylmercury contamination of fish (in Japan) and grain (in Iraq) produced well-documented fetal neurologic damage. Important possible but so far unproved teratogens include lead and polychlorinated biphenyl compounds (PCBs). Following the widespread use of the herbicide Agent Orange as a defoliant in Vietnam, there were many claims that the compound caused malformations in the offspring of exposed individuals. The widespread presence of dioxin as a contaminant in Agent Orange clouded the issue considerably, and both substances are teratogenic in animals. Intensive investigative efforts have thus far failed to demonstrate that Agent Orange is teratogenic in humans. Cigarette smoking during pregnancy is associated with low birth weight and premature birth but has not been demonstrated to cause malformations.

Many widely used and clearly efficacious pharmaceutical agents are known to be teratogenic in humans; their use in women of childbearing age requires the thoughtful balancing of therapeutic benefit and fetal risk as well as meticulous attention to appropriate contraceptive measures. Isotretinoin (13-*cis*-retinoic acid, a vitamin A analog) is a useful example of the complexity of problems of drug use in pregnancy. Isotretinoin is highly effective treatment for a severe and disfiguring condition called cystic acne. Used during the first trimester of pregnancy, it results in a high incidence of craniofacial, nervous system, and cardiac defects. This drug's fetal risk far outweighs its maternal benefit, necessitating carefully controlled prescription practices including pregnancy testing and contraceptive counselling, and placing great responsibility on the prescribing physician to educate his or her patient and to ensure compliance.

A different dilemma is posed by anticonvulsant medications; most of the widely used effective ones (diphenylhydantoin, trimethadione, valproic acid, and possibly phenobarbital) are known to be teratogenic. Equally clearly, prolonged or uncontrolled seizures pose a serious threat to both mother and fetus, and the use of these compounds in pregnant women is often unavoidable. Difficult and informed choices must be made by the physician and patient together. Similar considerations apply for the use of folate antagonists and alkylating agents in pregnancy; the risk of maternal neoplasia must be balanced with these drugs' known teratogenic effects. Aminoglycoside antibiotics, tetracycline, antithyroid drugs, and the anticoagulant warfarin are other examples of teratogenic drugs that may on occasion be indicated in pregnant women. At the other end of the scale is a group of drugs that either are not effective in the conditions for which they were used (diethylstilbestrol) or for which safe and effective alternates are available (thalidomide); these drugs should not be used at all. Finally, there is a group of drugs that have been investigated and found to have, in the usual therapeutic doses, no known teratogenic effect; this group includes aspirin, antihistamines, bendectin, cortisone, and vaginal spermicides. In general, no drugs that are not really necessary should be used during pregnancy.

As the use of crack cocaine has assumed epidemic proportions in most large urban areas, concern has increased about the deleterious fetal effects of maternal substance abuse. Because of the frequent coexistence of alcohol (and other substance) abuse, malnutrition, the social, economic, and psychologic characteristics of the study population, and a growing incidence of associated infectious diseases (HIV, syphilis, tuberculosis, and other sexually transmitted diseases), this has not been an easy question to answer. The data are most clear-cut for cocaine; this drug clearly causes abruptio placentae and preterm delivery, intrauterine growth retardation, functional neurologic defects, and a variety of congenital central nervous system and genitourinary tract anomalies, limb reductions, and intestinal atresias that almost certainly represent ischemic disruptions due to placental and fetal vascular disease. Heroin, marijuana, amphetamines, and the other drugs of abuse have not been demonstrated to be teratogenic, but do cause low birth weight, increased stillbirth, and neonatal withdrawal.

Ethyl alcohol remains the leading known environmental teratogen; the fetal alcohol syndrome is characterized by pre- and postnatal growth retardation, characteristic facial dysmorphism, and central nervous system dysfunction. Lesser degrees of severity can be demonstrated and are termed *fetal alcohol effect.* A dose effect appears likely, and most infants with the full-blown syndrome have frankly alcoholic mothers consuming eight to 10 drinks per day. Less severe involvement is detectable at four to six drinks per day. It is now apparent that these infants have lifelong neurologic dysfunction and maladaptive behavior. Incidence estimates range from 1 in 300 babies in Sweden to 1 in 1000 babies in the U.S. and France. The economic and social burden of this preventable group of birth defects is enormous.

Summary

Many conclusions and principles can be derived from this brief discussion of human teratogenesis; a summary of the important points would include these:

1. Although a definite etiology can be determined (as yet) in only a minority of cases, most congenital defects, properly diagnosed, are amenable to genetic counselling as to recurrence risk or, importantly, lack thereof. Many can be detected prenatally and prevented.

2. The evaluation of a patient must include careful family, preconceptional, and pregnancy history and meticulously thorough physical examination to arrive at a correct diagnosis.

3. History, physical examination, and appropriate imaging and laboratory data should be evaluated to determine timing of the insult and to uncover pathogenetic sequences that may shed light on the underlying etiology of the defect.

4. Abortuses, stillbirths, and lethally malformed fetuses and infants should be examined by individuals knowledgeable about developmental disorders so that complete and correct diagnoses can be made.

5. Conditions of varying and diverse etiology may produce similar phenotypes, and, conversely,

6. A single category of insult may give rise to a wide spectrum of changes.

7. Cause-and-effect relationships in human teratogenesis are difficult to establish and require carefully designed and interpreted studies. Thus, extreme caution should be exercised in ascribing causality.

8. Many congenital defects of known etiology are preventable with currently available means; these include embryopathies caused by rubella, alcohol, diabetes, and cocaine. The economic and social cost of this group warrants increased investment of resources for prevention.

Recommended Reading

Anderson, J. D., Thomas, E. E., and Cimolai, M. Infections and the Conceptus. In J. E. Dimmick and D. K. Kalousek (eds.), *Developmental Pathology of the Embryo and Fetus*. Philadelphia: Lippincott, 1992. Pp. 143–198.

Beckman, D. A., and Brent, R. L. Mechanisms of known environmental teratogens: Drugs and chemicals. *Clin. Perinatol.* 13:649–687, 1986.

Brent, R. L. The complexities of solving the problem of human malformations. *Clin. Perinatol.* 13:491–503, 1986.

Brent, R. L. Evaluating the alleged teratogenicity of environmental agents. *Clin. Perinatol.* 13:609–648, 1986.

Gilbert-Barness, E., and Opitz, J. Chromosomal Abnormalities. In J. T. Stocker and L. P. Dehner (eds.), *Pediatric Pathology*. Philadelphia: Lippincott, 1992. Pp. 41–72.

Gilbert-Barness, E., and Opitz, J. Congenital Anomalies and Malformation Syndromes. In J. T. Stocker and L. P. Dehner (eds.), *Pediatric Pathology*, Philadelphia: Lippincott, 1992. Pp. 73–115.

Hoyme, E. H. Teratogenically induced fetal anomalies. *Clin. Perinatol.* 17:547–567, 1990.

Jones, K. L. *Smith's Recognizable Patterns of Human Malformation*. Philadelphia: Saunders, 1988.

Hall, J. Developmental Defects in Stillborn and Newborn Infants. In J. E. Dimmick and D. K. Kalousek (eds.), *Developmental Pathology of the Embryo and Fetus*. Philadelphia: Lippincott, 1992. Pp. 111–142

Kalter, H., and Warkany, J. Congenital malformations. *N. Eng. J. Med.* 308:424–431; 308: 491–497, 1983.

Machin, G. A. The Causes of Malformation. In J. S. Wigglesworth and D. B. Singer (eds.), *Textbook of Fetal and Perinatal Pathology.* Boston: Blackwell, 1991. Pp. 307–338.

Mullick, F. G., and Moran, C. A. Effects of Maternal Drugs in the Fetus. In J. T. Stocker and L. P. Dehner (eds.), *Pediatric Pathology.* Philadelphia: Lippincott, 1992. Pp. 250–252.

Neave, C. Congenital malformation in infants of diabetic mothers. *Persp. Pediatr. Pathol.* 8:213–222, 1984.

Oakley, G. P. Frequency of human congenital malformations. *Clin. Perinatol.* 13:545–554, 1986.

O'Shea, P. A. Infections of the Fetus and Neonate. In J. T. Stocker and L. P. Dehner (eds.), *Pediatric Pathology.* Philadelphia: Lippincott, 1992. Pp. 203–218.

9

Fetal Physiology

Donald R. Coustan

The human fetus differs significantly from the human adult with regard to physiologic function. The differences are apparently "designed" to allow the fetus to grow and develop in an environment that would be relatively hostile to the free-living adult. In this chapter we shall explore these differences in order to arrive at a better understanding of fetal development and to lay the groundwork for an understanding of the transition from fetal to neonatal life.

The Placenta

The placenta is a fetal organ that has no single parallel in the adult. It performs for the fetus many of the functions normally carried out by the respiratory system, gastrointestinal system, liver, and kidneys of the free-living organism, and also acts as an endocrine gland. Along with its membranes, the placenta may be critically important in the initiation and maintenance of labor, and its expulsion may be necessary for the initiation of lactation.

Anatomy

The word *placenta* derives from the Latin term for *cake,* and is descriptive of the gross appearance of the human placenta, which is flat and round if it is spread out on a surface after delivery. The placenta at term weighs, on average, 500 g and is 15 to 20 cm in diameter and 2 to 3 cm thick. Placentae have been anatomically classified according to the number of tissue layers interposed between the maternal and fetal circulations. By this scheme, the human placenta is *hemochorial*, with three layers (trophoblast, connective tissue, and fetal capillary endothelium) being present. Most importantly, there is no maternal vascular endothelium; rather, maternal blood empties into the *intervillous space* that bathes the villi (Fig. 9-1).

Originally, the classification by number of interposed layers was believed to explain differences in placental transport of various substances between maternal and fetal compartments in different species. However, further investigations have revealed that placental transport is a much more complex process than originally postulated, and many factors in addition to the distances that substances must traverse have been shown to be important. Therefore, the designation of the human placenta as hemochorial has been relegated to mostly historical significance.

Early in placental development, primitive villi grow toward the maternal decidua. While some make contact with the decidua and become anchoring villi, the majority end in the intervillous space. These original stem villi branch repeatedly over the course of gestation, with finer and finer subdivisions emerging. The area of the placenta served by a stem villus and its arborizations is known as a *cotyledon*.

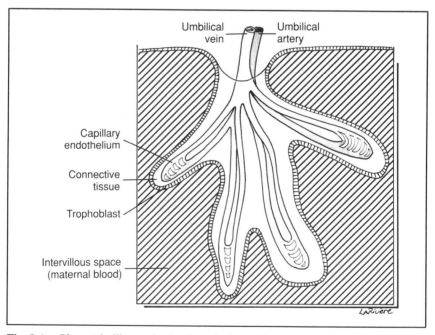

Fig. 9-1. Placental villus projecting into the intervillous space. Note the three layers of the hemochorial placenta (fetal capillary endothelium, connective tissue, and trophoblast), through which oxygen, carbon dioxide, and nutrients must pass to move between maternal and fetal blood.

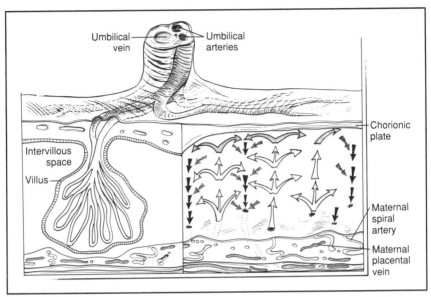

Fig. 9-2. Maternal and fetal circulations to the placenta. On the left is the villous circulation of the fetus. On the right is the maternal blood flow within the intervillous space. Note that maternal arterial blood enters the intervillous space from the spiral arteries, which run perpendicular to the myometrial wall. The arterial pressure carries the oxygenated blood to the chorionic plate, where it spreads out within the intervillous space and is collected within the maternal placental veins that run parallel to the myometrial surface.

The Uteroplacental Circulation

Under normal circumstances, blood in the maternal and fetal circulations is separate, and does not mix. Therefore, the placenta has two distinct circulations (Fig. 9-2).

Maternal Uteroplacental Circulation

Maternal arterial blood, bearing oxygen, nutrients, and other substances, travels via the hypogastric arteries to the uterine arteries. On entering the uterus, blood may supply either the uterine muscle (myometrium) or the placenta via the intervillous space. Animal data suggest that, in the nonpregnant condition, equal amounts of blood go to the myometrium and endometrium, but by the end of pregnancy 90 percent goes to the intervillous space. Since the uteroplacental blood flow in term human pregnancy represents 500 or more ml/minute, which is 10 to 20 percent of maternal cardiac output, it is apparent that a large proportion of maternal resources is shifted towards nurturing the developing fetus.

On entering the uteroplacental circulation, blood flows through the spiral arteries, oriented perpendicularly to the uterine wall, and enters the intervillous space at the basal (maternal) surface of the placenta. The arterial blood enters in spurts, propelled by the high head of pressure of the maternal systole. Each spurt travels upward toward the chorionic plate as a stream. As the head of pressure is dissipated, the stream broadens and the blood is dissipated laterally. Finally, when the pressure has totally dissipated, the blood flows back toward the basal plate, where it is taken up by maternal placental veins, which run parallel to the surface of the myometrium and drain into the uterine veins. The difference in orientation of spiral arteries and placental veins, along with the increased pressure in arteries compared to veins, allows for the maintenance of a supply of oxygen and nutrients in the intervillous space even when the uterus contracts during labor. Early in the uterine contraction cycle, the veins are occluded by increased myometrial pressure, which interferes with removal of the maternal blood from the intervillous space. As higher myometrial pressure is attained, the arteries are eventually occluded. In the meantime, more maternal blood has flowed into the intervillous space than has exited, ensuring a reserve to last throughout the contraction, under normal circumstances. Thus, the intervillous space is not emptied by each uterine contraction.

Fetal Placental Circulation
The fetal circulation to the placenta consists of two umbilical arteries and one umbilical vein, which travel in the umbilical cord supported by a matrix of Wharton's jelly. The presence of a single umbilical artery, found in slightly less than 1 percent of all umbilical cords, is associated with an increased likelihood of various malformations and other adverse pregnancy outcomes. The arteries carry deoxygenated fetal blood to the placenta, while the veins carry oxygenated blood from the placenta to the fetus. Although this situation is exactly the opposite of the normal adult systemic circulation, where arteries carry oxygenated blood and veins carry deoxygenated blood, it is analogous to the adult pulmonary circulation, and serves to emphasize that the placenta functions as a respiratory organ for the fetus. The two arteries tend to anastomose near the insertion of the umbilical cord into the placenta. The vessels branch when they reach the chorionic plate, spreading out to reach all cotyledons of the placenta, and ultimately supplying each of the villi. When the fetal surface of the placenta is viewed, the arteries are seen to lie superficial to the veins. Because the villi project into the intervillous space, bathed in maternal blood, fetal blood is carried into close approximation to, but not in continuity, with maternal blood.

Function of Placenta

Respiratory

As mentioned above, one of the primary functions of the placenta is to act as a respiratory system for the fetus, allowing the exchange of oxygen and carbon dioxide. One of the unique properties of the placental circulation is that the two systems flow *concurrently*, rather than in a countercurrent manner (Fig. 9-3).

Because highly oxygenated maternal arterial blood spurts as a stream almost to the chorionic plate before diffusing, fetal blood entering the villi from the umbilical arteries initially comes into approximation to maternal arterial blood. Fetal blood entering the umbilical venous circulation is in approximation to deoxygenated maternal blood that is about to enter the maternal venous circulation. Because of this arrangement, there is a steep gradient for oxygen and carbon dioxide at the beginning of the fetal villous circulation, but as fetal blood leaves the placenta its partial pressure of oxygen cannot be any higher than that in the maternal uterine veins. For this reason, the fetus exists in an environment wherein oxygen tension is relatively low, an environment that has often been compared to that atop a high mountain. However, the delivery of oxygen to the fetal tissues

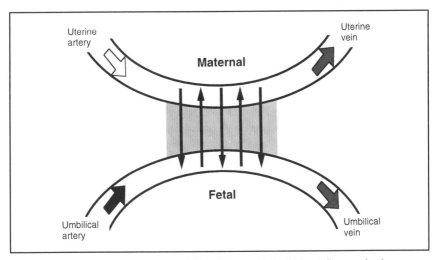

Fig. 9-3. Concurrent flow. Maternal blood flow and fetal blood flow go in the same direction at the placental interface. Fetal umbilical arterial blood (the lowest PO_2) first enters in close proximity to maternal uterine arterial blood (the highest PO_2). At the end of their close proximity, fetal umbilical venous blood is opposite maternal uterine venous blood. Thus the PO_2 in the umbilical vein can be no higher than that in the uterine vein.

is not a function only of the PO_2, but depends on total oxygen content and the ease with which oxygen can be liberated from its primary carrier molecule, hemoglobin.

The fetus is uniquely equipped to exist at low oxygen tensions. Fetal hemoglobin, which compromises 75 percent of the hemoglobin species even at term, manifests an oxygen dissociation curve that is to the left of maternal hemoglobin (i.e., fetal hemoglobin binds oxygen more avidly than adult hemoglobin at lower partial pressures of oxygen) (Fig. 9-4).

Fetal hemoglobin binds 2,3-diphosphoglycerate (2,3-DPG) less avidly than does adult hemoglobin, and thus has greater oxygen affinity at a given PO_2. This condition favors transfer of oxygen from mother to fetus. At a given PO_2 level, fetal hemoglobin has a greater oxygen content than does maternal hemoglobin. Because fetal hemoglobin concentrations are considerably higher than those of adults, and because the ventricles of the fetal heart, working in parallel rather than in series (see below) produce such a high cardiac output, oxygen delivery to fetal tissues is quite efficient despite the relatively low oxygen tension of the intrauterine environment.

The above system may best be illustrated by an example from clinical medicine. Increasing the mother's arterial PO_2 from a normal range of 90 mm Hg to a very high level, approximately 600 mm Hg, results in only a minimal rise in fetal arterial PO_2, perhaps from 12 mm Hg to 18 mm Hg. This might lead one to speculate that giving oxygen to the mother in situations in which fetal hypoxia is suspected is not very worthwhile. However, the oxygen content in the blood is the most important variable impinging on delivery of oxygen to the tissues. If, for example, we raise the mother's arterial PO_2 by 535 mm Hg, we may raise the arterial oxygen content by only 1.3 mM/liter, since at high oxygen tensions the mother is at a very flat part of her hemoglobin dissociation curve. If we assume that fetal oxygen extraction is unchanged by this process, we would expect that blood in the uterine vein would similarly have its oxygen content increased by 1.3 mM/liter. However, venous blood, with its lower oxygen tension, is at a steeper part of the hemoglobin dissociation curve, and thus the maternal uterine venous PO_2 would only increase by 11 mm Hg. Because the PO_2 in the fetal umbilical vein is limited by the PO_2 in the uterine vein, we could also anticipate that the fetal umbilical venous PO_2 would increase by 11 mm Hg. Since the fetal hemoglobin dissociation curve is quite steep at the relatively low oxygen tension found in utero, the fetal umbilical venous blood would increase its oxygen content by 2 mM/liter. Again, assuming that the fetal oxygen extraction is unchanged, fetal umbilical arterial oxygen content would increase by 2 mM/liter, an increase that is greater than twofold over the previous value, even though the PO_2 has only increased by 6 mm Hg! Thus, although marked increases in maternal PO_2 raise the fetal PO_2 only minimally, the effects on total oxygen content are quite dramatic (Fig. 9-5).

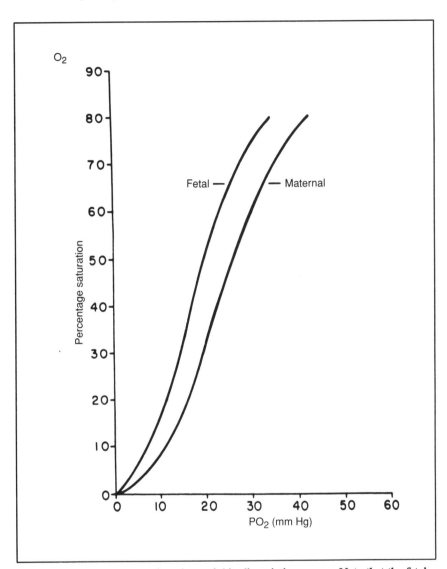

Fig. 9-4. Fetal and maternal oxyhemoglobin dissociation curves. Note that the fetal hemoglobin curve is "to the left" of the maternal curve, meaning that at a given PO_2 a higher proportion of oxygen is bound to fetal hemoglobin. (With permission, from Pritchard J. A., MacDonald, P. C., and Gant, N. F. (eds.). *Williams Obstetrics (17 ed.).* Norwalk: Appleton-Century-Crofts, 1985. P. 152. Adapted from Hellegers, A. E., and Schruefer, J. J. P. Normograms and empiric equations relating oxygen tension, percentage saturation, and pH in maternal and fetal blood. *Am. J. Obstet. Gynecol.* 81:377, 1961.)

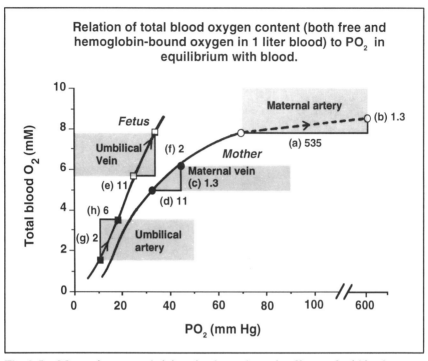

Fig. 9-5. Maternal oxygen administration has a dramatic effect on fetal blood oxygen content even though fetal PO_2 is changed relatively little. *Step a.* Oxygen therapy increases PO_2 of maternal arterial blood from 65 to 600 mm Hg. *Step b.* PO_2 increase leads to 1.3-mM increase of maternal arterial oxygen content. *Step c.* Because changes in maternal arterial PO_2 have no effect on maternal placental blood flow or rate of uterine oxygen consumption, maternal placental venous blood oxygen content also increases 1.3 mM. *Step d.* The increase in maternal venous oxygen content leads to an increase of 11 mm Hg in maternal placental venous PO_2. *Step e.* Fetal umbilical venous blood PO_2 increases by approximately the same amount (11 mm Hg). *Step f.* Because the fetal curve relating total blood oxygen content to PO_2 is steep, a small PO_2 increase is associated with a large total oxygen content increase, 2 mM, in the umbilical vein. *Step g.* Because umbilical blood flow is unchanged, the oxygen content of the fetal umbilical artery increases as much as the oxygen content of the umbilical vein (less if fetal oxygen consumption increases)—2 mM. *Step h.* The PO_2 in the umbilical artery increases by 6 mm Hg. (Adapted, with permission, from Meschia, G. How oxygen is transferred across the placenta. *Contemp. Ob/Gyn.* 14:152, 1979.)

Ranges of average values for various blood gases and acid-base characteristics of fetal and maternal blood are depicted in Table 9-1.

Nutrient Transport

If the function of pregnancy is to construct a baby out of simple raw materials, and the DNA and RNA are considered "blueprints" for this construc-

Table 9-1.   Fetal and maternal blood gases*

		Scalp blood	Cord blood	
			Venous	Arterial
Fetal blood gases				
PO$_2$ (mm Hg)	First-stage labor	17–24		
	Second-stage labor	14–18		
	At delivery		21–32	10–22
PCO$_2$ (mm Hg)	First-stage labor	33–50		
	Second-stage labor	39–51		
	At delivery		33–42	40–60
pH	First-stage labor	7.28–7.40		
	Second-stage labor	7.18–7.37		
	At delivery		7.27–7.40	7.20–7.39
Maternal arterial blood gases				
PO$_2$ (mm Hg)	First-stage labor	83–110		
	Delivery	91–118		
PCO$_2$ (mm Hg)	First-stage labor	22–32		
	Delivery	22–32		
pH	First-stage labor	7.41–7.50		
	Delivery	7.34–7.46		

*Source: Adapted from Huch R., and Huch, A. Maternal and fetal acid-base balance and blood gas measurement. In R. W. Beard and P. W. Nathanielz (eds.), *Fetal Physiology and Medicine* (2nd ed.). London: Marcel Dekker, 1984. Pp. 720–728.

tion process, one of the roles of the placenta is to serve as the materials management department, providing both fuels and building blocks for the project. Substances cross the placenta by a number of processes. Their ultimate concentration and availability in the fetus may be limited by factors such as protein binding on each side of the placenta, placental metabolism of substances as they "pass through," or lipid- and water-solubility.

Simple diffusion, in which substances travel from mother to fetus down a concentration gradient, follows physical chemical principles. Substances of low molecular weight, under 500 daltons, diffuse easily. Such substances include oxygen, carbon dioxide, water, and some electrolytes, as well as most anesthetic gases.

Facilitated diffusion, a process that is more efficient than simple diffusion and is responsible for transplacental glucose and lactate transport, is mediated by more or less specific carrier proteins that can be saturated such that, above certain maternal circulating substrate concentrations, further transport is not as efficient. This process is believed to be critical for ensuring a constant supply of glucose, the most important metabolic fuel to the fetus. It does not appear to be energy-requiring.

Active transport, an energy-requiring process by which substances are transferred against a concentration gradient, results in concentrations of substances in the fetal circulation that exceed those in the maternal circulation. Examples of substances undergoing active transport include many amino acids, ascorbic acid, iron, iodides, and possibly some fatty acids.

Endocytosis is a process by which some surprisingly large molecules may traverse the placenta. An example of this is immunoglobulin G, which by term is present in the fetal circulation in concentrations similar to those observed in the mother. Immunoglobulins A and M do not cross the placenta to any extent at all. Maternal IgG enters the fetal circulation and accomplishes the passive transfer of maternal immunity. Maternal IgG helps the neonate fight infections encountered in early life, but it also has implications in certain pathologic situations, such as red-cell isoimmunization and maternal-immune thrombocytopenic purpura, in which the IgG antibodies may have detrimental effects on the fetus in utero. Recent evidence suggests that insulin derived from animals, administered to mothers with diabetes, may cross the placenta to the fetus when bound to antibodies. The clinical significance of this finding is yet to be elucidated.

Waste Removal

The fetal liver and kidneys are relatively immature throughout gestation. The kidneys cannot concentrate the urine very effectively, and the urine enters the amniotic cavity, where it is swallowed by the fetus; this is a rather inefficient system for the removal of nitrogenous wastes. The liver is relatively poor at conjugation and excretion, and again there would be no escape for the waste products. Therefore, the placenta carries metabolic by-products back to the maternal circulation, where the mother's liver and kidneys can excrete them. The transfer of substances such as urea and bilrubin is bidirectional, so that pathologic maternal conditions such as uremia and hepatic failure may cause dangerous accumulations of these toxins in the fetal compartment. Thus, mothers undergoing hemodialysis during pregnancy may require more frequent treatments than they do in the nonpregnant state.

Endocrinology

The placenta is an active endocrine organ that produces a number of hormones. The major placental hormones are either proteins (human chorionic gonadotropin [hCG] and human placental lactogen [hPL], which is also known as human chorionic somatomammotropin [hCS]), or steroids (estrogens and progesterone). All hormones but hPL appear to be critical, at various stages of gestation, for the normal development and outcome of pregnancy.

The protein hormones, hCG and hPL, are analogous to the pituitary hormones luteinizing hormone (LH) and human growth hormone (hGH). They are produced in the syncytiotrophoblast of the placenta, which has been likened to the anterior pituitary gland. It has been postulated that the cytotrophoblast of the placenta is analogous to the hypothalamus, since hormones analogous to gonadotropin-releasing hormone (GnRH) and somatostatin have been found in these cells. Similarly, corticotropin-releasing hormone (CRH) and thyrotropin-releasing hormone (TRH) have been isolated in cytotrophoblast cells and adrenocorticotropic hormone (ACTH) and thyroid-stimulating hormone (TSH) are produced in the syncytiotrophoblast.

Human chorionic gonadotropin (hCG) is a glycoprotein hormone with a molecular weight of approximately 36,700 daltons. Roughly 30 percent of the molecule is carbohydrate, and it is composed of alpha and beta subunits. The alpha subunit is homologous to the alpha subunits of the pituitary glycoprotein hormones follicle-stimulating hormone (FSH), LH, and TSH, and so it is not immunologically specific to hCG. The beta subunit, which is immunologically specific to hCG, contains 147 to 149 amino acids. It is the carboxy terminal 24–30 amino acids that are unique to hCG. It is believed that GnRH produced in the cytotrophoblast cells is a regulator of hCG production or release, or both.

Human chorionic gonadotropin acts on LH receptors. In fact, exogenous hCG injections are used to induce ovulation in some infertility patients whose ovarian-hypothalamic-pituitary axis does not produce the normal midcycle LH surge. This hormone is responsible for maintenance of function of the corpus luteum during early pregnancy, particularly progesterone production. It also appears to promote testosterone production by the testes of the male fetus, which is important for male sexual differentiation. Human chorionic gonadotropin has thyroid-stimulating properties and is also believed to play a role in the relative immunosuppression of pregnancy. Methods of measurement of hCG, as well as the pattern of its secretion throughout pregnancy, are discussed in Chapter 11.

Human placental lactogen (hPL) is a single-chain polypeptide with a molecular weight of approximately 22,000 daltons. There are 191 amino acids in the chain, with a high degree of homology to the 188 amnio acids in human growth hormone, and to the approximately 190 amino acids in prolactin. The site of synthesis of hPL is the syncytiotrophoblast of the placenta, and the hormone is secreted almost exclusively into the maternal circulation, with little present in the fetus or amniotic fluid. First measurable in the maternal circulation by 3 weeks after conception, hPL levels rise progressively throughout pregnancy, reaching µg/ml levels during the third trimester. In fact, with its rapid half-life it is the most abundant polypeptide hormone known, with production levels reaching as much as a gram per day near term.

Although apparently normal pregnancies have been reported in which hPL levels were so low as to be undetectable, hPL appears to have profound effects on maternal metabolism. These effects are most easily visualized as diabetogenic, or anti-insulin, and include the enhancement of lipolysis and inhibition of gluconeogenesis and glucose storage. Teleologically, one can think of hPL as serving as a backup system in case of long-term starvation, such as might have been encountered in ancient times. Under such circumstances, lipolysis would allow the pregnant woman to utilize fat as fuel, sparing glucose for the conceptus. At one time, hPL measurements were used to monitor fetal-placental function. Such efforts have been generally abandoned, because the results were unreliable as predictors of pregnancy outcome.

The fetus and placenta are interdependent in the production of *steroid hormones*. The placenta is unable to convert acetate to cholesterol, and so converts preformed maternal cholesterol to pregnenolone, or utilizes fetal pregnenolone, to produce *progesterone* by the action of 3-β-hydroxysteroid dehydrogenase, an enzyme relatively lacking in the fetal adrenal gland. The progesterone may then be utilized by the fetus as a precursor for other steroid hormones or may be released into the maternal circulation. Because the placenta does not contain the 17-alpha-hydroxylase enzyme, any 17-hydroxyprogesterone present is likely to have come from the maternal ovaries, particularly during the first 8 weeks of pregnancy when corpus luteum progesterone production is responsible for maintenance of the pregnancy (Fig. 9-6).

Progesterone levels continue to rise throughout pregnancy, from about 25 ng/ml at 6 weeks to approximately 140 ng/ml at term. Progesterone production at term is about 250 mg/day. The functions of progesterone include its smooth muscle–relaxing effects, which may be important in preventing the untimely early onset of labor, as well as widespread effects on other maternal visceral organs such as the stomach, gall bladder, and urinary tract. It is a competitive inhibitor of aldosterone and causes increased urinary sodium loss, which in turn may lead to compensatory increases in aldosterone production. It is believed to be immunosuppressive, and complements the effect of hCG. Progesterone also contributes to the functional maturation of the breasts and preparation for lactation.

Estrogens are synthesized primarily by the placenta. As mentioned above, the placenta produces pregnenolone from maternal cholesterol. The fetal adrenals then convert the pregnenolone to dehydroepiandrosterone (DHA), which is used by the placenta as a precursor for estrone, first through the action of 3-β-hydroxysteroid dehydrogenase to produce androstenedione, then to estrone through aromatization, and finally to estradiol through the further action of 17-β-hydroxysteroid dehydrogenase. Another estrogen hormone, estriol, circulates in particularly high concentrations during pregnancy. Fetal DHA can be converted to 16-alpha-hydroxy-DHA in the fetal liver. It is then converted by the placenta to 16-hydroxy-androstenedione and then is aromatized to estriol. Huge amounts of estrogens are produced by the fetoplacental unit at term, with 1 day's output approximately equalling the results of 3 years' ovarian function in an ovulating nonpregnant woman (Fig. 9-7).

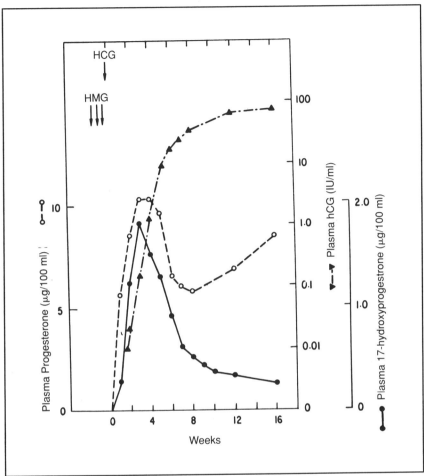

Fig. 9-6. Mean plasma levels of progesterone, 17-hydroxyprogesterone, and hCG of women with pregnancies resulting from induced ovulation. Day 0 is the day of ovulation. Note that ovarian 17-hydroxyprogesterone rises and then falls at approximately 4 to 8 weeks after ovulation, reflecting declining corpus luteum function. The transient fall in progesterone also reflects decreased ovarian production, with the subsequent rise being due to placental steroidogenesis. (With permission, from Yoshimi, et al. *J. Clin. Endocrinol. Metab.* 29:225, 1969.)

The functions of estrogens are myriad. They stimulate growth of the endometrium in preparation for pregnancy, cause hyperplasia of myometrial cells, increase uterine blood flow, and have other maternal effects described in Chapter 10. Estrogens appear to be involved in bringing about the chemical changes in the cervix known as "ripening," in preparation for labor. They also are important in preparing the breasts for lactation,

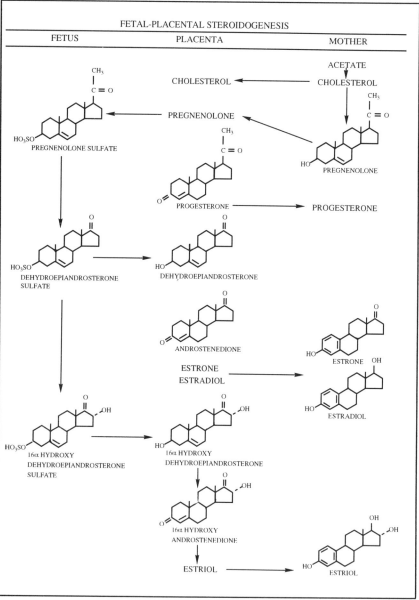

Fig. 9-7. Maternal, placental, and fetal contributions to synthesis of estrogens. Fetal liver is necessary for 16-hydroxylation to form the precursor of estriol. Placental sulfatase is necessary to cleave the sulfate prior to placental aromatization to produce estrogens.

and the abrupt fall in maternal estrogen levels after delivery is a signal for lactogenesis. Fetal ACTH appears important in regulating fetal estrogen precursor synthesis, since anencephalic fetuses who lack an anterior pituitary gland produce diminished amounts of estrogen. In the past, daily maternal urine or serum estriol measurements were obtained as a marker for fetoplacental well-being in high-risk pregnancies. These tests have been supplanted by biophysical testing such as nonstress tests, contraction stress tests, and biophysical profiles (see Chap. 16) because estriol measurements were cumbersome and imprecise expressions of fetal health.

Fetal estrogen precursors are sulfated, and the placenta must hydrolyze the sulfate prior to conversion to estrogens. When placental sulfatase activity is deficient, as in an X-linked condition that also includes ichthyosis, placental estrogen production is markedly diminished and the cervix may not undergo its usual "ripening" process, although the pregnancy tends to be otherwise uneventful.

The Fetus

Circulatory System

Fetal blood is oxygenated in the placenta and carried via the umbilical vein to the liver, where most enters the *ductus venous* and avoids the hepatic circulation (Fig. 9-8). The oxygenated blood then enters the inferior vena cava, traverses the right atrium, and enters the left atrium via the foramen ovale, avoiding the right ventricle and pulmonary circulation. This process is accomplished because the *foramen ovale* is directly opposite the termination of the inferior vena cava, so that the force of the stream of blood carries it directly through this opening into the left side of the heart. This highly oxygenated blood then enters the left ventricle, exits through the ascending aorta, and mainly supplies the brain and heart. Deoxygenated blood from the brain enters the right atrium via the superior vena cava, drains into the right ventricle, and is carried into the pulmonary artery. Approximately two-thirds of the pulmonary arterial blood traverses the ductus arteriosus to the descending aorta, and supplies the body and placenta.

This remarkable series of hydraulic shunts—the ductus venosus, foramen ovale, and ductus arteriosus—allows the fetal heart to work in parallel, with the right-sided cardiac output supplying relatively de-oxygenated blood to the placenta and fetal body, and the left-sided cardiac output supplying the brain and heart with relatively highly oxygenated blood. In contrast, the adult circulatory system works in series, with the entire output of the right heart going to the lungs for oxygenation before returning to the left heart for distribution to the systemic circulation. This approximate doubling of cardiac output, coupled with the relatively high fetal heart rate, increases oxygen delivery to the tissues as if to compensate for the

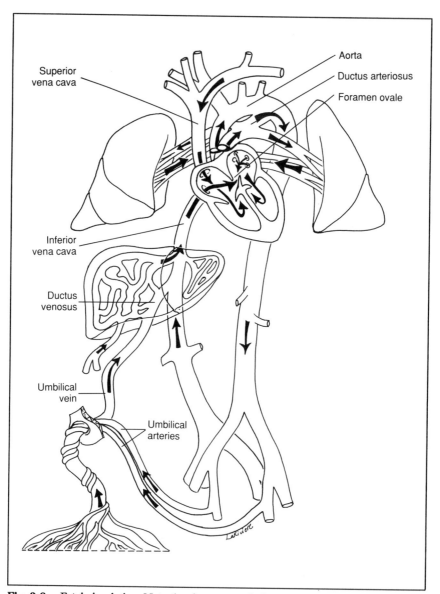

Fig. 9-8. Fetal circulation. Note the *foramen ovale* between the right and left atria, the *ductus arteriosus* between the pulmonary artery and aorta, the umbilical arteries and vein, and the *ductus venosus* from the umbilical vein to the inferior vena cava. These shunts enable the fetal circulatory system to function in parallel, bypassing the pulmonary circulation, with the right heart pumping the most oxygenated blood to the head and upper body, while the left heart pumps primarily de-oxygenated blood to the placenta and lower body.

relatively low oxygen content of fetal blood. The patency of the foramen ovale, a unidirectional flap valve, is maintained throughout fetal life because right atrial pressures exceed those in the left atrium. Flow through the ductus arteriosus is maintained by the influence of prostaglandin E, which is released locally in response to the low oxygen tensions present in fetal blood. This set of circumstances maintains high pulmonic vascular resistance as well.

When the newborn takes his or her first breath and expands the lungs, pulmonary vascular resistance falls markedly and oxygen tension increases. These changes cause a fall in right-heart pressures with closure of the foramen ovale, and a fall in pulmonary arterial pressure that results in increased flow through the pulmonary circulation (Fig. 9-9). As oxygen tension rises, prostaglandin E release is diminished in the ductus arteriosus, which allows constriction of this shunt. Functional closure of the foramen ovale and ductus arteriosus establishes the neonatal circulatory system in series rather than in parallel. Simultaneously there is a decreased demand for cardiac output as the placenta, which receives approximately 40 percent of fetal cardiac output at term, is removed from the circulatory system. Cessation of blood flow to the placenta after delivery results in the ultimate obliteration of these vessels that are so important to fetal life, with the umbilical arteries becoming the *hypogastric ligaments,* the umbilical vein becoming the *ligamentum teres,* and the ductus venosus becoming the *ligamentum venosum.* The atrophied ductus arteriosus becomes the *ligamentum arteriosum.*

Hematopoiesis
The first site of red blood cell production is the yolk sac, which is active during embryonic life. By the beginning of the second trimester hematopoiesis is active in the liver and spleen, while the bone marrow becomes increasingly important from midpregnancy onward. By term the bone marrow is almost exclusively responsible for red-cell production, but under conditions of stress, particularly with severe anemia, extramedullary hematopoiesis may persist in the liver and other sites.

During the embryonic period, primitive hemoglobins are produced, but by the end of the first trimester *hemoglobin F* (fetal hemoglobin) is the primary species present. The globin moiety of hemoglobin F is composed of two alpha and two gamma chains, as opposed to the two alpha and two beta chains in hemoglobin A (adult hemoglobin). Although the gamma chain differs from the beta chain at approximately one-fourth of its amino acid sequence, it is believed to be primarily the presence of serine instead of histidine at position 143 that causes decreased binding of 2,3-DPG to the fetal hemoglobin molecule; this provides greater oxygen affinity at a given oxygen tension, and moves the fetal hemoglobin dissociation curve to the left of that of adult hemoglobin (i.e., fetal hemoglobin binds oxygen more avidly than adult hemoglobin at lower partial pressures). Another

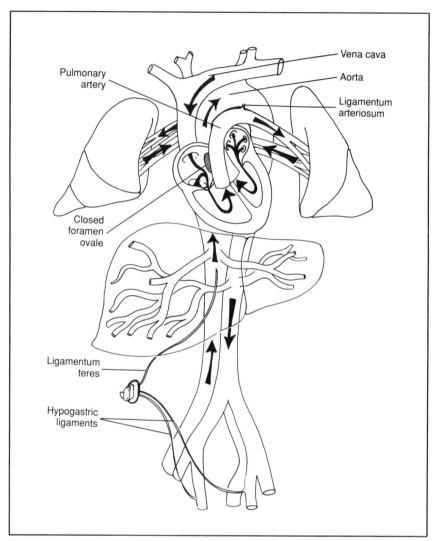

Fig. 9-9. Neonatal cardiovascular adaptations. Note that the circulation is now in series. The ductus arteriosus has closed and is now the *ligamentum arteriosum.* The foramen ovale has closed. The umbilical arteries have atrophied to become the *hypogastric ligaments* and the atrophied umbilical vein is now the *ligamentum teres.*

difference is that fetal hemoglobin is more resistant than adult hemoglobin to acid or alkali denaturation.

The beta chain, and thus hemoglobin A, begins to be produced at the end of the first trimester, and by term hemoglobin A comprises 25 to 30 percent of the hemoglobin present in fetal red blood cells. Hemoglobin concentration rises progressively in the fetus, reaching 18 to 20 g/dl at term. As mentioned earlier in this chapter, this relative plethora allows the fetus to deliver more oxygen to its tissues despite an intrauterine environment that contains a lower oxygen tension than that of the air-breathing organism. The total blood volume of the fetoplacental unit is approximately 125 ml per kilogram of body weight at term.

A clinical application of the above information is the estimation of the volume of fetomaternal hemorrhage that occurs at the time of childbirth. It is common for some fetal blood to enter the maternal circulation, presumably at the time of separation of the placenta. If the mother is Rh-negative and therefore does not carry the gene for D (one of the Rh blood group factors), and the fetus does carry this gene, Rh-positive fetal cells may incite an immune response by the mother's immune system, and antibodies against D may persist into future pregnancies, crossing the placenta and causing hemolysis of fetal red blood cells. This phenomenon can be prevented by passive immunization of the mother at the time of delivery with antibodies against the Rh D factor, called *Rh immune globulin.*

The dose of Rh immune globulin to be administered is determined by the volume of fetal red cells present in the maternal circulation. To quantitate this fetomaternal hemorrhage, a *Kleihauer-Betke test* is performed (Fig. 9-10). A thin smear of maternal blood, obtained shortly after delivery, is

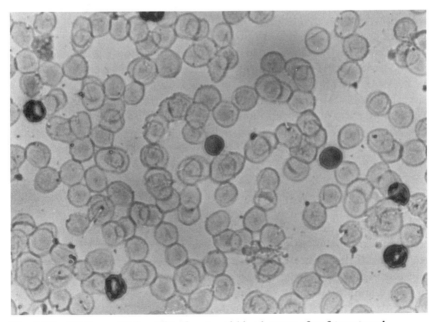

Fig. 9-10.   Kleihauer-Betke stain of maternal blood smear after fetomaternal hemorrhage (original magnification X450). There are seven fetal (dark-staining) cells among dozens of pale "ghost" maternal cells. (Courtesy of Dr. Don Singer.)

subjected to acid elution before staining. The relatively acid-resistant fetal hemoglobin retains its pink color, whereas adult hemoglobin gives a very pale appearance to the red cells. Fetal red cells are then counted and expressed as a proportion of each thousand total red cells.

Using an average value for the maternal red-cell volume, the volume of fetal red cells present in the maternal circulation can be estimated. Similarly, if a pregnant woman has been subject to abdominal trauma, as in a motor vehicle accident, and placental vascular disruption with fetomaternal hemorrhage is suspected, a Kleihauer-Betke stain can be performed with maternal blood and the volume of fetal red cells present in the maternal circulation can be expressed as a proportion of total fetoplacental blood volume lost, in order to estimate the potential for intrauterine fetal anemia. It is now also the usual practice to administer a dose of Rh immune globulin to Rh-negative mothers at approximately 28 weeks' gestation, in order to protect against the slight possibility of isoimmunization from spontaneous fetal-maternal hemorrhage during the third trimester. This passive immunization is also used in Rh-negative mothers who are undergoing amniocentesis.

Immune System

As discussed earlier in this chapter, maternal IgG antibodies cross the placenta to the fetus, and offer some passive protection against infectious agents encountered in the neonatal period. Every adult is a walking catalogue of infectious agents encountered in the course of a lifetime, inscribed in the form of circulating antibodies produced by clones of lymphocytes. At the time of birth, the fetus has most likely never encountered any infectious agents, and so carries no catalogue of lymphocytes and antibodies, only a poor copy of his or her mother's antibodies, written in "disappearing ink." These passively acquired maternal antibodies survive for 6 to 8 months, affording some protection, particularly against gram-positive bacteria and viruses.

Because maternal IgM antibodies do not cross the placenta, the fetus or neonate is afforded little passive protection against gram-negative organisms. If the fetus is exposed to infectious agents in utero, it is capable of responding by producing antibodies of the IgM class, and the presence of IgM antibodies is used clinically as a marker for fetal and neonatal infection. However, the normal transformation from IgM production to IgG production, which occurs in the adult within weeks of exposure to an antigen, does not occur in the fetus. This ability to produce IgG antibodies develops slowly in the newborn, and as the child encounters antigens in the environment he or she slowly increases the IgG catalogue, reaching approximately 60 percent of adult levels by 1 year of age (Fig. 9-11).

The transplacental transfer of maternal IgG antibodies is gestational age–dependent, and reaches its maximum in the last few weeks of gestation. Therefore, preterm neonates have significantly lower levels of passively acquired immunity than do infants born at term. These passively acquired

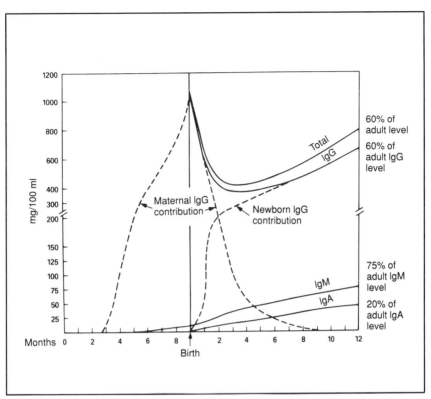

Fig. 9-11. Immunoglobulin levels in fetus and infant. Note that IgM production begins in utero, while IgG production does not begin until after birth. Passively acquired maternal IgG disappears rapidly during the first year of life. (With permission, from Scott, J. R. *The Female Patient*. Secaucus, N.J.: Core Publishing [subsidiary of Reed Elsevier] 1978. P. 93.)

IgG antibodies are not always helpful to the fetus. As mentioned previously, if the mother is Rh D–negative, and has produced antibodies against the D antigen *(isoimmunization)*, these antibodies may cross the placenta and attack the red blood cells of subsequent Rh-positive fetuses, causing hemolysis and the syndrome known as *erythroblastosis fetalis.* Details of diagnosis and management of this problem are discussed in Chapter 24.

Urinary System
Fetal urine production begins as early as 12 weeks after the last menstrual period, and after that time contributes increasingly to the formation of amniotic fluid. Although water and solutes can enter and leave the amniotic cavity via the membranes and umbilical cord, this exchange appears to be primarily passive, and is mediated by solute concentrations and osmolality. Fetal urine, however, is relatively hypotonic because of the poor

concentrating capacity of the immature kidneys, but contains high concentrations of urea and other nitrogenous wastes. Between 23 and 32 weeks, a new layer of glomeruli forms in the renal cortex weekly. Urine production increases from approximately 10 ml/hour at 30 weeks to approximately 27 ml/hour at term.

Recommended Reading

Beard, R. W., and Nathanielsz, P. W. (eds.). *Fetal Physiology and Medicine* (2nd ed.). New York: Marcel Dekker, 1984.

Bissonnette, J. Placental and Fetal Physiology. In S. G. Gabbe, J. R. Niebyl, and J. L. Simpson (eds.), *Obstetrics: Normal and Problem Pregnancies* (2nd ed.). New York: Churchill-Livingstone, 1991. Pp. 93–124.

Buster, J. E., and Carson, S. A. Placental Endocrinology and Diagnosis of Pregnancy. In S. G. Gabbe, J. R. Niebyl, and J. L. Simpson (eds.), *Obstetrics: Normal and Problem Pregnancies* (2nd ed.). New York: Churchill-Livingstone, 1991. Pp. 93–124.

Cunningham, F. G., MacDonald, P. C., Gant, N. F., Leveno, K. J., and Gilstrap, L. C. III. *Williams Obstetrics* (19th ed.). Norwalk: Appleton & Lange, 1993. Pp. 111–207.

10

Maternal Physiology

Donald R. Coustan

Human pregnancy lasts approximately 266 days, or 38 weeks, from ovulation and conception until delivery. By convention, because many women are unaware of the time of conception but most know the date of the beginning of their last menstrual period, "gestational age" is calculated from the commencement of menses, which makes the duration of pregnancy 280 days, or 40 weeks. During this interval, numerous maternal adaptations must occur in order to sustain the developing conceptus and allow the mother to withstand the challenges of pregnancy and delivery. A thorough appreciation of these normal changes is critical for the intelligent evaluation of a pregnant woman who is experiencing medical problems as well as for an understanding of normal pregnancy.

Genital Tract

Uterus
The uterus that has never sustained a pregnancy (i.e., *nulligravid*) weighs approximately 70 g; its cavity, which is a potential space, has a capacity of approximately 10 ml. By the end of pregnancy, the average uterus weighs 1100 g and contains 5 liters. This dramatic change is a result of both hyperplasia and hypertrophy. Hyperplasia, with increased mitotic activity that results in the formation of new cells, appears to occur mainly during the first 2 months of gestation and is believed to result primarily from increases in circulating estrogen levels. As progesterone levels rise, the proliferation of muscle cells declines, and hypertrophy supervenes. Individual muscle cells increase in length by approximately 10-fold, and in width by approximately fivefold (Fig. 10-1). This change is primarily a

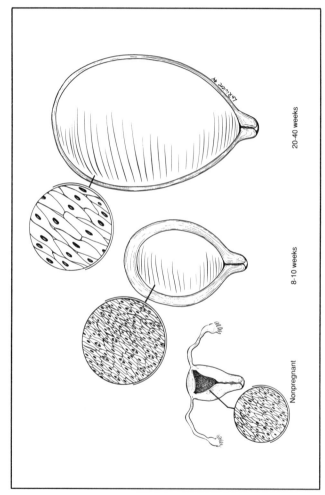

Fig. 10-1. Changes in uterine muscle during pregnancy. Insets represent myometrium in non-pregnant state *(left)*, at 8 to 10 weeks *(middle)*, and in the second half of pregnancy *(right)*. Hyperplasia, an increase in the number of muscle cells, occurs during the first 2 months under the influence of estrogen. Hypertrophy, eventuating in an increase in muscle-cell length by 10× and width by 5×, occurs later, presumably due to progesterone.

Nonpregnant   8-10 weeks   20-40 weeks

response to uterine distention, but appears to be enhanced by increasing progesterone levels.

Pregnancy is arbitrarily divided into trimesters, each lasting 13 weeks. During the first trimester, the uterus grows more rapidly than the gestational sac. The isthmus, or region between the anatomic internal os and the functional internal os, softens (Hegar's sign) but does not otherwise change during this period. However, between approximately 14 and 16 weeks' gestation, the isthmus unfolds from increasing pressure from the conceptus. The functional internal os moves downward and assumes responsibility for preventing the gestational sac from exiting the uterus (Fig. 10-2).

An important clinical correlate of this physiologic change is the possibility of a condition called "incompetent cervical os," which causes the pregnancy to be lost. In this syndrome there is dilation of the cervix that is usually described as painless, meaning that it is apparently not due to uterine contractions. Once the cervix has dilated to a certain point, contractions may begin and the process accelerates. This problem is believed by many to be a mechanical problem, since risk factors include previous forceful dilatation of the cervix, as in repetitive pregnancy terminations or cervical surgery such as cone biopsy, and possibly congenital cervical abnormalities, as might be seen with in utero exposure to diethylstilbestrol (DES). However, some cases occur in the absence of such a history, and the chemical changes responsible for cervical "ripening" may occur prematurely in such patients. The fact that isthmic unfolding does not usually occur until the fourteenth to sixteenth weeks of pregnancy thus becomes helpful information, since a pregnancy loss in the first trimester cannot be ascribed to an incompetent cervix. The late first trimester is an opportune time to place a cervical cerclage, a suture designed to prevent pregnancy loss in individuals identified as having cervical incompetence in a previous pregnancy.

The cervix itself undergoes changes during pregnancy, with softening and increased vascularity present early in the first trimester. The endocervical glands increase in size and number, and increase their production of mucus. Presumably because of the large amounts of progesterone in the circulation, cervical mucus secreted during pregnancy does not usually form a "fern" pattern when dried on a slide and viewed through a microscope, as is seen in nonpregnant individuals prior to ovulation. Another type of "ferning" is seen later in pregnancy when amniotic fluid, obtained from the vaginal pool of a patient whose membranes have ruptured, is allowed to air-dry on a microscope slide. This fern pattern is not due to cervical mucus, but is apparently the result of crystallization from the high saline content of amniotic fluid.

The squamocolumnar junction, where squamous and columnar epithelia meet, advances onto the vaginal portion of the cervix, and the reddened appearance of this glandular epithelium has given rise to the so-called cervical erosion seen in pregnancy, which is really not an erosion at all.

In addition to the increased uterine muscle mass, there is an increase in the fibrous tissue and elastic tissue that add strength to the uterine wall.

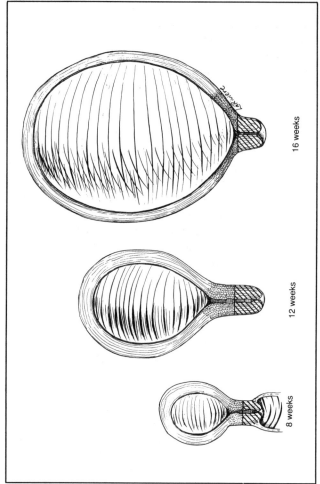

Fig. 10-2. Changes in cervix and lower uterine segment during the first half of pregnancy. Cervical tissue is cross-hatched and isthmus of uterus is stippled. Uterine muscle grows at a rate faster than the conceptus during the first trimester. By 16 weeks the conceptus has enlarged enough to put pressure on the isthmus, causing it to unfold. From this time on the cervix is responsible for containing the pregnancy. (Adapted from Danforth, D. N. The fibrous nature of the human cervix and its relation to the isthmic segment in gravid and nongravid uteri. *Am. J. Obstet. Gynecol.* 53:550, 1947.)

There is a marked increase in the size and number of both blood vessels and lymphatics. Uterine blood flow increases progressively throughout pregnancy, reaching approximately 500 ml/minute at term, or 10 times its nonpregnant level. By term the uterus is receiving 10 to 20 percent of total maternal cardiac output. The uterine arterial vasculature is normally maximally dilated, so that pharmacologic maneuvers are not successful at increasing uterine blood flow in normal pregnant women. However, uterine blood flow may be diminished by changes in maternal vascular tone and blood pressure, by pharmacologic means, and by changes in position (e.g., when a woman who is in the second half of pregnancy is supine, the uterine may rest on the vena cava [restricting venous return] or on the iliac vessels, or both, diminishing uterine perfusion). Such reductions in blood flow may then be corrected by pharmacologic agents, or by changes in maternal position (e.g., lying on her side).

The uterus contracts every 5 to 20 minutes throughout pregnancy, and even in the nonpregnant state. These contractions are irregular, not coordinated, and increase in frequency throughout the course of gestation. When they are perceived by the pregnant woman, they are called *false labor*. This phenomenon was described by Dr. John Braxton-Hicks in 1872, and thus such contractions have come to be known as *Braxton Hicks contractions*. There is often great difficulty in distinguishing between Braxton Hicks contractions and the contractions of preterm labor. The difference between the two lies primarily in the presence or absence of progressive cervical change; this topic will be covered more thoroughly in Chapter 17.

Ovaries

Ovulation does not occur during pregnancy; thus, superfetation (twins conceived during two separate ovulatory cycles) is highly unlikely. However, superfecundation (twins conceived in two separate sexual contacts during the same ovulatory cycle) has been proved by demonstrating with genetic markers that the two offspring had different fathers.

A corpus luteum of pregnancy is generally present on one or the other ovary. Ovarian steroid hormone production is evidently not critical for maintenance of pregnancy after the first trimester, since removal of the corpus luteum after this period does not result in spontaneous abortion. However, the ovary continues to secrete relaxin, a polypeptide hormone, throughout pregnancy. The function of relaxin is yet to be defined, but it may be involved in the chemical changes in the cervix that occur before the beginning of labor.

Vagina

During pregnancy, vaginal secretions increase in quantity and the pH becomes acidic. There is an increased susceptibility to vaginal candidiasis (moniliasis) during pregnancy. Approximately one-third of all gravidas are thought to harbor the causative fungus *(Candida albicans)* and over half of these women become symptomatic. The cause has been variously ascribed to the effects of high estrogen levels, the increase in glycogen deposition within the vaginal mucosal cells, and an altered immune state.

There is increased vascularity with hyperemia in the vaginal mucosa, which results in a characteristic violet-blue color (Chadwick's sign) that is often considered to be an indicator of early pregnancy. The vaginal connective tissue also softens and becomes increasingly distensible, perhaps in preparation for the descent and delivery of the fetus.

Metabolism

Weight Gain

A great deal of confusion has arisen over the years as to how much weight should be gained by a pregnant woman. In the not too distant past, obstetricians attempted to severely limit a patient's weight gain in the mistaken belief that the amount of weight gained was causally related to the likelihood of the development of a condition called preeclampsia, which will be discussed in Chapter 23. In fact, preeclampsia may cause excessive and rapid weight gain because fluid retention is one of the components of this disorder, but the converse appears not to be true. The Collaborative Perinatal Project, in which over 50,000 pregnancies in many centers around the United States were observed and data were systematically recorded, concluded that the average total weight gain throughout pregnancy is approximately 25 lb. Of this, approximately 2 to 6 lb is added during the first trimester, and 10 to 12 lb is added during each of the remaining two trimesters. For normally proportioned women, perinatal mortality rates gradually increased when weight gain was less than 15 lb, whereas for overweight women excessive weight gain was associated with a slight increase in adverse outcomes. The most striking increase in risk was seen in underweight women who gained less than 20 lb. During the siege of Holland in World War II, maternal starvation during the first half of pregnancy had little effect on birth weight, whereas starvation during the latter half was associated with marked reduction in the size of the neonates.

In 1990, the Institute of Medicine published the following recommendations for maternal weight gain during pregnancy that were based on a committee's review of the available literature. Weight gain should be based on the prepregnancy body-mass index (BMI), which is equal to weight (kg) ÷ (height [m])^2. To convert BMI calculated in lb/in.^{2} to metric BMI, multiply by 700. The woman's weight and height should be measured while she is not wearing shoes. The recommended total body weight gain ranges for pregnant women by prepregnancy BMI (based on mean weight gain for women delivering full-term babies weighing between 3 and 4 kg) are given in Table 10-1. The risk of maternal weight retention postpartum and fetal macrosomia may increase with higher weight gains in each range.

Table 10-1. Recommended weight gain ranges for pregnant women*

	Recommended total gain	
Prepregnancy weight-for-height category	(kg)	(lb)
Low (BMI < 19.8)	12.5–18	28–40
Normal (BMI 19.8–26.0)	11.5–16	25–35
High (BMI > 26.0–29.0)	7–11.5	15–25
Obese (BMI > 29.0)	at least 6.0	at least 15

*Source: Institute of Medicine. *Nutrition During Pregnancy.* Washington: National Academy Press, 1990. P. 10.

At term, the average fetus weighs 7.5 lb (3.4 kg), and the placenta, membranes, and amniotic fluid weigh approximately 3.5 lb; this accounts for 11 pounds of the weight gained. The uterus itself has gained about 2.5 lb, and the breasts have gained about 1 lb. Blood volume has increased by approximately 3.5 lb, and fluid and fat accretion account for the remaining weight, which is approximately 10 lb. It is thus easy to understand why women do not immediately lose all of their pregnancy weight gain in the process of delivery.

Fluid Accumulation
The fetus, placenta, and amniotic fluid account for a net gain of approximately 3.5 liters of water at term. Another 3 liters is added by the increased maternal blood volume, uterus, and breasts. The accumulation of interstitial fluid in the lower extremities, often 1 liter or more, results from increased venous pressure in the lower extremities and is associated with pitting edema in more than 50 percent of pregnant women.

Protein
Approximately 1 kg of protein, equally divided between the fetal-placental unit and the mother, primarily in the blood, uterus, and breasts, is accumulated during the course of pregnancy. The serum albumin level falls by approximately 22 percent, primarily due to dilution. However, globulins, fibrinogen, transferrin, and ceruloplasmin all increase during pregnancy. Maternal amino acid levels tend to be lower during pregnancy than in the nonpregnant state, presumably because these substances are actively transported to the fetus across the placenta against a concentration gradient.

Carbohydrate
Glucose, amino acids, and ketone bodies readily cross the placenta, whereas insulin and glucagon are not transferred to any appreciable extent. The placenta also utilizes metabolic fuels for its own very active functions. Fetoplacental glucose utilization appears not to be insulin-dependent, and thus the effect of pregnancy is similar to adding an extra glucose-consuming

organ. The fetus requires approximately 6 mg of glucose per kilogram of body weight per minute at term. Fetal circulating glucose levels are approximately 10 to 20 mg/dl lower than simultaneously measured maternal levels. Presumably as a result of this constant siphoning off of maternal glucose, pregnancy is characterized by a lowering of fasting plasma-glucose levels (Fig. 10-3).

As pregnancy progresses, maternal postprandial glucose levels tend to rise, presumably due to both central and peripheral insulin resistance. The rising postprandial glucose levels and *insulin resistance of pregnancy* are partially compensated for by an increase in insulin production and release. However, when a pregnant woman has deficient insulin production (as in type I diabetes), or exaggerated insulin resistance (as in type II diabetes and the transient hyperglycemic state known as gestational diabetes), requirements for exogenous insulin may be amplified. This amplification has been demonstrated in studies of the changing insulin requirements among pregnant individuals with diabetes (Fig. 10-4).

The postulated causes of this insulin resistance, also called the *diabetogenic effect of pregnancy,* are numerous. Human placental lactogen (hPL) is a polypeptide hormone that causes lipolysis and has an anti-insulin effect (see Chap. 9). Estrogen and progesterone are increased in pregnant women, and have diabetogenic effects under some circumstances. Free cortisol is

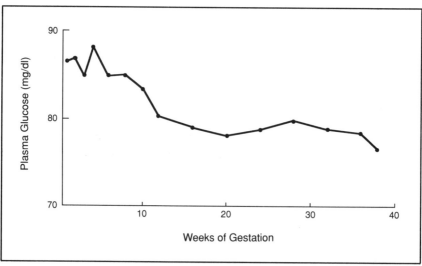

Fig. 10-3. Fasting plasma-glucose concentrations throughout normal pregnancy. Note that most of the fall occurs during the first trimester. (With permission, from Lind, T., and Aspillaga, M. Metabolic changes during normal and diabetic pregnancies. In E. A. Reece and D. R. Coustan (eds.), *Diabetes Mellitus in Pregnancy: Principles and Practice.* New York: Churchill-Livingstone, 1988. P. 77.)

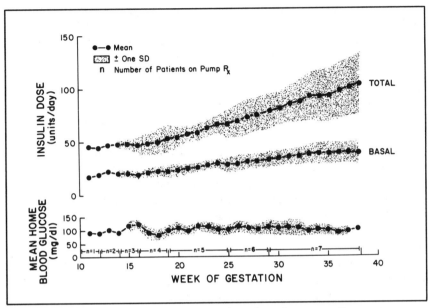

Fig. 10–4. Changes in insulin requirements throughout the course of pregnancy among women with type I diabetes. Since such patients have no endogenous insulin production, the trend in insulin requirement should be similar to the increasing insulin production in nondiabetic pregnant women. (With permission, from Rudolf, et al. *Diabetes* 30:893, 1981.)

also modestly elevated. Finally, the placenta appears to be capable of degrading insulin. The relative contributions of these various factors are unclear at present.

Lipids

The fall in fasting glucose levels occurs more rapidly during pregnancy than in the nonpregnant state, and is accompanied by increased fat breakdown and the early appearance of the ketone bodies, beta-hydroxybutyrate and acetoacetate, in blood and urine. This phenomenon is often referred to as the *accelerated starvation of pregnancy.*

Plasma cholesterol and triglyceride levels increase by about 50 percent and 200 percent, respectively. These changes are probably related to changes in specific lipid-binding proteins.

Cardiovascular System

Peripheral vascular resistance is decreased by pregnancy, probably as a result of arteriolar smooth-muscle relaxation related to the presence of high levels of progesterone, but possibly also due to shunting of blood through the uteroplacental circulation, a low-resistance circuit. Maternal blood pressure slowly falls, reaching a nadir at approximately 24 weeks' gestation, then rising again as term approaches, often reaching nonpregnant values (Fig. 10-5).

The maternal resting pulse rate increases slowly during pregnancy, and reaches a maximum of approximately 15 to 20 beats/minute above prepregnancy values in the third trimester. Cardiac stroke volume increases rapidly during the first trimester and remains elevated during the latter stages of pregnancy if measurements are made when the patient is in the lateral recumbent position rather than in a supine position. Blood volume increases to nearly 50 percent above nonpregnant levels by term, with the majority of the increase taking place during the first half of pregnancy. The net effect of increases in pulse rate and stroke volume is to increase cardiac output markedly during the first trimester and more slowly during the second trimester, with relatively stable levels in the third trimester at 30 to 50 percent above nonpregnant levels. Some studies have suggested a modest fall in cardiac output and stroke volume during the last month, but controversy exists as to the importance of these findings. During each

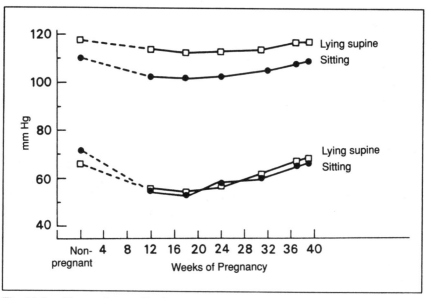

Fig. 10-5. Changes in systolic *(upper two curves)* and diastolic *(lower two curves)* blood pressure during pregnancy in primigravid women. Open boxes represent blood pressures taken with the patient in a supine position, and closed circles represent blood pressures taken with the patient in a sitting position. (With permission, from DeSwiet, M. The Cardiovascular System. In F. Hytten and G. Chamberlain (eds.), *Clinical Physiology in Obstetrics.* Oxford: Blackwell, 1980. P. 12.)

uterine contraction of labor, if the patient is supine, stroke volume and cardiac output increase by as much as 33 percent, presumably due to increased venous return when the contracting uterus rises off of its position atop the vena cava, as well as contraction-induced emptying of the uterine vasculature into the venous circulation. These changes are much less dramatic if the patient assumes the lateral position.

The heart must adapt to the above changes, and does so by myocardial hypertrophy and increased contractility. In addition, the enlarging uterus elevates the diaphragm, causing the heart to move upward and rotate to the left. This shift causes left-axis deviation on electrocardiogram and cardiomegaly on chest radiograph. On cardiac auscultation there is an accentuated splitting of the first heart sound and a loud, easily heard third sound. The majority of pregnant women have a systolic murmur audible along the left sternal border, which is believed to be related to increased flow across the aortic and pulmonic valves. A soft diastolic murmur has been heard in a small proportion of pregnant women, but most authorities suggest further evaluation if such a murmur is obvious. A continuous murmur may be heard in some patients along both sides of the sternum, and is believed to be due to increased flow in the blood vessels that supply the breasts. Many of the above cardiovascular changes are believed to be related to fetoplacental steroidogenesis, with increased estrogen causing cardiac hypertrophy and hyperfunction, progesterone causing smooth-muscle relaxation, and possibly increased aldosterone producing increased plasma volume.

When the pregnant woman assumes the supine position, the uterus may compress the inferior vena cava against the spine, which causes decreased venous return and consequently decreased cardiac output. The patient may experience a marked fall in blood pressure when lying on her back, and may develop symptoms of dizziness and, in extreme cases, loss of consciousness. This problem is called the *supine hypotensive syndrome,* and is easily relieved when the woman is moved to the lateral position. If the gravid uterus should compress the aorta rather than the vena cava, arterial blood pressure below the point of compression may drop, and flow to the uterus and lower extremities may be diminished. This problem may be difficult to diagnose, since arterial blood pressure measured in the brachial artery is unaffected, and the condition often is manifested by apparent fetal compromise found on the fetal heart rate monitor, with no obvious cause. This situation most often follows the administration of conduction anesthesia, since pharmacologic sympathectomy often results, with reduced vascular tone. For this reason, when fetal compromise is suspected, a change in maternal position should be one of the first responses. With uterine compression of the vena cava, venous pressure below the point of obstruction is increased, often to a level 3 times that in the upper extremities at term; this is one of the postulated causes of increased venous varicosities in pregnant women.

Respiratory Tract

Although the sensation of dyspnea is common during pregnancy, the respiratory rate does not change. There is a roughly 36 percent decrease in tracheobronchial resistance, believed to be mediated by progesterone-induced relaxation of bronchomotor smooth muscle, and a resultant increase in the caliber of the tracheobronchial tree. Tidal volume is increased by approximately 40 percent, a change that is also probably progesterone-induced, and is called the *hyperventilation of pregnancy*. The administration of exogenous progesterone to nonpregnant individuals increases respiratory drive by a mechanism that is probably centrally mediated. This increase in tidal volume leads to a similar increase in minute ventilation. Elevation of the diaphragm that results from the enlarging abdominal mass of pregnancy results in a 25 percent decrease in residual volume and functional residual capacity, but vital capacity remains unchanged, because the fall in expiratory reserve and inspiratory reserve is compensated for by the increased tidal volume (Fig. 10-6).

The increase in minute volume causes a mild decrease in PCO_2, and thus a slightly alkalotic pH. This alkalosis is compensated for by renal bicarbonate excretion, and thus results in a fall in serum bicarbonate levels to approximately 19 to 20 mEq/liter.

Urinary Tract

Hydroureter and hydronephrosis are commonly seen in pregnancy. There is a divergence of opinion as to whether this change is mechanical or hormonally induced. As the gravid uterus enlarges and rises out of the pelvis, the ureters are compressed against the pelvic brim, leading to relative obstruction and dilation above the point of compression. This view is supported by the observation that the hydroureter and hydronephrosis are generally more marked on the right, which coincides with dextrorotation of the uterus. In addition, the ovarian veins enlarge markedly, and cross the ureter on the right, possibly leading to compression. Finally, the sigmoid colon may provide some degree of protection to the left ureter against compression. The view that hormonal factors are important is supported by the generalized relaxation of smooth muscle brought about by progesterone, and by the fact that ureteral dilation may precede the time at which the enlarging uterus can cause mechanical compression. Also, removal of the primate fetus with the placenta left in place does not prevent further dilation of the ureters. In fact, both mechanisms are probably operative. Hydroureter and hydronephrosis may be associated with urine stasis, a proclivity toward pyelonephritis in pregnant women, and difficulty in interpreting intravenous pyelography during pregnancy. These changes disappear by 6 to 8 weeks postpartum.

Renal plasma flow increases markedly during early pregnancy, reaching levels 50 to 75 percent above nonpregnant norms by the end of the first

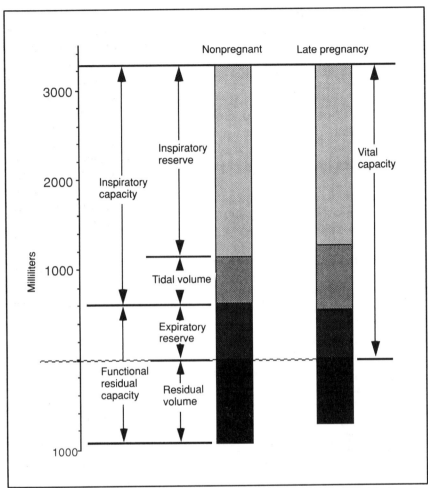

Fig. 10-6. Components of pulmonary function tests in nonpregnant individuals and during late pregnancy. Note that residual volume and expiratory reserve volume decreases, while tidal volume increases secondary to progesterone mediated "hyperventilation of pregnancy." (With permission, from Hytten, F. E., and Leitch, I. (eds.). *The Physiology of Human Pregnancy.* Oxford: Blackwell, 1964.)

trimester. This increase is sustained until the last month of pregnancy, when a mild decrease occurs, probably secondary to increased vascular resistance. The glomerular filtration rate (GFR) similarly increases by 30 to 50 percent in the first trimester, and this change is sustained to term. In clinical practice, GFR is estimated by creatinine clearance, which may increase to values approaching 200 ml/minute. Because creatinine is secreted by the tubules as well as filtered in the glomerulus, creatinine clearance is somewhat of an overestimation of GFR. Creatinine clearance is easily calculated by the following formula:

urine creatinine (mg/24°) ÷ 1440 (min/24°) ÷ serum creatinine (mg/100 ml)

$$\times 100 \ (ml/100 \ ml)$$

This formula provides an answer of units in ml (of serum filtered) per minute. Renal plasma flow and GFR decrease when a pregnant woman is supine, for the reasons outlined in the section on cardiovascular physiology.

Because of the increase in renal plasma flow and GFR, many solutes are presented to the nephron in quantities higher than in the nonpregnant state. As a result, blood urea nitrogen decreases to values below 10 mg/dl, serum creatinine falls to levels around 0.5 mg/dl, and the tubular maximum (T_{max}) for reabsorption of glucose is often exceeded, which leads to glucosuria.

Pregnancy is accompanied by changes in various serum electrolytes. For example, serum sodium falls by approximately 4 mEq/liter during the first trimester, and continues at that lower level throughout pregnancy. Although total body sodium increases by about 1000 mEq (including fetal-placental accretion), this change is more than offset by the increase in total body water. High levels of progesterone promote renal sodium loss, while increased levels of aldosterone, estrogen, and adrenal mineralocorticoids partially compensate; aldosterone is 2 to 3 times higher during the third trimester of pregnancy than in the nonpregnant state. This change is believed to be brought about by increases in plasma renin activity, renin substrate, and angiotensin. Although angiotensin sensitivity is reduced in normal pregnancy, high levels of this substance promote increased aldosterone production.

Serum potassium levels fall slightly during pregnancy, by approximately 0.2 mEq/liter. Total (bound plus free) serum calcium falls by about 1 mg/dl, from approximately 9.5 mg/dl to approximately 8.6 mg/dl, but this fall is related to falling serum albumin values, as 1 g of albumin binds 0.7 mg of calcium. Free, or ionized, calcium probably does not change during pregnancy. Serum magnesium levels fall slightly, and chloride remains unchanged. As mentioned in the section on respiratory physiology, the respiratory alkalosis of pregnancy, with PCO_2 levels falling to approximately 33 mm Hg, induces renal compensation, with a fall in serum bicarbonate levels to approximately 20 mEq/liter. Serum osmolality falls from 290 mOsm/kg water in the nonpregnant state to approximately 280 mOsm/kg water in early pregnancy, and this change is sustained throughout gestation; this is related to the fall in serum sodium and other anions. The pregnant woman does not respond to this fall in osmolality by diuresis, so the osmotic receptor system appears to be readjusted during pregnancy.

Gastrointestinal Tract

Nausea and vomiting commonly accompany early pregnancy. Although often called *morning sickness*, this type of distress is not confined to any particular time of day. The cause is not clear, although many believe the phenomenon to be related to increasing levels of progesterone or human chorionic gonadotropin (hCG), or both. There is evidence that such symptoms are a reassuring sign, since pregnancies unaccompanied by such symptoms have a somewhat poorer prognosis. In the severe form, hyperemesis gravidarum, this symptom complex can be a medical emergency, requiring hospitalization and parenteral hydration and, on occasion, hyperalimentation. Untreated, it can lead to dehydration, ketosis, electrolyte derangements, and liver and kidney damage.

Gastrointestinal tone and motility diminish as a result of the high levels of progesterone produced by the fetoplacental unit. This change results in a marked prolongation of the gastric emptying time, particularly during labor, when it is common to see undigested food vomited many hours after the last meal. Obstetric anesthesia is thus made somewhat more hazardous by the fact that every laboring patient must be considered to have a full stomach, no matter how long it has been since she has eaten. Vomiting and aspiration during general anesthesia used to be common causes of maternal mortality, but this problem is rare today, since endotracheal intubation during rapid sequence induction of anesthesia secures the airway from such sequelae. In addition, general anesthesia is no longer widely used for childbirth, except in emergency situations.

Dyspepsia, or heartburn, is a common problem in pregnant women, presumably due to relaxation of the gastroesophageal sphincter with reflux esophagitis. The gallbladder is hypotonic and distended, and the likelihood of later gallstone formation is increased with increasing numbers of pregnancies, possibly due to changes in the composition of bile secreted during pregnancy. Small and large bowel motility are decreased, and thus the stools become firmer with increased time for water reabsorption in the colon. Constipation is often a problem, and may be aggravated by the mechanical effects of the uterus compressing the colon. Venous pressure is increased in the vessels of the abdominal viscera, probably from both the progesterone effect and mechanical obstruction to venous return, which combined with constipation may be responsible for the increased frequency of hemorrhoids.

Hepatic blood flow appears to be unchanged during pregnancy, but some results of the laboratory tests usually used to distinguish abnormal liver function may be altered by pregnancy. Alkaline phosphatase rises to approximately double the nonpregnant norm, but most of this increase is from placentally derived heat-stable alkaline phosphatase. Amino-transferase enzymes (SGOT, SGPT) are unchanged by pregnancy, as is bilirubin. Serum albumin falls by approximately 30 percent, but other proteins produced by the liver such as the binding proteins for estrogen, thyroxine, and corticosteroids are elevated. Serum fibrinogen rises by approximately 50 percent, a change that is at least partially responsible for the marked increase in the erythrocyte sedimentation rate in pregnant women. To add to the confusion surrounding liver function testing, palmar erythema and spider angiomata, common signs of hepatic failure, are present in many normal pregnant women. This phenomenon is most likely related to high levels of estrogen in the circulation, due to increased production in pregnant women rather than to decreased detoxification as in patients with liver disease.

The appendix is displaced upwards and laterally by the enlarging uterus, so that by term it is located in the right upper quadrant (Fig. 10-7). This relocation can be a source of confusion in cases of appendicitis, particularly as to the site of incision for appendectomy.

Endocrine System

Pituitary

The anterior pituitary gland increases in size by about 20 percent during normal pregnancy, and increases in vascularity as well. The enlargement is due primarily to the increased size and numbers of lactotrophic cells, which are associated with the marked increase in serum prolactin that reaches levels averaging 10 times nonpregnant values (Fig. 10-8).

Growth hormone levels are unchanged during pregnancy, whereas the release of growth hormone in response to hypoglycemia and arginine stimulation are suppressed. Gonadotropin-releasing hormone levels are suppressed by the high levels of circulating sex steroids, and thus gonadotropic hormone levels are low. Thyroid-stimulating hormone (TSH) levels may fall slightly early in pregnancy, perhaps due to suppression by high levels of hCG, but are apparently unchanged later in pregnancy. Adrenocorticotropic hormone levels rise during pregnancy, presumably due to corticotropin-releasing hormone produced by the placenta (Table 10-2).

Antidiuretic hormone release from the posterior pituitary has not been found to undergo any particular change during pregnancy, despite the fall in serum osmolality. Circulating oxytocin levels increase throughout pregnancy with a further rise at term. The role of maternal oxytocin in initiating labor is unclear. It is likely that the uterus becomes more sensitive to oxytocin as term approaches, and there is evidence of an increasing frequency of pulsatile oxytocin release during the second stage of labor. However, labor occurs after posterior hypophysectomy, which suggests that pituitary release of oxytocin may not be critical. This finding should not be surprising, since oxytocin and vasopressin are produced in the hypothalamus and then are transported to the neurohypophysis. Since oxytocin levels are higher in the fetal umbilical artery than in the vein, it is possible that oxytocin derived from the fetal pituitary has some function during labor.

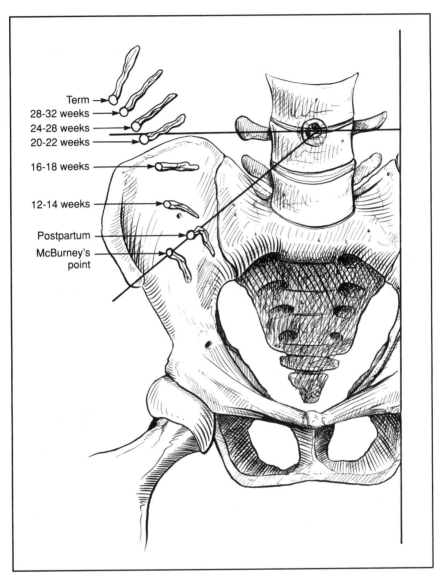

Fig. 10-7.   Changes in the position of the appendix as pregnancy progresses. (With permission, adapted from Baer, et al. Appendicitis in pregnancy. *JAMA* 98:1359, 1932.)

Thyroid

It has long been written that the thyroid gland increases in size during pregnancy. These observations were probably dependent on the presence of relative iodine deficiency in many pregnant women. Currently, with iodine supplementation widely practiced, goiter is a rare finding among

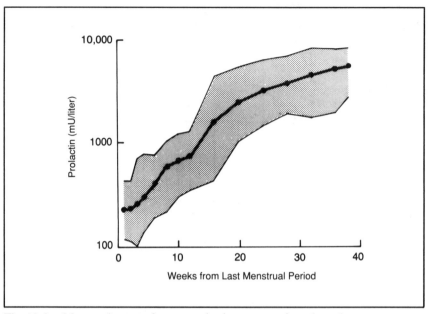

Fig. 10-8. Mean and range of serum prolactin concentrations throughout pregnancy. (With permission, from Lind, T. *Maternal Physiology*. Washington: Council on Resident Education in Obstetrics and Gynecology Basic Science Monograph Series, 1985, P. 66.)

pregnant women. However, marked changes in laboratory tests of thyroid function can be a source of confusion in evaluating gravidas. Because thyroid-binding proteins increase markedly under the influence of estrogen, tests of tri-iodothyronine (T_3) uptake detect the excess binding sites and may suggest hypothyroidism. However, the excess binding sites tend to tie up thyroxine, and the thyroid gland compensates by producing more thyroid hormone in order to maintain a stable level of free thyroxine, thus falsely elevating the total thyroxine (T_4). Since free thyroxine is unchanged, it is perfectly physiologic for pregnant women to have a "hypothyroid" T_3 uptake and a "hyperthyroid" total T_4. Thyroid-stimulating hormone has been reported to fall slightly during early pregnancy, presumably due to the TSH-like activity of hCG, but later in pregnancy TSH levels are similar to those seen in the nonpregnant state, and sensitive tests for TSH are most helpful in diagnosing subtle disorders of thyroid function.

Total T_4: high

T_3 uptake: low

TSH: Normal

Table 10-2. Pregnancy effect on anterior pituitary hormones

Prolactin	Growth hormone	Follicle-stimulating hormone, luteinizing hormone	Thyroid-stimulating hormone	Adreno-corticotropic hormone
Up	No change	Low	Low early, unchanged late	Up

The above changes are also present in patients taking estrogen-containing oral contraceptives. Thyroid hormone and TSH cross the placenta poorly if at all, whereas drugs such as propylthiouracil, which is used to treat hyperthyroidism, cross the placenta readily and can induce compensatory fetal goiter if used in high doses.

Adrenal

Primarily because of increasing production of cortisol-binding globulins under the influence of high estrogen levels, serum cortisol increases to almost double nonpregnant norms. Free cortisol, which competes with progesterone for intracellular binding sites in the hypothalamus and pituitary, is only slightly elevated and diurnal patterns of cortisol secretion are maintained. Aldosterone production is markedly increased during pregnancy, perhaps to compensate for the natriuretic effect of progesterone. Increases in renin substrate and angiotensinogen are probably the mechanism for this increase in aldosterone.

Hematologic System

The average blood loss at vaginal delivery is 600 ml and at cesarean section it is 1000 ml. Preparation for this blood loss is accomplished by expansion of the pregnant woman's total blood volume by nearly 50 percent by term. The plasma volume expands by 45 percent, beginning near the end of the first trimester and reaching a maximum in the middle of the third trimester. Red-cell mass increases continually throughout pregnancy, reaching a maximum of 20 to 30 percent above nonpregnant levels, depending on iron stores. Because plasma volume expands relatively more than red-cell mass, the hemoglobin and hematocrit fall, averaging approximately 11.5 g/dl and 34 percent at 30 weeks' gestation.

The definition of anemia must, therefore, be changed during pregnancy. Most authorities would not begin an anemia workup if the hemoglobin were above 11 g/dl and the hematocrit above 30 percent. Although possible teleologic explanations for this blood volume expansion are many, and include the anticipation of blood loss at delivery and the need to carry more oxygen to supply the developing fetus, the mechanism is unclear. For the above reasons, and also because of the need to supply iron to the growing conceptus, pregnancy is a time of markedly increased iron requirements. The average menstruating woman begins pregnancy with total body iron stores of only 2.0 to 2.5 g, as compared to 4 g in the average man. Pregnancy requires an additional 1 g of iron, or roughly 50 percent of iron stores. This amount can be divided into 300 mg to meet the needs of the fetoplacental unit, 200 mg to cover the obligatory excretion of iron, and 500 mg to cover the increased red-cell mass, since each ml of red blood cells requires 1.1 mg of iron. Most of these needs occur during the second and third trimesters. If the mother has approximately 24 weeks to absorb 1000 mg of iron, she must absorb approximately 6 mg per day. Since only approximately 10 to 20 percent of ingested iron is absorbed, she must ingest at least 30 to 60 mg per day. The average daily dietary iron intake is 18 mg. Therefore, the nonanemic pregnant woman usually is prescribed an iron supplement of at least 30 mg elemental iron per day, in the form of ferrous sulfate or ferrous gluconate. Thus a total of approximately 48 mg is ingested each day, and 4.8 to 9.6 mg is absorbed. If the mother has diminished iron stores, more supplementation is needed. Fortunately, maternal iron deficiency does not appear to diminish iron transport to the fetus.

Other formed elements in the blood are less dramatically changed by pregnancy. There is a modest rise in the leukocyte count from a nonpregnant average of 6000 to 7000/µl to 10,000/µl at term, but leukocyte counts in laboring women may go as high as 25,000/µl. The rise is primarily in neutrophils. The effect of pregnancy on platelet counts is controversial, but there may be a modest decline, perhaps as much as 25 percent, by term in some patients. This decline is believed to be due to increased destruction of platelets. Platelet size increases, which indicates younger platelets in the circulation.

Platelet counts may be quite low in women with immune thrombocytopenic purpura (ITP), an autoimmune disorder relatively common in women of childbearing age, in which antiplatelet antibodies cause rapid destruction of maternal platelets. This disease is of particular interest to obstetricians, since the antibodies are often of the IgG subclass, and may traverse the placenta, causing destruction of fetal platelets as well. Fetal thrombocytopenia has been associated, in case reports, with intracranial hemorrhage at the time of vaginal delivery. Although cesarean section used to be the standard delivery technique for these infants, to avoid even mild degrees of fetal head trauma, newer techniques for fetal evaluation such as scalp blood sampling during labor and percutaneous umbilical blood sampling prior to the onset of labor have now allowed the prenatal diagnosis of fetal thrombocytopenia, with cesarean section being reserved for those fetuses with markedly diminished platelet counts. Because intrapartum fetal hemorrhage from thrombocytopenia is unusual even in offspring of mothers with ITP, the need for fetal platelet counting prior to delivery is currently being reevaluated in some centers.

The clotting mechanism is augmented during pregnancy, which leads to a "hypercoagulable state." This increased coagulability may be necessary for the body to deal with frequent disruptions in the integrity of the vascular tree in the placental bed, so that abruptio placentae is not easily propagated. Fibrinogen levels increase markedly from a normal range of 200 to 400 mg/dl in the nonpregnant state to a level of 300 to 600 mg/dl in the third trimester. This increase in fibrinogen is responsible for the increase in the erythrocyte sedimentation rate (ESR) of pregnant women. The ESR test is useless in the evaluation of inflammatory conditions during pregnancy, since virtually all pregnant women have sedimentation rates that are distinctly abnormal by nonpregnant standards.

Clotting factors VII, VIII, IX, and X increase during pregnancy, while XI and XII decrease. Prothrombin time and partial thromboplastin time are unchanged or slightly shortened during pregnancy, and bleeding time and clotting time are unaffected. Fibrin degradation products are normally slightly increased.

Recommended Reading

Burrow, G., and Ferris, T. (eds.). *Medical Complications During Pregnancy* (4th ed.). Philadelphia: Saunders, 1984.

Coustan, D. R., and Plotz, R. D. The Laboratory in Diseases Associated with Pregnancy. In H. N. Mandell (ed.), *Laboratory Medicine in Clinical Practice.* Boston: John Wright PSG, 1983. Pp. 353–386.

Cruikshank, D. P., and Hays, P. M. Maternal Physiology in Pregnancy. In S. G. Gabbe, J. R. Niebyl, and J. L. Simpson (eds.), *Obstetrics Normal and Problem Pregnancies* (2nd ed.). New York: Churchill-Livingstone, 1991. Pp. 125–146.

Cunningham, F. G., MacDonald, P. C., Gant, N. F., Leveno, K. J., and Gilstrap, L. C. III. Maternal Adaptations to Pregnancy. In *Williams Obstetrics* (19th ed.). Norwalk: Appleton and Lange, 1989. Pp. 209–246.

Longo, L. D. Maternal blood volume and cardiac output during pregnancy: A hypothesis of endocrinologic control. *Am. J. Physiol.* 245:720, 1983.

11

Diagnosis of Pregnancy

Ray V. Haning, Jr.

Timely and accurate diagnosis of pregnancy is crucial to providing good health care to women. A false-positive diagnosis of pregnancy can lead to unnecessary emotional trauma and may result in unnecessary surgical procedures (e.g., laparoscopy to rule out ectopic pregnancy, dilatation and curettage [D&C] to rule out incomplete abortion, or suction D&C if the pregnancy is unwanted).

Failure to recognize pregnancy may lead to missing a potentially fatal ectopic pregnancy or to ordering administration of medications, treatments, or diagnostic studies that are, at best, unnecessary, or worse yet, harmful to the pregnancy or the woman. The key to successfully diagnosing pregnancy is to have a high index of suspicion and to apply sensitive and accurate tests for pregnancy whenever a suspicion of pregnancy arises. The pregnancy can then be evaluated with a careful history and physical examination. Other tests such as ultrasound and human chorionic gonadotropin (hCG) doubling time determinations can be used if further evaluation is needed.

Develop a High Index of Suspicion

Pregnancy is the most common cause of amenorrhea in the childbearing-age group. Pregnancy may occur in "infertile women" with many years of antecedent amenorrhea, women diagnosed as menopausal, and young girls who have denied sexual activity; even the presence of an intact hymen fails to exclude pregnancy since sperm can enter the vagina from ejaculation on the perineum.

A negative pregnancy test fails to exclude pregnancy entirely since approximately 1 week passes from the time of fertilization until implantation takes place, and the detection of hCG first occurs at approximately the time of the missed period even when a sensitive assay with an antibody directed against the beta-subunit of hCG is utilized. Less sensitive tests may not become positive until the patient is 2 weeks late for the expected period (1 month postconception). Physical examination or x-ray films can detect later pregnancies, but physical examination is unreliable in early pregnancy or in obese women, and the use of x rays in pregnant women should be avoided whenever possible. Ultrasound is useful for determining the location of early pregnancies and to determine their viability, but ultrasound cannot detect a normal intrauterine pregnancy until about 5 to 6 weeks after the last menstrual period (LMP). To avoid missing undiagnosed pregnancies, routine pregnancy testing is often performed prior to surgery or other medical procedures.

Symptoms of Pregnancy

The symptoms of pregnancy may include a late menstrual period, breast and nipple tenderness, abdominal bloating, urinary frequency, pelvic cramping sensations suggestive of an impending menstrual period, nausea, and vomiting. These symptoms can mimic a gastro-enteric illness, occasionally prompting extensive radiologic evaluations when the diagnosis of pregnancy has not been considered. Some pregnant women may have such severe vomiting that they must be hospitalized for intravenous therapy, but others have no symptoms. Even today women occasionally present to the emergency room in active labor at term without having ever recognized that they were pregnant.

Once the suspicion of pregnancy arises, pregnancy testing should be performed. All early tests for pregnancy are based on the detection of hCG in blood or urine. The hCG concentration in blood rises exponentially, doubling approximately every 2 days until about the eighth week of pregnancy and then continues to rise somewhat more slowly to a peak concentration at about the tenth week (Fig. 11-1). After the peak, hCG concentrations decline slowly and then become nearly constant throughout the remainder of pregnancy (see Fig. 11-1). Thus, very sensitive methods are required to detect hCG at the time of the missed period, whereas even crude methods such as bioassays using rabbits or frogs will work as the hCG concentrations near the 10-week peak. Bioassays are no longer performed, and essentially all contemporary methods for pregnancy testing rely on the ability of antibodies or luteinizing hormone (LH) receptors to recognize the hCG molecule.

Various detection systems are utilized. Hemagglutination inhibition or latex agglutination inhibition were used in the older less sensitive methods. The newer, most sensitive methods are based on radioimmunoassay or enzyme-linked immunoassay. Urine samples have the advantage that less specimen preparation is required prior to testing, but the variation in

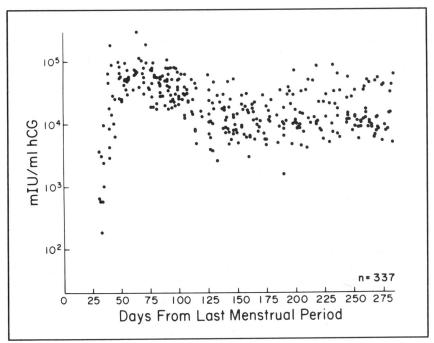

Fig. 11-1. Concentration of serum hCG in normal singleton pregnancies plotted on a log scale versus days from the last menstrual period on a linear scale. (Source: Haning, R. V., Jr., et al. Interrelationships among human chorionic gonadotropin (hCG) 17β-estradiol, progesterone, and estriol in maternal serum: Evidence for an inhibitory effect of the fetal adrenal on secretion of hCG. *J. Clin. Endocrinol. Metab.* 56:1188–1194, 1983; © The Endocrine Society.)

urea and electrolyte concentrations present in urine samples renders tests based on serum the most sensitive and reliable for providing quantitative determinations of the hCG concentration. Kits are available over-the-counter in most drug stores, so that the patient may test her own urine. Most such kits now use an enzyme-linked antibody to hCG to produce a color change that indicates whether or not the patient is pregnant. Many of these kits are now more reliable and sensitive than tests performed in hospitals only a decade ago. However, when performed by the untrained, emotionally involved patient, the result must be considered unreliable for medical diagnosis. Where the suspicion of pregnancy persists in the face of a negative test, the physician should not hesitate to repeat the test on another sample after waiting for 1 week, or to request a more sensitive assay if one is available.

Human chorionic gonadotropin, a glycoprotein hormone with a molecular weight of approximately 36,700 daltons, has the same alpha-subunit as thyroid-stimulating hormone (TSH), follicle-stimulating hormone

(FSH), and LH, and it shares many antigenic sites on its beta-subunit with the beta-subunit of LH. At the present time, the radioimmunoassay for hCG in serum using an antibody directed against the beta-subunit of hCG is the most sensitive and reliable means of detecting hCG. Because of the potential cross reactions of the antibody to hCG with elevated concentrations of LH, some pregnancy testing systems can give false-positives with women whose FSH and LH concentrations are elevated because of menopause or premature ovarian failure. Such false-positives can be detected by the alert physician by checking the serum FSH concentration, which should be low in pregnancy but which will be high in such patients.

Evaluating the Viability of Early Pregnancy

Because of the characteristic exponential rise in hCG, calculation of the doubling time of hCG based on samples obtained 2 or more days apart provides information on the viability of the pregnancy in its first few weeks. Once the pregnancy is advanced enough to allow detection of the heartbeat by ultrasound, the latter becomes the preferred means of determining both the location and the viability of the pregnancy. In 22 normal single pregnancies, the geometric mean doubling time was 2.3 days with 95 percent confidence limits of 0.89 to 6.0 days. The geometric mean progesterone concentration in 19 normal pregnancies was 15.5 ng/ml with 95 percent confidence limits of 4.5 to 54 ng/ml. Human chorionic gonadotropin concentrations that fail to increase normally or which fall in the first few weeks of pregnancy suggest loss of viability. A low concentration of progesterone increases the chance that the pregnancy is abnormal. Such findings may be seen in intrauterine pregnancies that will ultimately result in miscarriages or in ectopic pregnancies. Finding a normal rate of rise of hCG fails to rule out an ectopic pregnancy since some ectopic pregnancies have a normal fetus and a normal rate of rise of hCG production. Thus, ultrasound examinations must be used to determine the location of an early pregnancy when a suspicion of ectopic pregnancy exists.

Ultrasound

Sacs in the uterus can be located with an abdominal transducer by 6 weeks, and fetal heart motion can be visualized by 8 weeks from the LMP. Use of a vaginal probe sometimes allows earlier identification of the sac—at about 5 weeks—and earlier identification of the fetal heart activity—at about 6 weeks from the LMP. The combination of a high degree of clinical suspicion, the use of sensitive pregnancy testing, and ultrasound location of intrauterine gestations allows identification of pregnancies that need further studies to rule out ectopic pregnancy.

Ectopic Pregnancy

Ectopic pregnancy is the most frequent pregnancy-related cause of maternal death in the first trimester of pregnancy. It should be suspected in women with spotting or bleeding in early pregnancy and in those with a history of acute pain, a pelvic mass, or cardiovascular collapse. When the pregnancy cannot be located in the uterus on schedule, the diagnostic approach must be individualized depending on the availability of diagnostic procedures, whether the pregnancy is desired, and other risk-benefit information; this is covered in detail in Chapter 12.

Recommended Reading

Speroff, L., Glass, R. H., and Kase, N. G. (eds.). *Clinical Gynecologic Endocrinology and Infertility* (4th ed.). Baltimore: Williams & Wilkins, 1989. Pp. 329–332.

Yen, S. S. C. Endocrine Metabolic Adaptations in Pregnancy. In S. S. C. Yen and R. B. Jaffe (eds.), *Reproductive Endocrinology* (3rd ed.). Philadelphia: Saunders, 1991. Pp. 950–954.

Abortions, Miscarriages, and Ectopic Pregnancies

Gary Frishman

All pregnancies that end before the twentieth week of gestation are considered to be abortions. There are three general categories to be considered. Miscarriages, or spontaneous abortions, include all intrauterine pregnancies that end involuntarily whether the pregnancy was intended, desired, or not. The most common abbreviation of this term is *SAb* (spontaneous abortion). When counselling patients, it is important to be aware of the implication of the term *abortion,* even when used with the modifier *spontaneous.* Therapeutic abortions, commonly known as abortions, or terminations, consist of all pregnancies that are terminated intentionally. Common abbreviations of this term include *TAb* (therapeutic abortion) and *TOP* (termination of pregnancy). An ectopic pregnancy is any pregnancy that occurs outside the uterine corpus. A pregnancy is considered to be an embryo until the eighth week of gestation and a fetus thereafter. Regardless of location or timing, the tissue of the pregnancy is called the *products of conception* (POC).

Spontaneous Abortions

Incidence
The reported incidence of spontaneous abortion varies with the study design. Approximately 20 percent of all clinically recognized pregnancies

(when the patient is aware that she is pregnant) end in miscarriage. Studies that evaluate clinically silent pregnancies reveal significantly higher overall miscarriage rates. These investigations usually involve the routine testing of a woman's urine with a sensitive human chorionic gonadotropin (hCG) assay at the end of her menstrual cycle. This methodology allows the documentation of early pregnancies that would not normally be detected by the patient and leads to significantly higher reported miscarriage pregnancy rates of at least 40 percent. Of these miscarriages, over half are silent. The high rate of asymptomatic embryo wastage is confirmed by assisted reproductive technologies such as in vitro fertilization (IVF), in which although several embryos are transferred to the uterus, the national average of ongoing pregnancies that result is only 15 percent. Clearly there are factors at work in embryo implantation and viability that are, as yet, not understood.

Studies suggest that subgroups of women, such as those pregnant for the first time and women with a completely normal reproductive history, may be at a substantially lower risk of miscarriage than the numbers quoted above. It is also well established that the mother's age plays a major role in the risk of miscarriage (as well as congenital anomalies and birth defects). A woman older than 40 years has more than twice the risk of a miscarriage than a woman younger than 20 years old. Although not as dramatically associated, the chance for a miscarriage also increases with increasing paternal age and maternal parity. Because a relationship between paternal age and chromosomal problems in the offspring was recently delineated, the American Fertility Society has lowered its suggested upper age limit for men who donate sperm from 50 years of age to 40 years of age.

Eighty percent of all miscarriages occur in the first trimester. When dating a pregnancy (and a miscarriage) it is important to distinguish between the terminology used in embryology and that used in obstetrics. Embryologists date a pregnancy starting at ovulation, whereas obstetricians begin with the last menstrual period. Thus there will always be a 2-week discrepancy between the gestational age and the conceptional age. Prior to the routine availability of ultrasound, many earlier miscarriages were probably inadvertently diagnosed as late first-trimester and early second-trimester losses. There is usually a lag between when a pregnancy fails and when symptoms present so that the actual losses may have happened weeks before any signs or symptoms occurred. Once fetal heart activity has been detected by ultrasound the risk of miscarriage drops to as low as 2 to 7 percent.

With the widespread use of ultrasound in early pregnancy there has been recognition of a phenomenon called the *vanishing twin*. This takes place when two, apparently viable, pregnancies are visualized in the uterus. Despite discernible fetal cardiac motion, one pregnancy subsequently dies. There may be bleeding or no signs at all. Usually, the remaining pregnancy proceeds to term uneventfully. The incidence of vanishing twins has been estimated at up to 20 percent of all pregnancies. The vanishing twin may account for a small percentage of pregnancies that are accompanied by spotting but go on to a normal delivery.

Etiologies of Spontaneous Abortions

Genetic

The most common cause of spontaneous miscarriage is a genetic problem. Several large studies involving cytogenetic analysis of thousands of aborted pregnancies have documented that chromosomal defects account for approximately 50 percent of all miscarriages. Of these defects, the most common abnormalities are autosomal trisomies (of which the most common is trisomy 16) and monosomy 45,X, which respectively account for about 50 and 20 percent of these losses. Because of the different types of autosomal trisomies (of which trisomy 16, 13, 15, 21, and 22 are the most common), monosomy 45,X represents the most common single abnormal karyotype. As discussed above, maternal age is a significant risk factor for miscarriage with the risk of trisomy increasing dramatically with the mother's age.

Structural

Congenital structural abnormalities of the uterus, which may occur in between 1 in 200 and 1 in 500 women, are often a cause of second-trimester miscarriages. About 20 percent of women with congenital incomplete fusion of the uterine horns have difficulty becoming pregnant and with miscarriages once they are pregnant. The most common uterine anomalies include the septate uterus, the bicornuate uterus, and the unicornuate uterus (Fig. 12-1). Surgical correction may be readily performed for the septate uterus; this correction requires an outpatient endoscopic procedure (hysteroscopic cutting of the septum). Because a laparotomy is required and beneficial results are not assured, surgical correction of a bicornuate uterus is not commonly performed. The least common malformation, the unicornuate uterus, carries the highest incidence of spontaneous abortions (50%) and is not amenable to surgical repair.

When the uterine cervix is not able to hold a pregnancy and asymptomatically (without uterine contractions) dilates early, it is called an incompetent uterine cervix. Cervical incompetence leads to a loss of structural support of the gestation with expulsion of the pregnancy following. This cause of second- or third-trimester miscarriage or preterm delivery, which rarely if ever occurs prior to 16 weeks' gestation, can usually be treated with a suture called a *cerclage* placed circumferentially around the cervix (Fig. 12-2). With repeated second-trimester miscarriages, the presentation of an incompetent cervix can sometimes be differentiated from that of a uterine anomaly by the time sequence of the losses. A woman with an incompetent cervix will have her pregnancies lost sequentially earlier and earlier as the cervix becomes even more incompetent, whereas the

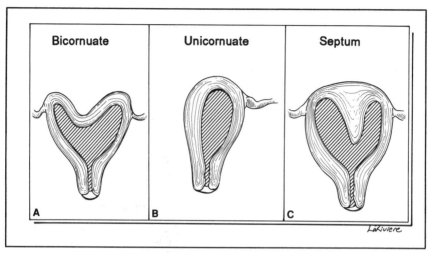

Fig. 12-1. Congenital uterine anomalies. (A) Bicornuate. (B) Unicornuate.
(C) Septum.

anomalous uterus will often stretch a little more with each subsequent pregnancy with these miscarriages occurring sequentially later and later. A leiomyoma (fibroid) is a surgically correctable benign tumor of the uterus that can occasionally be the cause of a miscarriage.

Diethylstilbestrol   Diethylstilbestrol (DES) is a synthetic estrogen that was used from the late 1940s until 1971 in up to 3 million pregnant women in the United States. Although DES was employed principally to decrease the risk of miscarriage and premature births, ironically its benefit for these conditions was never proven. When problems in the daughters of women who took DES during pregnancy became apparent, the Food and Drug Administration counselled against prescribing DES in pregnant women. Among the many syndromes attributed to DES, the two principle pertinent conditions are a significantly increased risk of a rare genital tract cancer (clear-cell adenocarcinoma of the cervix) and a constellation of abnormalities of the uterus including the classic "T-shaped" uterus. These uterine and tubal anomalies appear to significantly predispose affected women to infertility, miscarriage, and premature births. Unfortunately, there is no surgical treatment available for the majority of women with these conditions.

Intrauterine Adhesions (Asherman's Syndrome)   Intrauterine adhesions or synechiae usually result from surgically induced trauma to the endometrial lining of the uterus. This occurs most often from a dilatation and curettage (D&C) following a miscarriage or postpartum hemorrhage. The

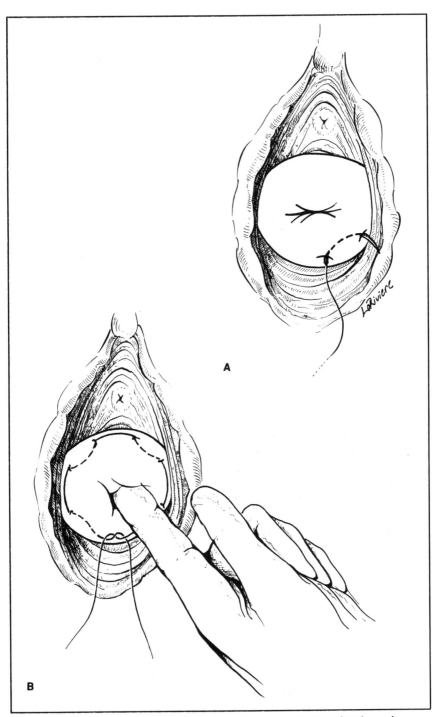

Fig. 12-2. Cervical cerclage. (A) First pass with suture. (B) Completed suturing.

adhesions can range from minimal with no resulting symptoms or problems to a total obliteration of the uterine cavity with complete amenorrhea. Intrauterine adhesions can lead to both infertility and miscarriage. Fortunately, the bands of scar tissue can often be treated effectively by hysteroscopic dissection.

Hormonal Causes

A deficiency of endogenous progesterone production by the ovarian corpus luteum cyst represents the primary endocrinologic cause of pregnancy loss, which usually occurs early in gestation. Treatment traditionally consists of either follicular phase stimulation (which causes the follicular cyst to produce a healthier corpus luteum cyst) with clomiphene citrate (Serophene, Clomid) or exogenous progesterone supplementation in the luteal phase and throughout the first trimester.

It is unlikely that diabetes mellitus (unless uncontrolled) or thyroid conditions are a major cause of miscarriage.

Environmental Causes

There is ongoing debate about the impact of the environment on the incidence of miscarriages and birth defects. There have been a number of studies with conflicting findings concerning a causal relationship between video display monitors and the electromagnetic fields that are associated with high-voltage power lines and electric blankets. Most reviews of this subject have concluded that the above phenomena do not play a meaningful role in reproductive wastage.

The study of the impact of environmental toxins and work-related exposures is a rapidly evolving field. One can imagine how difficult it is to isolate and confirm a relationship between any single agent or toxin among the many that patients (both men and women) are exposed to. However, it is likely that this field will ultimately demonstrate a cause-and-effect relationship between some environmental or work-related exposures and spontaneous abortions.

Toxins that have been identified by some investigators as a cause of miscarriage include cigarettes (heavy use) and alcohol. Radiation may lead to an abortion, especially exposure of the embryo around the time of implantation. As such, radiology departments routinely ask women who are to undergo radiologic procedures whether they are pregnant, and defer x-ray studies when they are not urgent and the possibility of pregnancy is significant.

Infections

Although infections are likely to play a role in the loss of some pregnancies, it is difficult to establish a causal relationship. It appears that some of the TORCH infections such as *Toxoplasma gondii* and particularly rubella, when first occurring during early pregnancy, may lead to an abortion.

However once the mother is infected, subsequent pregnancies should not be affected and these agents are not thought to play a role in sequential or habitual miscarriages.

Some investigators have concluded that cervical colonization with *Ureaplasma urealyticum* and *Mycoplasma hominis* increases the risk of miscarriage and that treatment with a tetracycline decreases this risk. However, these organisms are so pervasive and, because of their gastrointestinal reservoir, difficult to eradicate that it is difficult to draw meaningful conclusions. Most practitioners do not routinely screen for these agents until a women has suffered at least two sequential miscarriages. None of the sexually transmitted diseases are known to cause recurrent miscarriages.

Types of Spontaneous Abortions

There are many categories of spontaneous abortions. Although the age at which a neonate has any reasonable chance for survival has decreased dramatically over the past decade from approximately 34 weeks' gestational age to about 24 to 26 weeks' gestational age, it is unlikely that viability will be extended below this threshold. If a pregnancy aborts in the first trimester, it is referred to as an "early" abortion and a "late" abortion if it aborts after 12 weeks. The most common cutoff after which a late abortion is referred to as a fetal death or stillbirth is 20 weeks, although 500 g is also accepted as an endpoint. See Table 12-1 for the criteria used by different states.

Missed Abortion

A missed abortion occurs when the fetus has died 8 or more weeks prior to the diagnosis of its demise. With the advent of more sensitive pregnancy testing (see Chap. 11) and ultrasonography, this term has become dated since it is unusual for the nonviable pregnancy to undergo the 8 weeks of "silent" existence required for this definition. Some authors have suggested that the term "missed abortion" be modified to include any pregnancy that has become nonviable in the absence of symptoms.

Threatened Abortion

A threatened abortion occurs when bleeding with or without cramping occurs during the first half of pregnancy. Approximately 40 percent of all pregnancies produce some spotting or bleeding with up to half of these going on to miscarry. The chance of a miscarriage increases with the number of days of bleeding. Many pregnant women experience some spotting around the time of the first missed menstrual cycle. This spotting results from bleeding at the site of placental implantation and is harmless. Spotting associated with implantation is a common cause of misdating an early pregnancy because the patient believes that she has had a "light" period that month and conceived the following month. Cramping is a much more ominous sign and is associated with a substantially increased risk of mis-

Table 12-1. Reporting requirements for fetal death

20 weeks or more of gestation
  Alabama
  Alaska
  Arizona*
  California
  Connecticut
  Delaware
  Florida
  Guam
  Illinois
  Indiana
  Iowa
  Maryland*
  Minnesota
  Montana
  Nebraska
  Nevada
  New Jersey
  North Carolina
  North Dakota
  Ohio
  Oklahoma
  Oregon*
  Puerto Rico
  Texas
  Utah
  Vermont*
  Washington
  West Virginia
  Wyoming

20 weeks or more of gestation or birth weight of 350 g or more
  Idaho
  Kentucky
  Louisiana
  Massachusetts
  Mississippi
  Missouri
  New Hampshire
  South Carolina
  Wisconsin

Birth weight in excess of 350 g
  Kansas

20 weeks or more of gestation or birth weight of 400 g or more
  Michigan

(Continued)

Table 12-1.   *(Continued)*

Birth weight of 500 g or more
  New Mexico
  South Dakota
  Tennessee*

16 weeks or more of gestation
  Pennsylvania

20 weeks or more of gestation or birth weight of 500 g or more
  District of Columbia

All products of human conception
  American Samoa
  Arkansas
  Colorado
  Georgia
  Hawaii
  Maine
  New York
  Northern Mariana Islands
  Rhode Island
  Virginia
  Virgin Islands

*Specific modifiers apply.
Adapted with permission from the American College of Obstetricians and Gynecologists. Diagnosis
and management of fetal death. *ACOG Technical Bulletin #176.* Washington, 1993.

carriage. Cramping may be evidence of the uterus attempting to expel the
POC or extravasation of blood into the uterine cavity.

There are many causes of bleeding in the first half of pregnancy.
Nonobstetric causes include vaginal and cervical lacerations and erosions,
polyps, and vaginal infections. Obstetric causes include problems with placental implantation, insufficient production of progesterone from the corpus luteum (luteal phase defect), ectopic pregnancy, and the vanishing
twin.

Currently, there are no available treatment modalities to improve the
prognosis of a first-trimester pregnancy in which bleeding occurs. Despite
a paucity of evidence, given the lack of any other valid intervention, many
physicians prescribe reductions in physical activity or bed rest, or both, for
these patients. These pregnancies are usually followed closely with ultra-
sounds or serial pregnancy tests to determine viability. It was formerly
thought that if, despite a history of bleeding, a pregnancy continued, it was
at no greater risk of complications later in gestation. However, these pregnancies may be at somewhat greater risk for problems associated with the

placenta such as fetal distress in labor and intrauterine growth retardation. Nevertheless, the majority proceed to term without complications.

Inevitable Abortion
An abortion is considered inevitable when there is uterine bleeding and the cervix has begun to dilate, especially if there is rupture of the fetal membranes. There may be products of conception in the cervical os, but no tissue has been passed. There is often severe cramping associated with inevitable abortion, which is attributable to POC tissue in the cervix. Removal of this tissue usually dramatically relieves these symptoms. There is currently no technology or treatment that can increase the chance of these pregnancies continuing.

Incomplete Abortion
An abortion is considered incomplete when some, but not all, of the fetal tissue has been passed (the placenta is often the portion retained). The patient may or may not continue to have symptoms, usually bleeding and cramping. The treatment of choice remains a D&C to complete the process; this results in the immediate relief in symptoms.

Complete Abortion
When all POC (fetal and placental tissue) are expelled without the need for subsequent surgical intervention, the miscarriage is considered to be a complete abortion.

Septic Abortion
Septic abortion occurs when a pregnancy becomes infected, either spontaneously or secondary to instrumentation of the uterus. A septic abortion can be associated with a threatened, inevitable, or incomplete miscarriage and is usually polymicrobial in origin. These patients are generally quite ill and if antibiotic treatment and removal of the infected contents of the uterus is not effective, a hysterectomy may be required. With legalized abortion, septic abortions have become a relatively infrequent phenomenon.

Blighted Ovum
A pregnancy is considered a blighted ovum when only a gestational sac without a fetal pole or heartbeat is visualized via ultrasound. The production of hCG may mimic the rise seen with a normal viable pregnancy. This pregnancy may miscarry on its own or require a D&C but will not continue normally.

Habitual Abortion
Habitual abortion, also referred to as *recurrent abortion,* refers to any woman with three or more spontaneous pregnancy losses. This condition occurs in approximately 0.5 percent of women. Couples with the diagnosis of

habitual abortion often conceive readily, but consistently suffer a miscarriage, usually around the same gestational age in each pregnancy. Although women having one miscarriage statistically have no greater risk than the general population of miscarrying their next pregnancy, after three sequential miscarriages the risk of losing their next pregnancy is as high as 50 percent. Previous term pregnancies (especially if these occur between the miscarriages) substantially improve the prognosis. Common problems that contribute to habitual miscarriages include genetic abnormalities (e.g., balanced chromosomal translocations), hormonal deficiencies (e.g., inadequate production of progesterone by the corpus luteum cyst consistent with a luteal phase defect), structural abnormalities (e.g., uterine septum), and autoimmune disorders (e.g., antiphospholipid antibodies). However, approximately 50 percent of the time no specific etiology can be found.

Terminations of Pregnancy

Induced Abortion
When a pregnancy is intentionally terminated prior to 20 weeks' gestation, regardless of the method, it is termed an *induced abortion*. A therapeutic abortion is an induced abortion performed for health reasons such as when a pregnant woman's cardiac condition precludes her from safely carrying a pregnancy, whereas an elective abortion is performed as a matter of the woman's choice.

The percentage of pregnancies that end in an induced abortion varies with the age of the mother, her socioeconomic status, her marital status, and other variables. However, roughly 25 percent of all pregnancies in the United States are voluntarily terminated; this number is considered to be higher than the incidence of pregnancies that undergo spontaneous loss. There appears to be a trend towards an increase in the percentage of pregnancies that are ongoing compared to those that are terminated in the United States (Fig. 12-3). It is unclear whether this trend reflects an improvement in couples' education and ability to obtain contraceptive services or a decline in the accessibility of abortion counselling and services. Of the women who have abortions, approximately 75 percent are unmarried.

A termination of pregnancy is technically possible to perform during any trimester of pregnancy. However, it is illegal in most states to perform a third-trimester termination. States do vary somewhat in their laws governing the upper limit of gestational age at which an abortion may be performed. However, most states allow a termination to be performed up until about 20 weeks of gestational age, and roughly 90 percent of abortions are performed in the first trimester.

After the Supreme Court defined the stages of pregnancy at which states have a legitimate interest in regulating abortion, each state developed its

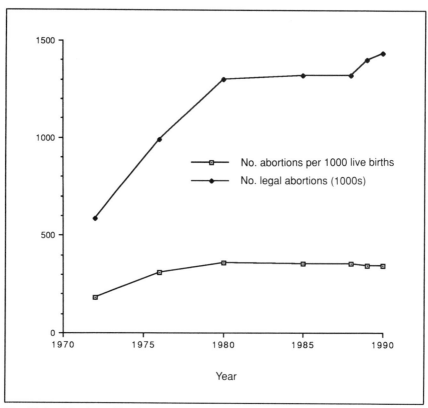

Fig. 12-3. Number of legal abortions compared to number of live births.

own set of statutes that dictate conditions such as whether a 24-hour waiting period is necessary, whether husband or parental notification or approval is required, and whether there are circumstances under which a termination may and may not be performed. With the legalization of abortion, the incidence of illegal abortions diminished dramatically. Prior to changes in legal status, the incidence of illegal abortions in the United States was estimated to be as high as more than 1 million in the 1960s. Abortions performed illegally were extremely dangerous and much more likely to result in hemorrhage, infection, and damage to the pelvic organs than a legal termination. The mortality associated with legal terminations of pregnancy declined from approximately 3.3 deaths per 100,000 procedures to less than 0.5 deaths per 100,000 procedures between the years 1973 and 1985 (Fig. 12-4).

First- and second-trimester abortions can be performed either medically or surgically. A surgical termination usually involves dilating the cervical canal and removing the POC. This procedure may require a device that produces suction, curettes, or other instruments. Risks of D&C include infection, incomplete evacuation of the uterus, damage to the uterus, bleeding, and the formation of scar tissue in the uterus (Asherman's syndrome). There are few long-term sequelae associated with legal abortions. There is no increased risk for miscarriage or premature cervical dilatation following a legal first-trimester abortion. There is probably little impact on future fecundity with carefully performed multiple abortions. Rarely, second-trimester abortions involve a laparotomy with the fetus being removed through an incision in the uterus (hysterotomy) or removal of the entire uterus (hysterectomy). Reliable medical termination of first-trimester pregnancies has become available in Europe with the progesterone antagonist RU-486 given in conjunction with a prostaglandin agent. Medical termination of second-trimester pregnancies involves the induction of labor with urea or prostaglandin $F_{2-\alpha}$ injected into the amniotic sac via amniocentesis.

Women who choose to have a termination in the second trimester of pregnancy usually fall in two categories: those who did not discover that they were pregnant until late in the gestation (because of normally irregular periods or lack of information) and women who have had abnormal results found with genetic testing of the fetus. Second-trimester terminations carry a slight increased morbidity compared with those performed in the first trimester. Furthermore, there is often an increased emotional

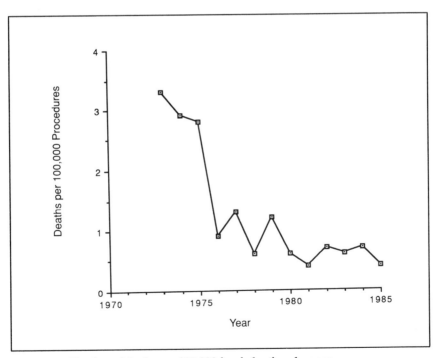

Fig. 12-4. Number of deaths per 100,000 legal abortions by year.

trauma associated with friends and relatives knowing that the patient is pregnant as well as a greater degree of "bonding" that has occurred between the parents and the fetus.

Ectopic Pregnancy

Definition

An ectopic pregnancy is defined as any pregnancy that results from the implantation of an embryo outside the uterine corpus. This is a more precise definition than "extrauterine pregnancy" since cervical and cornual pregnancies are also considered to be ectopic in nature. These latter relatively rare implantations are perhaps the most life-threatening ectopic pregnancies because of their typically delayed diagnosis and potential for intense hemorrhage with rupture.

Incidence

Ectopic pregnancies occur in between 1 in 80 and 1 in 300 of all pregnancies. In the United States, the incidence is roughly 1 in 100 pregnancies. Populations that are at risk for exposure to sexually transmitted disease are at greater risk for ectopic pregnancies. Since the Centers for Disease Control first started reporting statistics on ectopic pregnancies in 1970, there has been an approximately fourfold increase in the incidence (Fig. 12-5).

Mortality

Despite an increase in both the absolute number and the relative percentage of ectopic pregnancies compared to the number of pregnancies, there has been a roughly 10-fold decrease in the case-fatality rate in the United States since 1970 (Fig. 12-6).

Risk Factors

Tubal Damage

Tubal damage, which usually results from prior salpingitis (tubal infection), is probably the biggest single risk factor for ectopic pregnancy. With improved antibiotic therapy, women who previously would have become completely sterile may now have a fallopian tube that is functional enough to permit fertilization but still not allow for normal embryo transport and uterine implantation. Infections, most often from *Chlamydia trachomatis* or *Neisseria gonorrhoeae,* can lead to intraluminal tubal scarring, fibrosis, or narrowing with destruction of normal cilia function. These changes are often associated with peritubular adhesions that further increase the risk of an ectopic pregnancy.

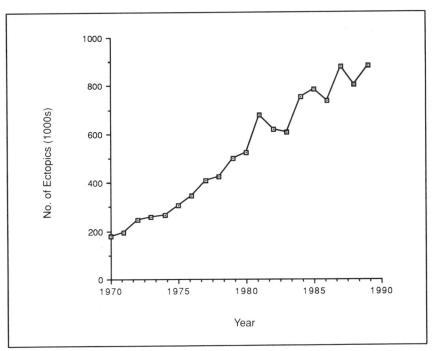

Fig. 12-5. Number of ectopic pregnancies per year.

Use of the Intrauterine Device

The intrauterine device (IUD), when properly used in the appropriate patient population, does not increase the risk of pelvic inflammatory disease and subsequent ectopic pregnancy. Data that quote a higher risk are based on earlier, poorly designed studies. However, the IUD only prevents intrauterine pregnancies. As such, although the overall chance of a pregnancy occurring is low, should a women become pregnant with an IUD in place, there is a much greater chance of the pregnancy being extrauterine in location.

History of Prior Tubal Pregnancy

A woman with a previous ectopic pregnancy has an approximately 15 percent risk of a repeat ectopic pregnancy with her next gestation. Whether this risk is related to the same risk factors and causative agents that led to the initial ectopic pregnancy, or the increased risk is based on the first ectopic pregnancy itself, tubal damage resulting from the ectopic pregnancy, or some other factor is not known.

Prior Tubal Surgery

Any tubal surgery increases the risk of an ectopic pregnancy, either by damaging a normal tube or elevating a completely nonfunctional oviduct

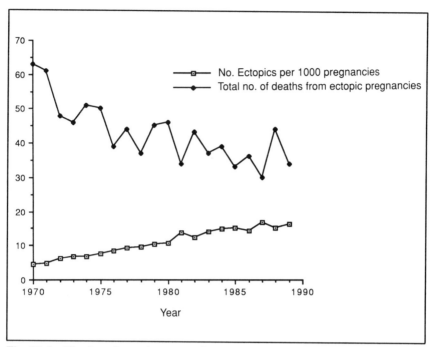

Fig. 12-6. Number of ectopic pregnancies per 1000 pregnancies and total deaths from ectopic pregnancies.

to an impaired but functional status. The greater the damage to the tube or the greater the surgical intervention, the greater the risk.

Like the IUD, a tubal ligation greatly reduces the overall chance of becoming pregnant. Similarly, any pregnancy that occurs after a tubal ligation has a much greater chance of being tubal in origin, although a normal intrauterine pregnancy can take place as well.

History of Infertility
A history of infertility, even in the absence of prior known salpingitis or tubal surgery, has been identified as a risk factor for a number of adverse reproductive sequelae including tubal pregnancy. Whether this represents a subclinical pelvic factor or other subtle processes is not known.

Pathology
There are many similarities between early intrauterine and ectopic pregnancies. Following a migration period, the embryo destined to become an ectopic undergoes implantation and attempts to receive a healthy vascular supply. There is some debate as to whether abdominal ectopic pregnancies arrive at their implantation site following an initial migration period or represent "tubal abortions," in which pregnancies are flushed or aborted

out of a fallopian tube and remain viable after implanting somewhere in the abdomen. Regardless of the process of migration and the location of the ectopic pregnancy, most of the time normal implantation and growth are not possible. Abnormal erosion of blood vessels at the site of implantation can cause bleeding. This bleeding may track down through the tubes and uterus and present as vaginal bleeding. Alternatively, the blood may escape into the abdomen and cause a local chemical peritonitis. If the blood irritates the diaphragm, referred shoulder pain via the phrenic nerve occurs. If the blood is trapped in the fallopian tube, a hematosalpinx results.

The hormonal changes associated with an ectopic pregnancy can mimic those of a normal gestation. Although most normal pregnancies manifest a doubling of the beta-hCG titer approximately every 2 to 3 days (see Chap. 11), only 15 percent of ectopic pregnancies follow this pattern.

With the production of hCG, the corpus luteum is stimulated and progesterone is produced. Although the progesterone levels achieved may approach those found in a normal pregnancy, investigators have found that a progesterone level below 5 ng/ml is indicative of a nonviable pregnancy. Unfortunately, there is no blood test to distinguish a nonviable intrauterine gestation from an ectopic one.

The Arias-Stella reaction, initially described in 1954, is a pathognomonic endometrial change that is associated with any pregnancy (whether intra- or extrauterine), consisting of cellular enlargement (Fig. 12-7) with significant hyperchromatosis, pleomorphism, and mitotic activity. These changes are usually localized and associated with decidual changes in the stroma and a hypersecretory pattern in the glands. These findings are not useful in determining the location of the pregnancy, but when found on an endometrial biopsy specimen, they serve as a warning that a pregnancy is present somewhere. Thereafter, if no pregnancy is found in the uterus, a diligent search for a possible ectopic pregnancy must be made.

With ultrasound, many diagnostic characteristics have been described for ectopic pregnancies, the majority of which directly correlate to the gestational age. However, the most significant ultrasonographic finding is the inability to identify an intrauterine gestation when the rising beta-hCG levels have reached the level where such identification is generally possible. An adnexal mass separate from the ovaries may be visualized as well.

Location of Ectopic Pregnancies

Most ectopic pregnancies occur in the fallopian tube (Fig. 12-8). An abdominal ectopic pregnancy can occasionally proceed to term. The diagnosis is often made when the patient does not go into labor and cervical dilatation or labor cannot be induced. The fetus is delivered by a traditional laparotomy. This procedure is not called a cesarean section because no uterine incision is made. When presenting at term, the most common problems associated with these babies are related to the lack of amniotic fluid and include lung hypoplasia and limb abnormalities. For the mother,

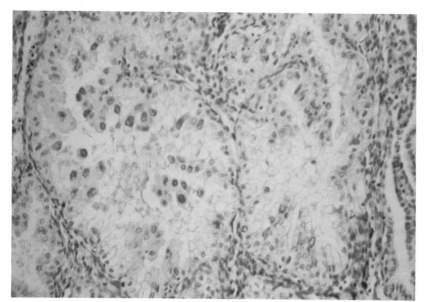

Fig. 12-7. Arias-Stella reaction.

the major problem associated with an abdominal pregnancy is the placenta, which is often attached to the bowel mesentary. Because of the risk of severe hemorrhage associated with attempted removal, the placenta is drained of blood and left intraabdominally in these cases.

Diagnosis

The classic triad of amenorrhea, pain, and spotting occurs in only 50 percent of patients with an ectopic pregnancy. Although spotting does increase the suspicion for an abnormal gestation, amenorrhea is not a useful sign other than to raise the question of a pregnancy being present. However, with improved diagnostic technologies and increased physician awareness of the risk of ectopic pregnancies, many women are completely asymptomatic at the time of diagnosis. Unfortunately, many women present with a ruptured ectopic pregnancy without any history of significant symptoms.

For an optimal outcome (specifically an unruptured fallopian tube), it is necessary that the diagnosis and treatment be made early. This can only be done with a high degree of clinical suspicion. As such, whenever a patient of reproductive age presents with amenorrhea, a pregnancy test should be performed. In any patient with risk factors for an ectopic pregnancy, sequential serum beta-hCG pregnancy tests should be obtained with an ultrasound scheduled to determine the location of the pregnancy.

There have been several recent noteworthy improvements in ultrasound technology. The use of a vaginal ultrasound probe is far superior to the older abdominal models in its ability to determine the location and viability of a pregnancy at an early gestational age. The probe of the vaginal ultrasound allows the transducer to be placed closer to the uterus and adnexal structures, thus affording better visualization at an earlier gestational age. More recently, color Doppler has provided improved delineation of the blood flow in the adnexa and uterus by demonstrating relative amounts and directions of flow, and may have application in the diagnosis of ectopic pregnancy.

After amenorrhea and spotting, the most common presenting symptom of an ectopic pregnancy is pelvic pain. This pain may have many etiologies, but commonly arises from stretching of the fallopian tube's lumen by an expanding hematoma or irritation of the peritoneum of the abdomen resulting from free blood. Referred shoulder pain may result from blood irritating the diaphragm and being perceived in the shoulder via the phrenic nerve. Significant abdominal pain or hypotensive symptoms (nausea, vomiting, diaphoresis, and syncope) are generally ominous in that they may represent imminent or current tubal rupture and hemorrhage. All of these symptoms may be transient or intermittent, or both. Although significant internal bleeding requiring emergency surgery and blood transfusions still occurs, less than 40 women die each year in the United States from ectopic pregnancies.

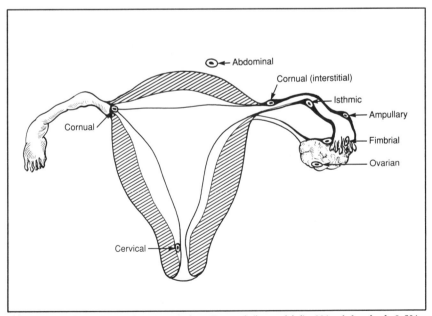

Fig. 12-8.   Sites of ectopic pregnancies. Cornual (interstitial), 2%; abdominal, 0.5%; ovarian, 0.5%; cervical, 0.1%; tubal, 97% (ampullary, 55%; isthmic, 25%; infundibulum and fimbria, 18%; interstitial, 2%).

Unfortunately, other than blood counts and serum pregnancy levels, there are few other accepted laboratory tests that aid in the diagnosis of ectopic pregnancy. One notable exception is the serum progesterone level. If this value is less than 5 ng/ml, then there is virtually no chance that a viable intrauterine pregnancy exists. Therefore, a careful D&C may be performed to search for a nonviable intrauterine gestation. If none is found, then the index of suspicion for an ectopic pregnancy increases dramatically.

The physical examination is often misleading in the search for an ectopic pregnancy. A pelvic mass is palpated in only approximately 50 percent of the cases. Furthermore, this mass may be palpated on the opposite side from the ectopic gestation since the corpus luteum is in the contralateral ovary in more than 15 percent of cases. The physical examination should be gentle in nature because an exuberant search for an ectopic pregnancy may rupture it. Because of hormonal stimulation, the uterus is usually uniformly enlarged in an early ectopic pregnancy similar to a normal intrauterine gestation. Asymmetric enlargement should raise the index of suspicion for a cornual pregnancy although other pathology, such as a fibroid tumor, may be the cause.

If there are significant changes in the patient's vital signs consistent with blood loss (tachycardia, hypotension, etc.) then the decision to proceed with a surgical exploration is already made for the physician. Otherwise, further diagnostic studies may proceed. A culdocentesis is a procedure in which a needle is placed transvaginally into the abdomen via the posterior cul-de-sac (Pouch of Douglas) (Fig. 12-9). It is a relatively straightforward and painless procedure that demonstrates the presence of nonclotting blood (indicating an older hemorrhage) or fresh blood. If there is old nonclotting blood with a hematocrit of ≥ 15 percent, then surgery is still indicated, even if a ruptured corpus luteum cyst represents the source of the blood. Major problems with culdocentesis include the invasiveness of the procedure and the high false-negative rate. Patients with no blood aspirated may still have significant intraabdominal bleeding.

Ultrasound has replaced the need for culdocentesis in many cases by clearly demonstrating either an intra- or extrauterine gestation. Although it is not able to quantify the type or source of fluid, ultrasound is excellent for determining the presence of free fluid in the pelvis. Patients with an ectopic pregnancy may have a "decidual cast" in their uterus. This structure represents a collection of blood or secretory changes, or both, in the endometrial lining related to hormonal influence that may be difficult to distinguish from the early gestational sac of a normal intrauterine pregnancy.

Besides ultrasonography, laparoscopy represents a major improvement in the diagnosis and treatment of an ectopic pregnancy. With this modality, both diagnosis and treatment can be performed at the same time, but laparoscopy carries a 5 percent false-positive and false-negative rate.

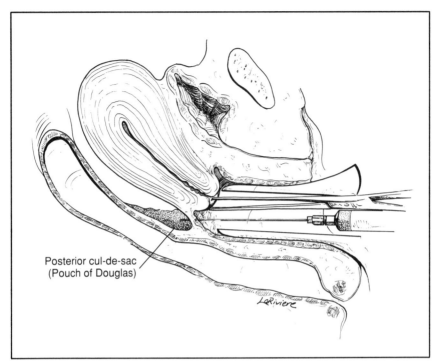

Posterior cul-de-sac
(Pouch of Douglas)

Fig. 12-9. Culdocentesis.

Treatment of Ectopic Pregnancies

Observation

Most ectopic pregnancies will resolve without intervention via a tubal abortion or other phenomenon. However, given the excellent treatment modalities available and the difficulty in deciding which patient is a candidate for observation alone, nonintervention is rarely used for a known ectopic pregnancy. Nevertheless, in a patient with declining serum beta-hCG values, a paucity of symptoms, absence of a large ectopic pregnancy by ultrasound, no fetal heart motion detected, and a desire for nonintervention, observation (with instructions on warning signs, informed consent, and ready access to surgery should it be needed) is acceptable.

Surgery

Surgical intervention is the standard treatment of ectopic pregnancies. There have been a number of prospective randomized studies documenting equivalent outcomes between ectopic pregnancies treated via laparoscopy compared to laparotomy. Since laparotomy results in a significantly greater morbidity and mortality, increased risk of postoperative adhesion formation, and increased costs, an increasing proportion of ectopic pregnancies are currently managed with laparoscopy instead of laparotomy given adequate training and equipment.

Prior surgical treatment for a tubal gestation used to consist of removing the affected tube (salpingectomy) with the thought that this would decrease the risk of future ectopic pregnancies in the damaged tube. Furthermore, to increase the chance of ovulation occurring on the side with the remaining fallopian tube, the (completely normal) ovary on the affected side was also removed (oophorectomy). It is now known that 50 percent of subsequent ectopic pregnancies occur in the contralateral tube. Thus, the ectopic pregnancy may be removed while leaving the tube in situ provided that it is not severely damaged by prior disease or tubal rupture. Occasionally it is possible to remove only part of the affected tube (partial salpingectomy) in the hopes of permitting a reconnection (anastomosis) to be performed at a future time. Because approximately 15 percent of intrauterine pregnancies occur via the contralateral ovary releasing the egg, and because of the advent of IVF (in which the fallopian tubes are completely bypassed), undamaged ovaries are no longer routinely removed. A good rule of thumb is to perform the most conservative organ-sparing procedure possible.

Medical Treatment

Many medical regimens are used both as a primary treatment and as a therapy for a persistent ectopic pregnancy. Medical treatments can be divided into two groups consisting of locally and systemically administered medications. Locally delivered medications are injected (either transvaginally or via laparoscopy) directly into the ectopic pregnancy and include prostaglandins, methotrexate, hyperosmolar glucose, potassium chloride, and other caustic agents. Although effective, these treatment regimens are not widely used because of the surgical procedure required and the safety and efficacy of systemic medications. Methotrexate is the drug of choice for the systemic medical treatment of ectopic pregnancy. Methotrexate is a folic acid antagonist that has a long history of use in the treatment of gestational trophoblastic disease. Methotrexate is given as a single intramuscular dose following a screening evaluation of liver and hematologic laboratory tests in appropriately screened patients with an intact ectopic pregnancy. Serial beta-hCG measurements are followed with a repeat dose of methotrexate given if an appropriate decline is not seen. Although relatively new, methotrexate treatment appears to be highly effective and safe. For ectopic gestations that are in highly vascular locations (such as cervical or ovarian pregnancies), medical treatment represents a highly desirable alternative to surgical intervention. Persistent ectopic pregnancy occurs when some viable hCG-producing trophoblastic tissue remains following surgical treatment. Persistent ectopic pregnancies carry the risk of tubal rupture and hemorrhage. Fortunately, methotrexate is also excellent for treating this entity and has replaced surgery in most cases.

Future Fertility
Women who have been treated for an ectopic pregnancy have an approximately 15 percent chance of a subsequent ectopic gestation with their next pregnancy. Although up to 49 percent of women who have had an ectopic pregnancy may not be able to conceive on their own, IVF represents an excellent option. However, despite placing the embryos in the uterine cavity and bypassing the oviducts, 10 percent of patients still develop ectopic pregnancies with IVF. Therefore, some authors advocate removing the fallopian tubes in women with known tubal damage prior to an IVF cycle.

Rh-negative women who experience abortions, ectopic pregnancies, or bleeding during pregnancy should be given anti-D globulin within 72 hours unless her partner is known with certainty to also be Rh-negative.

Recommended Reading

Grimes, D. A. Surgical management of abortion. In J. D. Thompson and J. A. Rock (eds.), *TeLinde's Operative Gynecology* (7th ed.). Philadelphia: Lippincott, 1992. Pp. 317–343.

Mishell, D. R. Abortion. In A. L. Herbst, et al. (eds.), *Comprehensive Gynecology* (2nd ed.). St. Louis: Mosby Year Book, 1992. Pp. 425–456.

Mishell, D. R. Ectopic Pregnancy. In A. L. Herbst, et al. (eds.), *Comprehensive Gynecology* (2nd ed.). St. Louis: Mosby Year Book, 1992. Pp. 457–490.

Rock, J. A. Ectopic Pregnancy. In J. D. Thompson and J. A. Rock (eds.), *TeLinde's Operative Gynecology* (7th ed.). Philadelphia: Lippincott, 1992. Pp. 411–437.

13

Antepartum Care

Cydney I. Afriat

Few areas of health care focus as heavily on the essentially healthy individual as does prenatal or antepartum care. In fact, obstetric care, unlike other specialty areas, always has placed emphasis on preventive care. The recently developed objectives for prenatal care as described by the Expert Panel on the Content of Prenatal Care are differentiated into three distinct groups: the pregnant woman, the fetus, and the family.

The objectives of prenatal care for the pregnant woman are:

1. To increase her well-being before, during, and after pregnancy and to improve her self-image and self care;
2. To reduce maternal mortality and morbidity, fetal loss, and unnecessary pregnancy interventions;
3. To reduce the risks to her health prior to subsequent pregnancies and beyond childbearing years; and
4. To promote the development of parenting skills.

The objectives of prenatal care for the fetus and the infant are:

1. To increase well-being;
2. To reduce preterm birth, intrauterine growth retardation, congenital anomalies, and failure to thrive;
3. To promote healthy growth and development, immunization, and health supervision;
4. To reduce neurologic, developmental, and other morbidities; and
5. To reduce child abuse and neglect, injuries, preventable acute and chronic illness, and the need for extended hospitalization after birth.

The objectives of prenatal care for the family during pregnancy and the first year of the infant's life are:

213

1. To promote family development, and positive parent-infant interaction;
2. To reduce unintended pregnancies; and
3. To identify for treatment, behavior disorders leading to child neglect and family violence.

These objectives are met through frequent prenatal visits during which key components of maternal and fetal well-being are evaluated.

In 1912 the United States Congress established the Children's Bureau, which conducted a study of infant deaths. They determined that the infant death rate was approximately 124 per 1000 live births. During the analysis of their data they identified a clear link between infant health and maternal health during the pregnancy. The bureau then expanded their study to maternal mortality rates and established the importance of early and continuous prenatal care in reducing both maternal and infant mortality. In 1941, the United States Department of Labor's Children's Bureau stated that "Adequate care before, during and after childbirth is the right of every mother." Up to that time it was not unusual for a woman to have one interview with a physician during the pregnancy and then not be seen again until labor. This was deemed to be inadequate prenatal care.

Pregnancy outcome is assessed in terms of maternal, neonatal, and perinatal mortality and morbidity rates. *Maternal mortality* is defined as the number of maternal deaths, indirect or direct, per 100,000 live births within 42 days of the termination of the pregnancy irrespective of the duration and site (intrauterine versus extrauterine) of the pregnancy. *Indirect maternal death* is death that occurs during the obstetric period but is not directly due to obstetric causes. It may be attributable to a preexisting disease or a disease that developed during pregnancy, labor, or postpartum but it was nonetheless aggravated by physiologic changes due to the pregnancy. *Direct maternal death* is death that results from an obstetric complication, i.e., postpartum hemorrhage. *Fetal death* or *stillbirth* is usually defined in the United States as the death of the fetus at or beyond 20 weeks' gestation. Internationally a gestational age of 28 weeks is often used. The *neonatal mortality rate* is the number of deaths of newborns delivered at 20 weeks (28 weeks internationally) or more within the first 28 days of life per 1000 live births. The *perinatal mortality rate* combines both fetal and neonatal deaths up to 6 days of life per 1000 births. In 1986 the perinatal mortality rate in the United States was 13.3/1000.

An *infant death* is the death of a live-born infant at any time from birth to the end of the first year of life. The *infant mortality rate* is the number of infant deaths per 1000 live births. In 1989, the infant mortality rate was 9.8 infants per 1000 live births in the United States. This was the lowest rate ever recorded in United States history. However, when this rate was further analyzed by race, the infant mortality rate for the white population was 8.1/1000 live births as compared with 18.6/1000 live births for the black population. The National Commission to Prevent Infant Mortality, which was founded by Congress in 1987, determined that the United States had fallen to twentieth place among developed nations that are attempting to decrease infant mortality rates.

Numerous studies have shown that infant outcome is better for those women who receive prenatal care during their pregnancies than for those who do not. Specific, definable reasons have remained elusive and are still being explored. There is concern that these perinatal and infant mortality and morbidity rates may worsen as poverty, infectious disease, and drug and alcohol abuse increase coupled with a decrease in access to health care, primarily prenatal care. The commission has called on government and private industry to guarantee universal access to early maternity and pediatric care. As late as 1986, it was estimated that 25 percent of pregnant women received inadequate (less than three visits per pregnancy) or no prenatal care at all.

Preconception Counselling

Ideally, the initiation of antepartum care should begin with preconception counselling of the woman or, preferably, the couple. During this counselling session, the health care provider elicits pertinent information that includes (1) historical information including but not limited to medical, family, and genetic history; (2) obstetric history; (3) gynecologic history; (4) surgical history; (5) social history including use of caffeine, alcohol, and recreational drugs; (6) current medical problems and treatments; (7) nutrition; (8) psychosocial history; and (9) sexual history (Table 13-1).

Table 13-1. Preconception or first visit

I. Historical information
  A. Demographic information
    1. Age
    2. Ethnicity
    3. Religion
    4. Genetic history
    5. Exposures to environmental toxins or hazards
  B. Medical history
    1. Childhood illnesses
    2. Immunizations
    3. Chronic illnesses
    4. Resolved illnesses
    5. Current and past medications
    6. Allergies
    7. Blood transfusions

(Continued)

Table 13-1 *(Continued)*

        8. Exposures to contagious diseases
    C. Surgical history
        1. Accidents and traumas
        2. Operations
        3. Operations related to reproductive tract
    D. Gynecologic history
        1. Menarche
        2. Cycle length and regularity
        3. Contraceptive use
        4. Pelvic infections and sexually transmitted diseases
        5. Sexual exposure to intravenous drug abuser
        6. Sexual history
    E. Obstetric history
        1. Prior pregnancies
            a. Term, preterm, abortions
            b. Obstetric outcome
                (1) Large for gestational age
                (2) Small for gestational age
                (3) Handicaps or retardation
                (4) Multiple gestation
                (5) Hemorrhage
        2. Location of prior births
        3. Birth weights
        4. Type of delivery
 II. Nutrition history
    A. Daily intake
    B. Food restrictions
III. Exercise history
    A. Type, duration
    B. Physical restriction
IV. Birth plan
    A. Childbirth education
    B. Support person
    C. Location of birth (hospital or birth center)
    D. Choice of analgesics, anesthetics
    E. Overall expectations
 V. Review of systems
VI. Physical examination
    A. Head, eyes, ears, nose, and throat
    B. Heart
    C. Lungs
    D. Abdomen
    E. Pelvic area
        1. Speculum examination
            a. Pap smear
            b. Cultures

(Continued)

Table 13-1   *(Continued)*

      c. Wet mount
        2. Bimanual examination
            a. Uterine size
            b. Uterine consistency
            c. Adnexae
            d. Clinical pelvimetry
        3. Auscultation of fetal heart rate
      F. Extremities and reflexes
 VII. Laboratory studies
      A. Urinalysis
      B. CBC, blood type, antibody screen
      C. Rubella titer
      D. Rapid plasma reagin test or Venereal Disease Research Laboratory test for
         syphilis
      E. Hepatitis-B surface antigen
      F. Human immunodeficiency virus
      G. Other
VIII. Nutritional counselling
  IX. Social service counselling
   X. Genetic counselling

By obtaining such information, the health care provider can guide the couple in planning their obstetric care and can be aware at the earliest possible stage of which special test or evaluation tool might provide the best outcome. In addition, in some cases, this is the ideal time to make appropriate referrals and recommendations. For instance, the woman with diabetes in anticipation of pregnancy would be able to make certain that her diet is appropriate and her blood glucose is in adequate control and to arrange to see an obstetrician with expertise in diabetes in pregnancy.

Terminology
Specific terminology for quantifying a woman's obstetrical history has been devised in order to enhance communication among providers. The suffix *gravida*, or gravidity (G), refers to the number of times a woman has been pregnant regardless of the gestational age achieved in any given pregnancy. Therefore, this category includes all abortions whether spontaneous, elective, or induced. A *primigravida* is a woman who is pregnant for the first time and a *secundigravida* is a woman who is pregnant for the second time. Women who are pregnant and have been pregnant more than one time are *multigravidas*.

The suffix *para*, or parity (P), refers to the number of pregnancies that completed the twentieth week of gestation or weighed a minimum of

500 g at birth. A multiple birth is a single parous experience. A primipara is a woman who has given birth for the first time to one or more newborns and a multipara is a woman who has given birth more than once.

Parity is often further differentiated into five subcategories. *Term* (T) pregnancies are defined as a gestation greater than 37 completed weeks. *Preterm* (P) is a gestation between 20 and 38 weeks. *Abortions* (A) include all gestations prior to 20 weeks or weighing less than 500 g. *Living* (L) includes all those children currently alive. Some clinicians add a fifth category for *multiple births* (M). For example, a woman who is a G5P21120 has been pregnant 5 times, delivered 2 term infants, 1 preterm infant, had 1 abortion, and now has 2 living children, none of whom were multiple births. This notation also indicates that she is currently pregnant. Many individuals find a mnemonic helpful to remember such complicated nomenclature. "*Texas Power And Light*" serves that purpose.

An alternate method of describing pregnancies and outcome is by enumerating gravidity, parity (all-inclusive), abortions, and living children. Using the same example as listed above, the woman would be a G5P3Ab1L2.

Diagnosis of Pregnancy

The accurate diagnosis of pregnancy is based on three types of findings: presumptive signs, probable signs, and positive signs. *Presumptive signs* of pregnancy (Table 13-2) are based on maternal physiologic changes that the woman experiences. The most typical presumptive signs include abrupt cessation of menses, nausea or vomiting, breast enlargement, increased urinary frequency, and elevation of basal body temperature for more than 14 days.

Probable signs of pregnancy include maternal physiologic and anatomic changes that are detected on examination and documented by the examiner. These signs include enlargement of the maternal abdomen, palpation of the fetal outline, enlargement of the uterus, softening of the uterine isthmus (Hegar's sign), cervical softening (Goodell's sign), and a bluish hue of the vulva, vagina, and cervix (Chadwick's sign). A positive pregnancy test is considered a probable sign of pregnancy rather than a positive sign since other maternal factors aside from pregnancy, such as tumors that produce human chorionic gonadotropin (hCG), can contribute to both a positive serum or urine pregnancy test.

Positive signs of pregnancy are directly attributable to the fetus but are detected and documented by the examiner. These include auscultation of the fetal heart sounds with a Doppler stethoscope or visualization of the fetal heart motions with ultrasonography (see Table 13-2).

Determination of Gestational Age

The normal or average length of a pregnancy is 10 lunar months, 40 weeks, or 280 days from the first day of the woman's last normal menstrual period

Table 13-2. Signs of pregnancy

Presumptive	Probable	Positive
Abrupt cessation of menses	Abdominal enlargement	Auscultation of fetal heart
Nausea and vomiting	Palpation of fetal outline	Visualization of fetal heart movement by ultrasound
Breast changes (tingling, tenderness, nodularity, enlargement)	Ballottement	
	Perception of fetal movement	
Urinary frequency	Enlargement of uterus on pelvic examination	
Fatigue		
Montgomery's tubercles (hypertrophied sebaceous glands in areola)	Piskacek's sign (uterine irregularity due to ovum implantation in cornua)	
Continued elevation of basal body temperature	Hegar's sign (softening of uterine isthmus)	
Expression of colostrum		
Ptyalism	Goodell's sign (cervical softening)	
Chadwick's sign (bluish vulva, vagina, cervix)	Braxton Hicks contractions: palpable by examiner	
Quickening		
Skin changes (chloasma, striae, linea nigra, vascular spiders, palmar erythema)	Positive urine or serum hCG pregnancy test	

(LNMP). This is the gestational or menstrual age of the pregnancy and is used by all obstetric health care providers to ensure dating consistency. Other biologists or scientists may use ovulatory or fertilization age (from conception), which is 2 weeks less than the menstrual or gestational age. Most women tend to begin counting based on conception and need to be reeducated.

Three methods may be used to determine gestational age (GA) and the estimated date of delivery (EDD). The oldest method is known as Nägele's rule, which involves determining the month and day of the last menstrual period (LMP), adding 7 days to the day and subtracting 3 months from the month. Therefore, if a woman's LMP was June 6, her EDD would be March 13.

The second method of determining gestational age is by using a manu-
factured pregnancy dating wheel. Many pharmaceutical and medical supply companies make these wheels and, therefore, some variation may exist
among them, altering the weeks' gestation or EDD by a day or two. Since
precise knowledge of this information is needed, care should be taken to
consistently use the same wheel for evaluating the pregnancy. The appropriate unit of measure of gestational age is number of weeks completed in
the pregnancy.

The third, and more technically advanced method of calculating gestational age is with ultrasonography, also known as sonography, which has
been employed since the mid-1970s. A gestational sac may be seen as early
as 5 weeks' gestation, fetal heart motion may be seen at 6 to 8 weeks' gestation, and a crown-rump measurement can also be obtained at that same
time. The crown-rump length obtained during the first trimester can accurately date a pregnancy to within 5 days.

In some cases, the woman may not recall her LMP or the clinician may
note that the size of the woman's uterus and her LMP are not consistent.
A sonographic estimate of fetal age may be done at that point and if
the sonographic dating of the pregnancy differs from the LMP dating by
more than 2 weeks, the EDD may be changed to the date based on the
ultrasonographic information. The new EDD is considered the "corrected
EDD."

Because of the neonatal implications of delivering either a premature
or a postdates pregnancy, dating the pregnancy is of critical importance.
Therefore, the American College of Obstetricians and Gynecologists has
established guidelines for dating of pregnancy prior to performing elective procedures at term, such as an elective cesarean delivery. One of the
following must be met:

1. Fetal heart tones must have been documented for 20 weeks by
    nonelectronic fetoscope or for 30 weeks by Doppler stethoscope.
2. It has been 36 weeks since a positive serum or urine hCG
    pregnancy test was performed by a reliable laboratory.
3. An ultrasound measurement of the crown-rump length, obtained
    at 6 to 11 weeks, supports a gestational age of greater than or
    equal to 39 weeks.
4. An ultrasound, obtained at 12 to 20 weeks, confirms the gesta-
    tional age of greater than or equal to 39 weeks determined by
    clinical history and physical examination.

Pregnancy is divided into three equal "trimesters," each consisting of
approximately 13 weeks. Common discomforts of pregnancy as well as complications of pregnancy are conventionally grouped into each of these trimesters. For instance, it is more common for a woman to experience frequency of urination during the first and third trimesters because during
the first trimester, the uterus is still a pelvic organ and places pressure on

the bladder and in the third trimester, the fetal presenting part descends back into the pelvis and again places pressure on the bladder. However, during the second trimester, the fetal-uterine unit is an abdominal organ and does not affect the bladder.

Initial Antepartum Visit

Ideally, prenatal care should begin shortly after the first missed menstrual period in order to permit accurate dating of the pregnancy and to develop an adequate data base of maternal historical information including obstetric testing, baseline laboratory values, and vital signs. However, regardless of the gestational age at the time of the first visit, a complete history and physical examination is done along with specific laboratory studies. The historical information should include prior and current medical history; surgical history; allergies to medications; blood transfusions; current medications; psychosocial history (use of drugs and alcohol, cigarette smoking, support mechanisms, family situation); obstetric, gynecologic, and sexual history; and work environment (with possible exposure to toxins). Included in the gynecology history should be documentation of the date of the first day of the LMP and LNMP (if the LMP was abnormal in length, flow or timing), length of cycles, and regularity. Additionally, the method of contraception used prior to pregnancy should be noted.

A complete physical examination includes a thorough pelvic examination. The pelvic examination includes attention to probable signs of pregnancy; performance of a Pap smear and appropriate cultures such as for gonorrhea and possibly chlamydia and a bimanual examination to determine uterine size and the presence or absence of adnexal masses. Finally, a clinical pelvimetry should be performed to assess the size, shape, and adequacy of the pelvis.

Laboratory testing includes, but is not limited to: (1) urinalysis; (2) complete blood count; (3) maternal blood type, Rh factor, and antibody testing; (4) rubella immunity detection; (5) hepatitis B antigen test; and (6) testing for syphilis. Additional testing based on ethnicity and historical information may include sickle-cell prep, Tay-Sachs test, hemoglobin electrophoresis, viral titers for toxoplasmosis, cytomegalovirus, and human immunodeficiency virus testing.

After the history and physical examination are completed and the laboratory work is reviewed, the health care provider determines the "risk" classification or category of the woman. If any prior medical, surgical, or obstetric historical factors suggest that the pregnancy is at increased risk of an adverse outcome, the woman is then determined to be "high-risk." If no high-risk factors are evident, then the pregnancy is determined to be "low-risk" until such time as a condition change occurs.

In general terms, a woman who is considered to be high-risk will require increased surveillance of her pregnancy and may be referred to a perinatologist for this care. Common situations that merit classification as high-risk include diabetes, chronic hypertension requiring medical management, multiple gestation, and severe pregnancy-induced hypertension.

Revisits

With the initial visit and completion of all the laboratory testing, the woman enters into a structured program of prenatal visits throughout the rest of the pregnancy. The 1989 guidelines as described by the Public Health Service Expert Panel on the Content of Prenatal Care recommend nine visits for the healthy nulliparous woman and seven for the healthy parous woman. These numbers include one preconception visit. This departure from traditional monthly, biweekly, and weekly visits has been suggested in order to best utilize limited resources and health care providers. The at-risk woman will require a greater number of visits, as does the lower-risk woman who has a change in maternal or fetal condition. This increased frequency of visits has been shown to improve maternal and perinatal outcome in the at-risk group.

The traditional scheduling of visits was designed to detect developing problems as early as possible by increasing the frequency of the visits as the pregnancy advanced toward term. This scheduling was based on the premise that the risk of both maternal and fetal problems increased toward full gestation. In retrospect, however, it has been noted that developing problems can be identified with less frequent visits. With less visits required, more prenatal visits can be provided to a larger group of women utilizing the same or similar resources.

For the nulliparous woman, the prenatal visits begin between 6 and 8 weeks' gestation with the second visit occurring within 4 weeks of the first visit. The multiparous woman will be seen between 6 and 8 weeks' gestation but may simply have phone contact with her health care provider for the next visit. As a minimum, the remaining visits for both groups will be between 14 and 16 weeks and then between 24 and 28 weeks followed by visits for the nulliparous at 32, 36, 38, 39, 40, and 41 weeks with the multiparous woman being seen at 32, 36, 39, and 41 weeks' gestation.

Each revisit begins with a review of the maternal records to refresh the memory of the health care provider. The history and physical examination findings are reviewed, as well as all laboratory data and findings from each prenatal visit. For example, if at the initial visit it is determined that the woman is Rh-negative, the results of the test may be reviewed with her at her current visit and the plan for the use of Rh immune globulin may be discussed with her.

At each revisit, the gestational age of the fetus is calculated. This knowledge is used as a cue as to the appropriate teaching that should be done at that visit. The teaching should include fetal growth and development, common maternal discomforts for this stage and the coming stage of pregnancy, signs and symptoms of complications, and any other appropriate counselling and support that may be warranted.

Special Laboratory Testing

During the preconception or initial prenatal visit it is determined if an indication for fetal chromosomal analysis exists. Possible indications for fetal genetic studies include advanced maternal age or maternal or family history of genetic defects or anomalies.

Currently, the most common method of obtaining genetic studies is by obtaining an amniotic fluid sample via amniocentesis. This procedure involves inserting a needle transabdominally into the gestational sac while an ultrasound machine provides direct guidance. The sample of fluid is then sent to the laboratory for the studies to be performed. Amniocentesis is generally done at approximately 16 weeks' gestation, but may be performed at some centers as early as 13 to 14 weeks. The risks of the procedure include rupture of membranes, infection, preterm labor, and fetal, maternal, or placental trauma. The currently reported overall risk of poor outcome from the procedure itself is 0.6 to 0.9 percent.

Results of the genetic studies may take from 10 days to 2 weeks to be reported back to the attending physician. The delay in the turnaround time as well as the inability to perform the procedure during the first trimester prompted researchers to investigate other methods of obtaining fetal cells for analysis. Chorionic villus sampling (CVS) has recently become available. Chorionic villus sampling is done between 10 and 12 weeks' gestation, once again under the direct visualization and guidance of ultrasound. Diagnostic analyses are performed on the villi without having to wait for the cells to grow. Therefore, karyotyping results are available within a few days. The primary advantage of CVS over amniocentesis is that it is done in the first trimester, prior to "showing" and prior to feeling fetal movement. However, the relative risks of CVS are not entirely established at the present time.

Maternal Serum Alpha Fetoprotein

A widely utilized screening program for neural tube defects involves analyzing maternal serum for the amount of alpha fetoprotein (AFP) present. In 80 to 90 percent of pregnancies with open neural tube defects such as anencephaly, the amount of AFP in the maternal serum is greater than 2.5 multiples of the mean. Therefore, the maternal serum alpha fetoprotein (MSAFP) has been deemed a worthwhile screening test to be offered to all pregnant women whose families do not have a history of neural tube defects. Alpha fetoprotein is the major protein produced by the fetus that can be measured in maternal serum. The greatest accuracy of MSAFP screening occurs between 15 and 18 weeks' gestation. Elevated AFP may be due to a host of factors, open neural tube defect being of greatest concern. Several other factors may cause the AFP to be falsely elevated, such as incorrect gestational dating or multiple gestation. Such MSAFP testing is a screening tool and not diagnostic. The high level of false-positive results demands that appropriate counselling be given to the pregnant woman prior to obtaining serum for analysis. An ultrasound examination of the fetus or an amniocentesis, or both, may be offered to the patient to further evaluate fetal condition.

First Trimester (0–13 Weeks' Gestation)

Physical Changes
Whether the pregnancy is a much-awaited planned pregnancy or not, the first trimester is a period of physical and emotional adjustment for all women. All aspects of the woman's body are affected. Increased levels of estrogen and progesterone are responsible for breast, skin, and uterine changes. Breast enlargement may cause tingling or discomfort. The nipples enlarge, and the production of colostrum begins. Total blood volume increases and causes the pulse to increase 10 to 15 percent. The diaphragm rises and increases the woman's awareness of her breathing. As the uterus increases in size, the pelvic ligaments stretch.

Psychosocial Changes
The first trimester is a period of transition and may produce some degree of ambivalence, even in the long-awaited planned pregnancy. The shift in hormonal levels may create an emotionally labile state. The pregnant woman may develop a fear of death for herself and for her child, perhaps through fear of the unknown. She may seek out new support from other pregnant women or women with children. Pregnant women may tend to focus on themselves and their bodily changes and discomforts, not knowing what to expect in terms of normal changes versus signs of complications. Sexual desires vary from individual to individual. Some women experience heightened sexual desires, others experience a decrease in libido. Open communication between spouses is essential in making a smooth transition.

Awareness of the hormonal and physical changes that transpire during the first trimester allows the health care practitioner to provide appropriate support and counselling. It is important for the practitioner to provide education and information about the physical and emotional changes that are occurring, and to convey reassurances that what the woman is experiencing is normal. If support and education do not seem to adequately reassure the patient, then professional counselling may be indicated.

Common Discomforts
Early pregnancy may be an uncomfortable time for a woman. Some of the discomforts commonly noted are fatigue, nausea, vomiting, frequency of urination, and breast tenderness. Because maternal perception of fetal movement has not yet transpired and the pregnancy is not apparent to

friends and family, the woman may not be getting emotional support and the pregnancy may not seem "real."

Reassurance should include an explanation of the normalcy of these complaints. The bladder frequency may be due to a urinary tract infection, but most likely it is caused by increased bladder pressure from the gravid uterus. The fatigue, nausea, and breast tenderness are most likely caused by the increased level of progesterone and generally resolve by the second trimester. Communicating this information to the patient will help her in coping with these normal, albeit uncomfortable symptoms.

Second Trimester (13–27 Weeks' Gestation)

Physical Changes
Evaluation of the pregnant woman during the second trimester is designed to detect any subjective or objective indications of developing problems or discomforts. At each revisit, direct communication about maternal and fetal well-being should include specific questioning about potential problems including dysuria, headaches, back pain, fetal movement, and pain (Table 13-3).

Maternal blood pressure is evaluated at each visit and should be taken with the woman's arm at the same level as her heart. The blood pressure reading is compared with those previously taken, especially with the baseline blood pressure reading taken at the first prenatal visit.

A urine specimen is obtained at each visit and is tested for the presence of protein, glucose, and nitrites. This simple screening evaluation helps in determining the need for further testing to diagnose the presence of preeclampsia, diabetes, or asymptomatic bacteriuria respectively.

Part of the physical examination at each revisit consists of measuring with a tape measure the fundal height in centimeters from the symphysis pubis to the top of the fundus. The fundal height should equal the number of weeks' gestation plus or minus 2 cm when the pregnancy is between 20 and 31 weeks. If a discrepancy is noted, then further evaluation is indicated to determine why the size is greater than or less than dates. Table 13-4 describes the most common causes of size-dates discrepancy.

An abdominal examination is done to evaluate abdominal muscle tone; to assess uterine irritability, tone, and tenderness; to check for the consistency and presence of contractions; to detect fetal movement; and to perform Leopold's maneuvers. These maneuvers are done to assess fetal lie, presentation, position, variety, and engagement. They are performed by standing at the mother's side while she is in the semiprone position. The abdomen is palpated first by moving both hands along the sides of the uterus to determine which fetal part is in the fundus, on which side the back lies, on which side the small parts are palpated and, finally, which fetal part is in the pelvis.

Table 13-3. Data to be gathered at return visit

I. Subjective information
   A. Presence of fetal movements
      Note date of quickening
   B. Complaints of
      1. Headaches, dizziness, visual disturbances
      2. Contractions or abdominal pain
      3. Vaginal bleeding, discharge, leakage of water
      4. Bladder frequency, urgency, dysuria
      5. Problems with bowels
      6. Edema
      7. Other
   C. Plan for childbirth education
   D. Discussion of circumcision
   E. Discussion for breast or bottle-feeding
   F. Birth plan
   G. Plan for contraception
   H. Review of nutrition and exercise
   I. Social service

II. Objective information
   A. Vital signs
   B. Urine dipstick for protein, glucose, nitrites
   C. Maternal weight
   D. Review recent laboratory and ultrasound data
   E. Calculate gestational age
   F. Fundal height measurement
   G. Auscultation of fetal heart rate
   H. Leopold's maneuvers
   I. Presenting part
   J. Deep tendon reflexes
   K. Other

III. Assessment
   A. Size-dates relationship
   B. Gestational age
   C. Other

IV. Plan
   A. Indicated laboratory studies
   B. Return visit
   C. Other

Fetal *lie* is the relationship of the long axis of the fetus to the long axis of the mother. The lie will be longitudinal, transverse, or oblique. The fetal *presentation* is that portion of the fetus that is in the pelvic inlet. The presentation will be cephalic, breech, or shoulder. The *position* of the fetus is the relationship of the fetal presenting part to the right and left sides of the mother's pelvis. The *variety* indicates the fetal relationship to the anterior, transverse, or posterior portion of the pelvis. Therefore, if the fetal vertex is in the pelvis with the occiput at the transverse plane of the right side of the mother's pelvis, the description is as follows: the lie is longitudinal, the breech is in the fundus, the back is on the mother's right, the small parts are on the mother's left, the presentation is cephalic, the position of the fetal head is right occipital transverse. Although this information may not be of extreme importance until the end of the third trimester, it will aid in the size-dates evaluation and in determining the best location for auscultation of the fetal heart rate (FHR).

The fetal heart rate may first be auscultated with a Doppler or ultrasound stethoscope at about 8 to 12 weeks' gestation. If a DeLee-Hillis (nonelectronic) stethoscope is being used, the FHR will first be heard at approximately 18 to 20 weeks' gestation. A chart notation should always be made as to the first time the FHR is heard with each method in order to aid in dating documentation of the pregnancy.

Another factor used to assist in dating a pregnancy is the notation of the date of "quickening." Quickening is the first time the woman feels fetal movement. Although fetal movements are present as early as 6 to 8 weeks, the primigravida usually does not perceive fetal movement until approximately 20 weeks. The multigravid woman usually notes quickening earlier, around 16 to 18 weeks, since her prior experience with fetal movement makes her more aware of the sensation. After quickening is felt, at each visit the woman is questioned and notes are recorded about fetal movement since the presence or absence of movement may be an indication of fetal well-being.

Finally, deep tendon reflexes may be evaluated as part of the prenatal visit. The presence of brisk reflexes combined with the presence of excessive edema, proteinuria, or blood pressure elevation may be an indication of developing preeclampsia.

Table 13-4. Size-dates discrepancy

Size < dates	Size > dates
Rule out:	Rule out:
Incorrect dating	Incorrect dating
Fetal demise	Multiple gestation
Rupture of membranes	Macrosomia
Oligohydramnios	Presence of fibroids
Fetal malposition	Polyhydramnios
Intrauterine growth retardation	Floating presenting part
Small for gestational age	
Lightening or engagement	
Fetal anomaly	

Laboratory Studies

As described earlier, because of maternal age or genetic history, fetal chromosomal studies may be indicated or offered. If maternal AFP serum screening yields either a low or high result, an amniocentesis may be offered as a follow-up diagnostic test to evaluate fetal chromosomes and amniotic fluid AFP levels. Other laboratory tests that are generally performed in the second trimester include a repeat complete blood count and a screening test for gestational diabetes at approximately 24 to 28 weeks' gestation. Also, if the woman is Rh-negative, a repeat antibody screen (ABS) will be done. If the ABS is negative, a prophylactic dose of Rh-immune globulin is given at 28 weeks' gestation to protect against exposure to Rh-positive fetal cells during the third trimester.

Common Maternal Discomforts

The second trimester involves fewer discomforts for the woman and has been described as being a period of "radiant health." Quickening has indicated the reality of the pregnancy and women are generally free of nausea and early pregnancy symptoms. Additionally, the uterus has gone from being a pelvic organ to an abdominal organ, thus alleviating direct pressure on the bladder.

Weight gain generally is not excessive during this time and with the return of the feeling of well-being, productive energy returns. It may also be a time of vivid dreams and the return of sexual interest. During this time, however, women may note round ligament pain as the uterus grows. The round ligaments are attached to either side of the uterus just in front of and below the fallopian tubes and cross the broad ligament in a fold of peritoneum. They then pass through the inguinal canal and insert in the anterior portion of the labia majora on either side of the perineum. In order for the uterus to grow, the round ligament must stretch. As the uterus rises in the abdomen, the ligament increases in length. Round ligament pain is thought to be secondary to this stretching. When a patient presents with abdominal pain, the differential diagnosis will include round ligament pain, appendicitis, cholycystitis, and gastric ulcer. One feature common to round ligament pain that is not common to the other conditions above is the extension of the pain into the inguinal area. Also, ligament pain is generally alleviated by the prone position with the knees slightly flexed. Since this ligament has stretched in the first pregnancy, it may not be as supportive with future pregnancies; the greater the number of pregnancies, the greater the amount of ligament discomfort. A supportive girdle, rest with a heating pad, and pelvic tilt exercises may help alleviate some of the discomfort.

Third Trimester (27–40 Weeks' Gestation)

Physical evaluations during prenatal revisits in the third trimester are essentially the same as in the second trimester, with few exceptions. Visits become weekly during the last month of the pregnancy. As the fetal presenting part lowers into the pelvis, measurement of the fundal height may be discrepant with the weeks' gestation. It also becomes essential in the third trimester to determine the presenting part. If the breech is in the pelvis, an external cephalic version may be done to turn the fetus into the more favorable vertex presentation. A version is done by manually turning the fetus from the breech to the vertex presentation under ultrasound guidance.

A pelvic examination may become part of the process during this time to evaluate vaginal lesions and to assess for sexually transmitted disease, ruptured membranes, or cervical dilation. Some practitioners routinely perform a digital examination every week during the last month of pregnancy to determine the early phases of cervical ripening or to aid in predicting the onset of labor. The Public Health Service Expert Panel on the Content of Prenatal Care recommends doing a digital cervical examination at the first visit and then again at 41 weeks to assess the cervix for induction of labor.

Physical and Emotional Changes

As the pregnancy advances and weight gain continues, the third trimester brings with it a greater level of discomfort as the pregnancy approaches full term. Round ligament pain may increase as a direct result of the strain placed on the supportive musculature. As the pregnancy utilizes more abdominal space, other common discomforts that may occur include shortness of breath, constipation, and fatigue. Toward the end of the third trimester, especially in the first pregnancy, there may be *lightening*, or the return of the fetal presenting part into the pelvis. Thus, there may be the resurgence of bladder pressure and urinary frequency experienced during the first trimester. Difficulty with sleeping may also occur and is directly related to the increasing discomfort and bladder pressure. The increasing level of discomfort has been associated with the process of "getting ready" for labor and birth. The woman's focus shifts to the process that is soon to begin and she may become hungry for more knowledge related to the inevitable experience. It is during this trimester that childbirth education usually begins.

Laboratory Studies

If a medical complication has developed, such as diabetes, pregnancy-induced hypertension, or blood dyscrasia, other laboratory follow-up studies may be indicated during the third trimester. In the essentially normal pregnancy, a routine Venereal Disease Research Laboratory test or rapid plasma reagin test for syphilis and complete blood count may be repeated. In some populations, cervical cultures for gonorrhea, chlamydia, and group B beta-hemolytic Streptococcus are performed.

Special Testing

If the pregnancy exceeds the estimated date of delivery by 10 to 14 days, fetal evaluation may be necessary. Perinatal morbidity and mortality increase with late pregnancies, so further information concerning fetal well-being is warranted. This testing may include the non-stress test (NST), the contraction stress test (CST), and the biophysical profile (BPP). Another method of assessing fetal well-being is by maternal assessment of fetal movement, known as *kick counts*. There are several types of kick counts, but generally, the woman is instructed to count fetal movements for 30 to 60 minutes each day, 2 or 3 times daily. If she counts less than three movements in an hour or less than 10 movements in 2 hours, this signals the "movement alarm system." The patient then contacts her health care provider and further fetal assessment is conducted, generally with the NST.

Nutrition and Maternal Weight Gain

Lack of consensus regarding recommendations for weight gain during pregnancy and vitamin-mineral supplementation during pregnancy led the Bureau of Maternal and Child Health Services to request that the National Academy of Sciences conduct a study of maternal nutrition. Thus, The Committee on Nutritional Status During Pregnancy and Lactation was formed and subcommittees were appointed to investigate specific issues and devise recommendations. The conclusions and recommendations that resulted were based on healthy women within the United States. Application of these results to women in less developed countries or women who have recently emigrated to the United States from these countries has not been evaluated.

Recommendations for maternal weight gain once were applied to all pregnant women regardless of height and preconception weight. In the 1970s, it was commonplace to restrict a woman's weight gain during pregnancy. However, during the 1980s an increase in gestational weight gain occurred as a result of an increase in the number of women receiving early prenatal care and the successful initiation of the Special Supplemental Food Program for Women, Infants, and Children. This upward trend in maternal weight gain occurred simultaneously with a decrease in infant mortality rates, an increase in average birth weights, and a decrease in low birth weights. However, there was no change in incidence of very low birth-weight infants. Due to this improvement in neonatal outcome, dietary recommendations have been reassessed.

The current recommendations for weight gain result from the investigations of the Subcommittee on Nutritional Status and Weight Gain During Pregnancy. The recommendations are based on the body mass index, which is defined as weight (kg) divided by height (cm) squared (Table 13-5). Women should be advised to gain enough weight to achieve at least the minimum noted in their weight-for-height category. The general recom-

Table 13-5. Classifying maternal prepregnancy weight-for-height status

Weight-for-height status	Body mass index (BMI) (kg/m^2)	1959 MLI (%)*
Very low	< 16.5	< 80
Low	16.5–19.7	80–90
Normal	19.8–26.0	91–120
High	> 26.0–29.0	121–135
Very high	> 29	> 135

*From Metropolitan Life Insurance Company (1959). Expressed as percent of desired body weight.

mendation is that women of normal prepregnancy weight-for-height with a single fetus gain between 11.5 and 16 kg (25–35 lb). This breaks down into approximately 0.4 kg (1 lb) per week in the second and third trimesters of pregnancy or 0.75 lb per week during the entire pregnancy. The target weight for obese or underweight patients must be assigned on an individual basis.

The Subcommittee on Dietary Intake and Nutrient Supplements During Pregnancy concluded that an evaluation of the pregnant woman's dietary pattern should be accomplished by using a food history or food frequency questionnaire. Protein intake is one area that needs to be assessed. Pregnant women should consume 10 g/day of protein over the recommended dietary allowance of 60 g/day, or a total of 70 g/day of protein. After the health care provider reviews the questionnaire, further specific information may be required concerning special problems or conditions that might affect dietary needs and the possible need for supplementation. The subcommittee also concluded that iron is the only known nutrient for which requirements cannot be met reasonably with diet alone. Supplements of 30 mg of ferrous iron daily are recommended during the second and third trimesters. Women should be advised that absorption of oral iron is best between meals or at bedtime on an empty stomach. Ascorbic acid does not enhance absorption of iron.

Recommendations for Supplementation of other Minerals and Vitamins

Calcium
Six-hundred mg daily of a calcium supplement should be added for women younger than 25 years of age if their daily dietary calcium intake is less than 600 mg. There is no evidence that older pregnant women have a special need for supplemental calcium intake. Increasing dietary calcium generally involves increasing the daily intake of dairy products. This increase

may be more of a challenge than in prior years because of the current emphasis on restricting fat intake to less than 30 percent of daily caloric intake. Most dairy products are comprised of a high percentage of fat. Another area of concern is with those women who have lactose intolerance and cannot ingest dairy products. Alternative sources of calcium must be found. Professional nutritional counselling may be indicated if diets cannot be easily altered.

Folate
Routine folate supplementation is not recommended. However, if inadequate dietary folate intake is suspected in the woman who does not ingest fruit, juices, whole-grain or fortified cereals, and green vegetables, then supplementation with 300 µg/day may be given.

Multivitamins
For women who are determined to have an inadequate diet and for women in high-risk categories, a daily multivitamin-mineral combination is recommended beginning in the second trimester. The recommended dosage can be found in Table 13-6.

Special Circumstances

Vitamin D
Vegans (vegetarians who consume no animal products at all), others with low intake of vitamin D–fortified milk, women in northern latitudes in the winter, and others with minimal exposure to sunlight (such as those who are hospitalized for extended periods of time) will need 10 µg (400 IU) of vitamin D daily.

Vitamin B_{12}
Vegans need 2.0 µg daily.

Table 13-6. Multivitamin and mineral supplements for pregnant women who do not ordinarily consume an adequate diet and for those in high-risk categories[a,b]

Iron	30 mg	Vitamin B_6	2 mg
Zinc	15 mg	Folate	300 µg
Copper	2 mg	Vitamin C	50 mg
Calcium	250 mg	Vitamin D	5 µg

[a]The supplements should be taken on an empty stomach between meals or at bedtime to promote absorption.
[b]From: Nutrition During Pregnancy. Institute of Medicine, National Academy of Sciences, 1990.

Zinc and Copper

If iron supplementation is being given to treat anemia, then approximately 15 mg of zinc and 2 mg of copper are needed because the iron may interfere with the absorption and utilization of those trace elements.

Exercise During Pregnancy

Within the last two decades, research into the safety of exercise during pregnancy has increased. The general advice that is given is that exercise routines performed prior to the pregnancy may be continued during the pregnancy with care taken not to exceed the resting maternal heart rate by 30 percent. If the maternal heart rate with exercise is less than or equal to 148 beats per minute, the FHR is unlikely to be effected. Pregnancy is not the appropriate time to begin a new form of strenuous exercise. The woman who has had a sedentary lifestyle may benefit from a closely monitored exercise class specifically designed for pregnant women or may enjoy long brisk walks. This decision should be discussed with her health care provider. If any deviation from normal exercise occurs during the pregnancy, the woman's level of exercise should be evaluated and discussed prior to her continuing.

Childbirth Education

Most women are very receptive to learning about their pregnancy. Although the ideal time to begin childbirth education is during preconception counselling, the vast majority of women present for health care after the pregnancy has been conceived. During the first trimester, an "early bird" class may be offered by the hospital education department or by an independent childbirth educator. The course content usually includes the "do's and don'ts" of pregnancy, basic exercises, nutrition, common discomforts, and an introduction into the expectations for the remaining months of pregnancy. Psychoprophylaxis in childbirth began in an effort to offer alternatives to analgesics for pain management during labor. Several methods of "breathing" were developed from the Bradley method to the Lamaze method. More recently, however, the childbirth education classes have evolved into a more eclectic approach with some educators teaching a combination of the breathing techniques plus discussing physical and emotional changes during pregnancy and preparation for labor and birth. The emphasis is on providing complete information to the couple about the process of pregnancy and birth so that they can then make educated decisions along with their health care provider. Cesarean birth is discussed as well as vaginal birth after cesarean section for the woman who has had a cesarean section in the past. Newborn care is generally included in most course curricula as well as infant cardiopulmonary resuscitation. Some courses include an exercise component.

Conclusion

The importance of prenatal care has been well established by both the scientific and political community. Only by accepting the challenge of providing access to prenatal care for all women and by constantly improving the scope of prenatal care can health care providers attain the goal of ensuring the best possible outcome for both the mother and fetus.

Recommended Reading

ACOG Committee Opinion. Fetal maturity assessment prior to elective repeat cesarean delivery. Number 98, 1991.

Cunningham F. G., MacDonald, P. C., Gant, N. F., Leveno, K. J., and Gilstrap, L. C. III. *Williams Obstetrics* (19th ed.). Norwalk: Appleton and Langer, 1993. Pp. 247–272.

Institute of Medicine. *Nutrition During Pregnancy.* Washington: National Academy Press, 1990.

Nagy, D. The content of prenatal care. *Obstet. Gynecol.* 74(3–2):516–528, 1989.

National Center for Health Statistics. *Monthly Vital Statistics Report.* 40(20): 9–11, 1992.

Public Health Service Expert Panel on the Content of Prenatal Care. *Caring for our Future: The Content of Prenatal Care.* Washington: Public Health Service, 1989.

Varney, H. *Nurse Midwifery.* Boston: Blackwell, 1990.

Prescribing During Pregnancy

Donald R. Coustan

Prior to the 1960s the placenta was widely viewed as a "barrier," protecting the fetus from compounds encountered by the mother. Thalidomide, a sedative widely prescribed in Europe and other parts of the world, was noted to be teratogenic in 1961. This prompted a shift in the prevailing view of the placenta to that of a "sieve," allowing all substances ingested by the mother to reach the fetus. Although neither view is entirely accurate, the latter is probably closer to the truth. This chapter shall discuss pharmacologic principles governing maternal-fetal drug interactions, outline some issues involved in decision making for prescribing medications during pregnancy, and then describe some of the more commonly needed drugs and the issues surrounding their use.

Principles of Pharmacology

The pregnant woman can best be considered using a "multicompartment system" model, with compartments consisting of the mother, placenta, and fetus. Pregnancy-related increases in maternal plasma volume, total body water, and adipose tissue may increase the volume of distribution for various drugs, and may lead to the need for higher doses to achieve therapeutic plasma levels. Changes in binding-protein levels, the pregnancy-related increase in renal plasma flow, and alterations in enterohepatic recirculation may affect maternal pharmacokinetics. The fetus may metabolize a particular drug via a different pathway from that of the mother. Alternatively, the drug or its metabolic product may be bound more avidly in the fetal compartment, either because of differences in protein binding or pH, with the fetus being marginally more acidemic than the mother. This may result in accumulation of the drug or its metabolite in the fetal compartment, as is the case with meperidine, an analgesic agent often used during labor, and its metabolic product normeperidine. Such accumulation in the fetus is often referred to as a "deep compartment" effect.

Not all agents cross the placenta with similar ease. Factors that predispose to transplacental passage include low molecular weight, high lipid solubility, preferential binding to fetal proteins, and relative absence of a highly ionic state. Heparin, for example, is large and highly charged, and thus crosses the placenta poorly if at all. Salicylates, however, are highly bound to albumin, which is in relatively high concentration in the fetal compartment; this results in higher fetal than maternal levels.

Assigning Teratogenicity

Physicians and patients are concerned about teratogenicity when a drug is prescribed during pregnancy. As discussed in Chapter 8, a teratogen is a compound that causes fetal structural malformations when administered during pregnancy. Since organogenesis occurs during the first trimester, it is believed that most teratogenic drugs exert their effects during early pregnancy. However, there are exceptions. For example, tetracycline can stain the fetal teeth only later in pregnancy, and warfarin anticoagulants may be associated with microcephaly and optic atrophy when administered in the second and third trimesters.

It is difficult to determine that a drug is teratogenic, and it is virtually impossible to determine with absolute certainty that a drug is unequivocally safe to prescribe during pregnancy. The reason for the difficulty is that one cannot ethically perform randomized toxicity trials, using untested drugs, in otherwise healthy human pregnancies. Therefore, new drugs are usually tested in pregnant animal species. Typically, rodents are used because of their rapid gestation and small size, which makes them convenient and inexpensive test models. Although there are many similarities between rodents and humans, and tentative conclusions are often drawn from rodent studies, great care must be exercised in making extrapolations to humans. The early testing of thalidomide in rodents failed to show teratogenicity. It was not until the drug was tested in larger animal species that the typical phocomelia or amelia observed in humans was noted.

Thalidomide embryopathy also demonstrates a number of other important principles. The timing of thalidomide exposure was critical. Only those human embryos exposed between approximately 3 and 6 weeks after conception were affected, with earlier exposure more likely to shorten the upper extremities and later exposure the lower extremities. No dose-response relationship could be established. Thalidomide proved to be one of the most potent known human teratogens, with approximately

20 percent of appropriately exposed pregnancies being affected. However, it was because the particular defects involved were quite unusual that thalidomide was rapidly identified as teratogenic. If thalidomide instead had caused one of the more common congenital cardiac defects, or perhaps a neural tube defect, it likely would have taken much longer for epidemiologic studies to reveal the association, with correspondingly greater numbers of infants affected.

There are a number of other potential pitfalls in assigning teratogenicity when the use of a drug is associated with a birth defect in case reports or even in case series. For example, a drug might be customarily prescribed for an illness that is "teratogenic," and thus be wrongly incriminated. Adrenal corticosteroids are commonly prescribed for autoimmune diseases such as systemic lupus erythematosus. It is now well known that the fetus of a mother with lupus is at particular risk for congenital heart block, particularly if the mother's serum contains the R_o antibody, which is suspected of attacking the conduction system of the fetal heart. If one were unaware of this association, the data might lead to the mistaken conclusion that maternal treatment with prednisone causes congenital heart block in the offspring.

A particular malformation might cause maternal symptoms that are then treated with a medication. When the baby is born, and the malformation becomes apparent, the drug may be blamed. For example, esophageal atresia interferes with the ingestion of amniotic fluid by the fetus, resulting in a condition known as *hydramnios,* an excessive amount of amniotic fluid. At one time, hydramnios was treated by administering diuretics to the mother in the hope of reducing the excess fluid. This treatment was not effective, but it is possible that diuretics might have been blamed for the esophageal atresia if attention were not paid to the timing of the formation of the esophagus, and the fact that the hydramnios was present before the diuretics were taken.

A third possibility could be that a drug inhibits the spontaneous abortion of an already malformed fetus. It is now clear that the majority of first trimester spontaneous abortions are associated with major structural malformations or karyotypic abnormalities. The so-called blighted ovum, in which no formed fetus is present, is the most extreme manifestation. At one time progestational agents were used to prevent spontaneous abortion in patients with a history of repeated miscarriages or with bleeding in the present pregnancy. It is now clear that such treatment is totally ineffective except in the rare situation of *inadequate luteal phase,* in which the corpus luteum fails to provide adequate progesterone production in the first 8 to 10 weeks of pregnancy to support the growing conceptus. Had progesterone compounds been effective in preventing abortion, there likely would have been an epidemic of malformed babies, and the progestational drugs might have been assumed to be teratogenic. Diethylstilbestrol (DES), a synthetic estrogen compound once used to prevent spontaneous abortion, is not a good example to use for this hypothetical phenomenon because it was truly teratogenic. In fact, the biggest tragedy of DES is probably not the fact that it caused clear-cell carcinoma in approximately 1 in a 1000 exposed offspring, but rather that it was totally ineffective in preventing abortion. If it had been effective, we might take some solace in knowing that the children would not have been born had their mothers not received this drug, and we could balance the risk of vaginal carcinoma against the benefit of preserving human lives. Unfortunately, DES was all risk and no benefit.

If a particular drug is often prescribed in combination with another drug which is truly teratogenic, the wrong drug might be blamed for causing the birth defects. Alternatively, there might be common risk factors for the use of a drug and the occurrence of congenital anomalies. For example, karyotypic abnormalities such as trisomy 21 are known to occur with increasing frequency as maternal age advances. Since most infertility specialists advise couples to attempt conception for a minimal interval, often 1 year, before evaluation and treatment are initiated, couples undergoing infertility treatment are likely to be, on average, older than those who conceive spontaneously. Thus, if corrections are not made for maternal age, it could be easily demonstrated that ovulation-inducing agents such as clomiphene citrate or gonadotropins are associated with an increased incidence of Down syndrome.

Finally, the very design of studies evaluating the effects of drug use in pregnancy can lead to false conclusions. When a large survey is conducted to correlate maternal medication use with birth defects in a population, one would expect that, by chance alone, one of every 20 medications included will show a statistically significant correlation with one or more congenital anomalies at the 0.05 significance level. This prediction is inherent in the use of statistics; the 0.05 level means that there is a 5 percent chance that this correlation could be spurious. When one asks a single question of the data set, finding a "yes" answer at the 0.05 level is highly meaningful. However, when one asks 20 questions, it is expected that at least one will be answered "yes" even though no association exists. The more questions asked, or associations looked for, the greater the likelihood of a spurious association emerging as significant. For this reason, such large open-ended studies should be considered useful only for generating hypotheses. When associations are found, they should serve only to direct future studies in other populations, in which limited numbers of questions are asked and issues of multiple comparisons are thus avoided. An example of the hypothesis-generating type of large population-based study is the Collaborative Perinatal Project of the National Institute of Neurological and Communicative Disorders and Stroke, a multicentered observational study involving 12 institutions and more than 50,000 pregnancies during the early 1960s. Several hundred drugs were reported to have been ingested by the mothers. Birth defects were evaluated blindly with respect to drug ingestion, and several hundred relative risk calculations were made. Heinonen, Slone, and Shapiro, the authors of the book that emerged from this study, were careful to point out the limitations of the study design, and the first few chapters of the book contain a lucid description of the problems inherent in such studies. For this reason the book is included in the reading list at the end of this chapter.

Another potential problem with study design is the difficulty of establishing true exposure to a drug when exploring prescription records. One study linked spermicide procurement during the 10 months prior to conception with a number of birth defects in the offspring, but when other investigators studied other populations no such association was found. Unfortunately, publication of the initial study led to a rather large award to the parents of an exposed and malformed baby, despite the Food and Drug Administration's (FDA) finding that spermicides were not teratogenic, and despite the multitude of evidence to the contrary. This event led to the appearance of the term "litogen," which was defined in the *New England Journal of Medicine* as "a drug that does not cause malformations but does cause lawsuits. . . ."

Another famous "litogen" story involves the formulation with the trade name Bendectine. This was a combination of doxylamine (an antihistamine) and vitamin B6 (pyridoxine). It also contained dicyclomine (an antimuscarinic) prior to 1976, but this was removed because it did not enhance efficacy. Bendectine was approved by the FDA for the treatment of nausea and vomiting of pregnancy and was, in fact, the only such approved drug. A 1979 study designed to explore the relationship between hormonal agents and congenital cardiac defects incidentally noted that mothers of babies with heart defects reported taking Bendectine almost twice as often as did mothers of normal babies. This phenomenon may well be an example of "recall bias," the phenomenon by which mothers of adversely affected offspring are more likely to report drug use than are mothers of normal offspring, presumably because the former mothers have searched their memories for explanations of the bad outcome. Despite the fact that more than 14 subsequent studies found no association between Bendectine use in pregnancy and congenital malformations, many lawsuits were filed against the manufacturer. This may be understandable, since approximately 3 percent of the general population give birth to infants with malformations (presumably by chance alone), and approximately 20 percent of pregnant women used Bendectine during the 1970s. Thus, even though Bendectine is not teratogenic, there are many children with birth defects whose mothers happened to have taken the drug. Although the overwhelming majority of cases were won by the manufacturer of the drug, Bendectine was voluntarily removed from the market in 1983 because of the tremendous costs of defending the suits. Consequently, there is no approved, safe, and effective drug currently available to treat nausea and vomiting in pregnancy.

Counselling

Although it would seem safest to recommend that pregnant women take no medications at all, thus eliminating any possible risk, this advice is neither practical nor always appropriate. Pregnant women, like any individuals, may have chronic or acute conditions that require treatment for survival, or for improved quality of life. Decision making requires a careful balancing of risks and benefits. It is clearly impossible to provide absolute assurance that a perfect pregnancy outcome will occur, given the background risk for birth defects of approximately 3 percent in the general population. None of the medications that may be prescribed (perhaps with the exception of insulin in the case of a diabetic woman planning pregnancy) is known to prevent congenital anomalies, so patients taking medications must contend with at least the background risk. Counselling is an important function of every health care provider, and should be individualized depending on the question being asked.

When counselling a couple with an anomalous child, the physician is likely to be asked "Did a drug that I took cause this baby's problem?" It is important to remember the stages of grieving, particularly the fact that anger and guilt invariably occur. It will not help a grieving couple to be told, simply, "Don't worry about it." The question must be taken seriously. The name of the medication and the time of its administration should be ascertained. If the drug is not known to be teratogenic, or the time of administration is remote from the time of occurrence of the anomaly, this information should be conveyed to the parents in an understandable fashion. It may be necessary to repeat the information on a number of occasions, since grieving parents may not remember things explained to them during the early stages of grief. If the counsellor is not certain as to the possibility of a causal relationship, it is best to explain to the couple that more information is necessary before an answer can be provided. A number of references are available, and many are listed at the end of this chapter. One very helpful resource is an on-line data base called Reprotox, which provides up-to-date information on a variety of medications. The parents should be given whatever information is available as soon as is practical in order to help them in their grieving process. Since considerably less than 5 percent of structural abnormalities are known to be caused by teratogenic medications, in most cases the answers provided will help to alleviate any sense of guilt.

A second type of question typically comes from a pregnant woman who has taken a particular medication before she knew that she was pregnant. "What should I do now?" means either "Should I have an abortion?" or "Can you give me any reassurance?" As with the previous question, counselling should start with a description of the population risk for birth defects of approximately 3 percent. Information should be obtained and conveyed as to any known risks associated with the agent in question. Counselling should be nondirective. Even with thalidomide, which was one of the most powerful known teratogens, the risk was in the range of 20 percent, so 80 percent of the time appropriately exposed fetuses were unaffected. Although many would opt for termination of pregnancy with such a risk, others would not and the decision must be considered to be a personal one. Fortunately, for most medications the known risks, if any, are not nearly as high as those posed by thalidomide, and the counselling is usually perceived as reassuring. The list included in Chapter 8 contains the names of fewer than a dozen medications and drugs known to be teratogenic. Of course, it must be made clear to the patient how difficult it is to be certain that a drug is entirely safe. It is also useful to point out that an unknown risk as high as 1 percent would probably be unrecognizable against the background population risk. Nevertheless, a couple facing the background risk of 3 percent does not usually opt to terminate the pregnancy; would it make sense to do so when the increase in risk is to 4 percent? While it is easy to advise pregnant women not to use medications, this is not the equivalent of recommending extreme measures when they do so.

The third type of question is usually the most straightforward, and typically comes from a physician. When confronted with a clinical situation, the question asked is "Which drug should I prescribe?" The counsellor should go to the literature, determine which drugs are most effective with the least risk, and provide the answer. Again, however, it is important that the patient be told of any known or suspected risks, and also of the background risk and the fact that no one can be guaranteed a perfect baby.

Specific Medications
The remainder of this chapter is devoted to describing selected commonly used or clinically important medications, and their specific effects on the pregnant mother, fetus, and newborn. Space limitations do not permit a thorough consideration of each drug that might be encountered, so the reader is referred to various standard reference works listed at the end of the chapter for other compounds or more detailed information regarding those that are discussed.

Salicylates
Aspirin is regarded by many patients as something other than a drug. It is available without a prescription in supermarkets, airports, and hotels, and is contained in many nonprescription combination products. Estimates of its use among pregnant women vary from as low as 10 percent to as high as 80 percent, with the lower figures generally coming from more recent studies. Evidence accumulated as of this writing does not support a teratogenic role for aspirin. However, aspirin can prolong hemostasis in the mother and the fetus, if taken in doses as low as 5 to 10 grains (325–650 mg) within 5 days prior to delivery. Intracranial hemorrhage has been reported to occur with greater frequency among preterm neonates whose mothers ingested such doses of aspirin within 1 week of delivery. These effects on

maternal and fetal hemostasis are believed to be due to inhibition of cyclooxygenase, which is responsible for the production of thromboxane, which activates platelets. Other effects reported, but not clearly established, with aspirin taken at the usual adult doses include prolongation of labor, prolongation of pregnancy, and premature closure of the fetal ductus arteriosus. All of these putative effects are presumably related to inhibition of prostaglandin synthesis. For these reasons pregnant women are usually advised to avoid taking adult doses of aspirin, even in the first and second trimesters prior to potential neonatal viability, since maternal bleeding might be increased by salicylates. However, the concept of risk and benefit must be taken into consideration. For example, a patient with rheumatoid arthritis whose existence may be utterly miserable without chronic ingestion of large doses of salicylates should be informed of the potential risks, but may opt to continue her treatment, given her perception that the likelihood of a preterm birth is statistically low enough to make the benefit outweigh the risk. Switching to nonsteroidal anti-inflammatory agents, about which much less is known, may not be a reassuring alternative. Drugs such as acetaminophen may not be acceptable because they do not have the anti-inflammatory effects of aspirin, and so are unlikely to be effective.

As of this writing, there is a good deal of interest in the use of low-dose aspirin (approximately 65 mg/day) as a means to lower the likelihood of preeclampsia and possibly intrauterine growth retardation. The proposed mechanism is, again, reduction of thromboxane production with lowering of the ratio of thromboxane A_2 to prostacyclin, which in turn is believed to favor vasodilation over vasoconstriction. At this low dose there appears to be no measurable effect on maternal or fetal coagulation. Initially, randomized studies suggested benefit in high-risk populations such as those with chronic hypertension, or a history of severe hypertensive complications in one or more previous pregnancies. Subsequent randomized trials of lower-risk populations, such as nulliparous women, also demonstrated slight reduction of preeclampsia, but one study suggested an increased risk of placental abruption. Currently many obstetricians prescribe low-dose aspirin for high-risk gravidas, but benefits of this potential prophylaxis against preeclampsia in the general population are not yet established.

Acetaminophen

Acetaminophen has not been shown to be teratogenic. One study found that acetaminophen ingestion was associated with decreased urinary prostacyclin excretion in pregnant women, but clinical data presently available do not suggest an adverse effect on maternal or fetal coagulation. Although in one study daily usage has been implicated as a cause of chronic renal disease, acetaminophen is considered the analgesic and antipyretic of choice during pregnancy, should such an agent be needed.

Narcotic Analgesics

Narcotic analgesic medications can be addicting to mother and fetus, and neonatal withdrawal has been reported after chronic maternal ingestion. However, the need for short-term narcotic analgesia arises with some frequency in medical settings and such drugs should not be withheld arbitrarily. All narcotic analgesics cross the placenta, and neonatal respiratory depression is a concern. Morphine, the prototypic narcotic, is rarely used during labor because of a widespread clinical impression (not proven) of greater neonatal depression than is seen with other narcotics. Meperidine, which is one of the most popular narcotics administered during labor, is metabolized to normeperidine in the fetus, and this derivative tends to accumulate in the fetal circulation. This accumulation may be responsible for respiratory depression and lower psychophysiologic test scores in neonates exposed during labor. Clearly one would not want to administer such a drug needlessly. However, primate studies have demonstrated that even mild maternal pain and anxiety are associated with decreased uterine perfusion, so that a patient whose labor is causing her distress may derive greater benefit than risk from narcotic analgesia.

Anticoagulants

Anticoagulation may be necessary during pregnancy to treat deep vein thrombosis, for prophylaxis in patients with artificial heart valves, or as treatment in women with antiphospholipid antibodies. Warfarin derivatives, such as coumarin, cross the placenta readily and have been associated with cases of fatal fetal hemorrhage in all trimesters. In addition, a fetal warfarin syndrome has been described. With first-trimester exposure, nasal hypoplasia and chondrodysplasia puctata (a stippled radiologic appearance of bones) are found in an estimated 5 percent of cases. Exposure in the second and third trimester has been associated with microcephaly, optic atrophy, and mental retardation. Although some authorities recommend using warfarin compounds during midpregnancy only, many suggest that the use of warfarins be avoided altogether in pregnant women. Heparin, the other available form of anticoagulation, is a large and highly charged molecule that does not cross the placenta to any appreciable extent, and thus has no direct fetal risks. For the same reason, it must be administered parenterally. Maternal risks include hemorrhage when coagulation times become more prolonged than is desirable, and the possibility of osteoporosis with long-term use. Nevertheless, heparin is considered to be the anticoagulant of choice during pregnancy.

Anticonvulsants

A number of medications such as phenytoin, valproic acid, and trimethadione, which are used to treat various forms of epilepsy, have been associated with specific types of congenital anomalies. Pregnant women with epilepsy often require these agents in order to be seizure-free, and hypoxia associated with grand mal seizures may pose a greater threat to mother and fetus than does the drug treatment. Thus, informed decisions must be made jointly by patients and caregivers.

Alcohol

Fetal alcohol syndrome, which consists of growth retardation, a pattern of abnormal features of the face and head, and evidence of central nervous system abnormality, is seen in between 2.5 and 10 percent of "heavy drinkers." *Heavy drinking* is variously defined, but most definitions include chronic, daily drinking of at least 3 oz of absolute alcohol (6 mixed drinks, cans of beer, or glasses of wine) per day. A dose-response relationship probably exists, with parts of the full-blown syndrome (called *fetal alcohol effects*) seen with lower rates of alcohol consumption. Since alcohol has no apparent therapeutic benefit for pregnant women, it is best to advise abstention. However, no adverse effects have been demonstrated for a single episode of alcohol consumption. Women who seek advice regarding a previous "binge" should not be counselled toward drastic responses such as termination of pregnancy.

Vitamins

Multiple vitamin preparations have traditionally been prescribed for pregnant women. Little evidence exists to support this practice, with the exception of folic acid. A number of controlled trials have demonstrated that daily supplementation of maternal folic acid intake, in various doses, during the month prior to conception and throughout the first trimester, can substantially reduce the likelihood of neural tube defects (anencephaly and spina bifida) in the offspring. Such regimens are effective in mothers with previously affected children, and also in the general population. In 1993 the Centers for Disease Control recommended that all women of childbearing age who are capable of becoming pregnant consume 0.4 mg of folic acid per day in order to reduce their risk of having an affected baby. It was suggested that women not ingest more than 1 mg per day because of the potential for masking vitamin B_{12} deficiency, and the possibility of other, as yet unknown, risks.

In general, the use of excessive amounts of water-soluble vitamins has not been associated with specific adverse effects in pregnancy, presumably because these substances are efficiently cleared by the kidneys. Fat-soluble vitamins, which can be stored in maternal adipose tissue and released over time, appear to pose considerable risks when taken in excess. For example, a syndrome of subaortic stenosis and craniofacial anomalies has been described in humans and animal models exposed to large amounts of vitamin D in utero. For this reason, it is recommended that pregnant women take no more than the usual 400 IU of vitamin D per day. Isotretinoin, a vitamin-A derivative used to treat chronic cystic acne, is one of the most powerful teratogens known, with severe facial and ear anomalies resulting from its use. Excessive use of vitamin A (retinol) has not been conclusively linked to adverse effects in human pregnancies, but a number of animal studies and indirect human evidence suggest a possible association with urogenital abnormalities and central nervous system defects.

Aspartame

Aspartame is a nonnutritive sweetener composed of the amino acids phenylalanine and aspartic acid. Because individuals with an inborn metabolic error, phenylketonuria (PKU), are unable to metabolize phenylalanine, and high maternal levels of phenylalanine are toxic to the developing fetus, there was some initial concern that aspartame might be harmful when used during pregnancy. The FDA has set a toxic threshold for phenylalanine of 100 µM/dl in adults. Because amino acids are actively transported across the placenta, a level of 50 µM/dl was set for pregnant women. In order to reach that level, the average 60-kg woman would have to consume 24 liters of aspartame-sweetened beverage at one sitting, a dose that is highly unlikely. Mothers with PKU should avoid aspartame during pregnancy, and they should avoid all food containing phenylalanine. If an individual consumed aspartame in greater amounts than did 99 percent of the population, her overall daily phenylalanine intake would increase by only 6 percent. The FDA considers aspartame safe to use during pregnancy.

Recommended Reading

Aranda, J. V., Hales, B. F., and Reider, M. F. Developmental Pharmacology. In A. A. Fanaroff and R. J. Martin (eds.), *Neonatal-Perinatal Medicine* (5th ed.). St. Louis: Mosby Year Book, 1992. Pp. 123–146.

Berkowitz, R. L., Coustan, D. R., and Mochizuki, T. K. *Handbook for Prescribing Medications During Pregnancy* (2nd ed.). Boston: Little, Brown, 1986.

Berlin, C. M., Jr. Pharmacologic considerations of drug use in the lactating mother. *Obst. Gynecol.* 58 (Suppl):17S–23S, 1981.

Briggs, G. G., Freeman, R. K., and Yaffe, S. J. *Drugs in Pregnancy and Lactation* (4th ed.). Baltimore: Williams & Wilkins, 1994.

Centers for Disease Control. Recommendations for use of folic acid to reduce number of spina bifida cases and other neural tube defects. *J.A.M.A.* 269:1233–1238, 1993.

Coustan, D. R. Nonprescription drugs and alcohol: Abuse and effects in pregnancy. In E. A. Reece, et al. (eds.), *Medicine of the Fetus and Mother.* Philadelphia: Lippincott, 1992. Pp. 317–327.

Heinonen, O. P., Slone, D., and Shapiro, S. *Birth Defects and Drugs in Pregnancy.* Boston: John Wright PSG, 1977.

Levy, G. Pharmacokinetics of fetal and neonatal exposure to drugs. *Obstet. Gynecol.* 58 (Suppl):9S–16S, 1981.

Mills, J. L., and Alexander, D. Occasional noted: Teratogens and "litogens." *N. Engl. J. Med.* 315:1234–1236, 1986.

The Fetus as Patient: Prenatal Diagnosis and Treatment

Patricia A. O'Shea

In the latter half of the twentieth century, enormous transformations have occurred in reproductive medicine brought about by a constellation of socioeconomic changes, basic science advances, and application of a host of new technologies to the study of the developing fetus. For the first time, we have the capability to observe the developing fetus closely, to study his or her genetic makeup, physiology, metabolism, and morphogenesis, and increasingly, to intervene to change the course of prenatal development.

Changes in economic forces, the demographic restructuring of the work force and family, concern for the consequences of overpopulation, and the availability of effective and safe contraception have led to smaller families and increased concern for the outcome of each desired pregnancy. That direct study of the human fetus was both feasible and productive was demonstrated in 1955, when Riis and Fuchs, working in Copenhagen, showed that the sex of a fetus could be determined by study of the cells found floating in the amniotic fluid. These cells are fetal in origin, derived from the amnion, and therefore contain a full complement of fetal DNA and express many (but not all) fetal antigens and metabolic pathways. Riis and Fuchs also were able to determine fetal ABO groups, because ABO antigens are expressed on amniocytes. Although fetal sex determination and blood grouping appear by modern standards to be relatively simple tests, their success led these investigators to predict that many genetic and metabolic diseases might be identified prior to birth by examination of the amniotic fluid and cells. Rapid advances in biochemistry, cytogenetics, molecular genetics, and ultrasonography have made evaluation of fetal well-being both feasible and relatively safe. Thus, prevention, early diagnosis, and therapeutic intervention on behalf of the fetus are now realities.

The current polemic centering on the legality and availability of abortion serves to focus attention, particularly in the lay press, on the role of prenatal diagnosis in detecting fetuses with abnormalities that cause debilitating conditions, mental retardation, and early death, so that these pregnancies can be terminated. Of equal importance is the role of prenatal diagnosis in identifying fetuses who can benefit from dietary or pharmacologic manipulation, preterm delivery, or potentially from intrauterine surgical intervention. Finally, the availability of safe and accurate prenatal diagnosis means that reassurance is possible for couples known to be at risk for genetic or metabolic disease and for older women who might otherwise choose not to undertake pregnancy at all.

Many techniques are available for assessing the well-being of the fetus in utero; second-trimester amniocentesis for detection of metabolic diseases like Tay-Sachs disease and for detection of trisomy associated with advanced maternal age formed the largest early experience with prenatal diagnosis. In the past decade, however, emphasis has shifted to earlier first-trimester diagnosis, to early detection of structural defects made possible by high-resolution ultrasonography, and to the direct and detailed study of ever smaller portions of the genome made possible by increasingly sophisticated molecular genetic techniques.

In the antepartum period, noninvasive diagnostic modalities include imaging studies (ultrasound, fetal echocardiography), chemical determinations performed on maternal serum, and measurements of the fetal physiology and fetal response to stress. Invasive methods include amniocentesis, chorionic villus sampling (CVS), percutaneous umbilical blood sampling (PUBS), and direct visualization of the embryo or fetus (embryoscopy or fetoscopy) for purposes of structural diagnosis, biopsy of fetal tissues, or therapeutic intervention.

Imaging Studies: Looking at the Fetus

Prior to the development of obstetric ultrasound, diagnostic imaging of the fetus was limited by the risk posed by exposure of the fetus to ionizing radiation. Pelvic x-ray films provided only relatively crude estimates of fetal skeletal development and feto-pelvic size relationships, and that at the price of exposure of the fetus to rather high doses of radiation. Invasive techniques, like amniography, added little useful information with the further risk of introducing foreign bodies and contrast media into the amniotic fluid. The diffusion of CT scans greatly increases image quality, but some radiation risk is still present. Magnetic resonance imaging produces images of exquisite clarity and detail without any currently recognized risk to the patient, but its potential for routine use in pregnancy has thus far been limited by tremendous expense and also by artifacts resulting from fetal movement. Additionally, the effects of a strong magnetic field on fetal development are largely unknown. Few would contest that the application of improved ultrasonographic imaging to obstetrics has wrought a revolutionary change in obstetric practice, or that recent technologic advances in digital technology, Doppler analysis, and color flow mapping portend even greater changes. Fetal ultrasound examination can be performed at low cost in a reasonable period of time in an office or clinic setting. The equipment is not prohibitively expensive and there is no risk to fetus or mother, so repeated examinations are feasible.

Diagnostic ultrasound takes advantage of the observation that sound travels at variable velocity depending on the molecular density of the medium in which it is propagated. Gases, including air, are poor conductors of sound waves; liquids are better, and dense substances like metal and bone are best. When sound waves traveling through one medium encounter another of different density, some of them are reflected. This phenomenon is called an *acoustic interface,* and the reflected sound waves are echoes. The human ear can hear sounds and echoes in the 20 to 20,000 Hz frequency range. The frequency of the sound waves used in diagnostic ultrasound is from 1 to 20 million Hz, or 1 to 20 MHz. This very high-frequency sound is produced by a transducer that converts electrical energy to sound energy (waves), directed at the area to be examined. When the waves meet an acoustic interface (between amniotic fluid and fetal skull, for instance) some waves are reflected back to the transducer where they are converted back to electrical energy and displayed on a monitor. The denser the structure reflecting the echo, the louder it will be; in so-called B-mode (brightness) sonography, the reflected sound wave is displayed as a spot on the screen with a brightness that is proportional to the amplitude (loudness) of the echo. By moving the transducer, one can build up a two-dimensional image of the acoustic interface. In real-time sonography, multiple images are created and compounded so rapidly that the fetus appears to be moving. As with other imaging methods, the resolution of fine structural detail is inversely proportional to the wavelength of the energy, in this case sound. High-frequency sound waves therefore give clearer images; tissue penetration, however, is better at lower frequencies, so a compromise must be made for imaging deep structures.

Doppler ultrasound is a modification based on the Doppler principle: sound waves are "compressed" to higher frequency when the echogenic interface is moving toward the transducer and "stretched" to lower frequencies when the interface is going away from the transducer. By using two transducers (one to emit and one to record) one can detect the direction and amplitude of motion of a target by recording the changes in frequency of the echo. Fetal heart rate and umbilical blood flow velocity are measured with this technique. Doppler ultrasound measures changes in frequency of *sound* waves; by displaying this sound energy as light energy of proportional wavelength (color), and combining Doppler measurements with real-time ultrasound, one can compound a colored image that in effect uses the Doppler data as "contrast media" for the two-dimensional ultrasound image.

An ultrasound imaging study can be a basic general physical examination of the fetus or a targeted in-depth examination of a particular feature or system. The basic ultrasound examination is appropriate for most routine or uncomplicated pregnancies and will detect most significant anomalies. Such an examination should include determination of fetal number, size, and viability, determination of gestational age and amniotic fluid volume, and location of the placenta. Anatomy of all major organ systems can be examined, and, if abnormalities are identified, more detailed targeted imaging or other confirmatory diagnostic studies like amniocentesis, CVS, or PUBS can be done. These detailed studies should be performed in a center where there is experience and expertise in the detection, diagnosis, and treatment of congenital disorders and where facilities and personnel for genetic counselling and parental support are available.

The types of structural defects detectable by ultrasound, and some examples, are listed in Table 15-1 and Fig. 15-1. The identification of any anomaly should lead to detailed targeted study by an experienced ultrasonographer for associated anomalies which, though they may be subtle, may permit a definitive diagnosis. Duodenal atresia, for example, is a common form of congenital bowel obstruction, amenable to surgical correc-

Table 15-1. Ultrasound diagnosis of structural anomalies

Absence of a structure normally present
  Anencephaly
  Acardia
  Limb reduction defects
Fetal masses not normally present
  Teratoma
  Polycystic renal disease
  Cystic hygroma
  Congenital neuroblastoma
  Encephalocele, meningomyelocele
Abnormal surface contours
  Facial clefts
  Hyper- or hypotelorism
  Gastroschisis
Herniation
  Diaphragmatic hernia
  Omphalocele

(Continued)

Table 15-1   *(Continued)*

Obstruction or dilatation
  Intestinal atresia
  Hydrocephalus
  Urinary tract obstruction
Disproportionate growth
  Intrauterine growth retardation
  Skeletal dysplasias
  Microcephaly
Abnormalities of fetal motion
  Congenital myopathies
  Arthrogryposis

tion. About one-third of cases occur in Down syndrome; other features of Down syndrome demonstrable on ultrasound include increased nuchal skin fold, shortened femur, clinodactyly, hypotonia, and various cardiac malformations including septal defects. Parental counselling and management of the pregnancy would clearly be influenced by the finding of these associated anomalies.

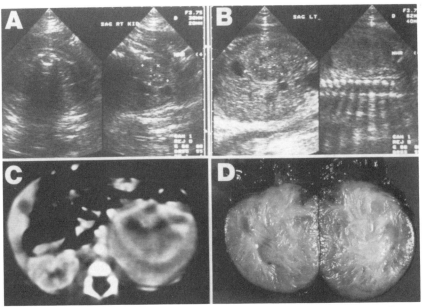

Fig. 15-1.   An abdominal mass discovered on routine prenatal ultrasound. Panels A and B are sagittal images of a normal right *(A)* and enlarged left *(B)* kidney. The infant was delivered uneventfully at term and a large left renal mass was confirmed on CT scan *(C)* and removed shortly after birth. Panel D shows the cut section of the benign congenital renal tumor, a congenital mesoblastic nephroma.

As of this writing, most antenatal ultrasound diagnosis has been carried out via transabdominal ultrasound in the second trimester. Recent advances in transvaginal probes have resulted in enhanced resolution of very small structures and now permit evaluation of first- and early second-trimester fetuses. The detailed images obtained can be used to compare developmental milestones of the embryo and early fetus with well-established normals, thus permitting accurate determinations of gestational age and earlier diagnosis of anomalies. Many major anomalies (anencephaly, spina bifida, and many renal anomalies) may be accurately identified in the first trimester. For those patients who choose to terminate the pregnancy, first-trimester abortion is both safer and less costly than second-trimester abortion.

Maternal Biochemical Determinations as a Reflection of Fetal Physiology

The placenta functions as both a barrier and a route of exchange between mother and fetus, and it is therefore reasonable to expect that fetal metabolic events will be reflected at least in part in maternal biochemical determinations. The possibility of applying this concept for prenatal diagnosis first emerged in 1972, when Brook and Sutcliffe reported that mothers of fetuses with open neural tube defects (spina bifida, meningomyelocele, and anencephaly) had elevated serum values of a protein known to be produced by the fetus. Alpha fetoprotein (AFP) is a glycoprotein of MW 70,000 produced by the fetal liver and yolk sac and secreted into the fetal blood. It constitutes the major fetal serum protein during the second trimester, reaching peak fetal blood levels at 13 weeks of gestation and declining thereafter toward term. Under normal circumstances, AFP reaches the amniotic fluid via the fetal urine and crosses the placenta to enter maternal blood. Maternal serum levels rise gradually with increasing gestational age (Fig. 15-2). In situations of increased fetal proteinuria, of abnormal transudation of protein into the amniotic fluid, or of abnormal communications between fetal intravascular space and amniotic cavity or maternal circulation, the maternal serum AFP (MSAFP) is elevated (Table 15-2). MSAFP may also be elevated, for reasons that are not at the present time clear, in pregnancies destined to be complicated by intrauterine growth retardation or unexplained fetal death.

Because the normal range of MSAFP varies with gestational age (see Fig. 15-2), MSAFP levels are uninterpretable without accurate dating of the gestation. In addition to gestational age, normal values must be corrected for maternal age, race, and presence of diabetes. The test is reported in multiples of the median (MOM) for a given gestational age, and the appropriate first response to abnormal levels (more than 2.5 MOM) should always be to check the gestational age. If the dates are accurate and a second determination is abnormal, the next step is either a careful ultrasonographic

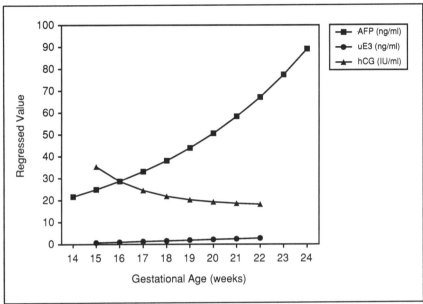

Fig. 15-2. Variation in alpha fetoprotein (AFP), estriol (uE3), and human chorionic gonadotropin (hCG) with advancing gestational age. Using these three maternal serum biochemical measurements and maternal age, it is possible to predict a specific risk of Down syndrome for each pregnancy. This permits selection of high-risk pregnancies for amniocentesis and cytogenetic confirmation, and minimizes the number of amniocenteses done in women at low risk. (Data provided by Dr. Jacob Canick, Prenatal AFP Laboratory, Women and Infants Hospital of Rhode Island. These normal values are continually revised as the laboratory's experience increases.)

Table 15-2.   Conditions associated with elevated maternal serum alpha fetoprotein

Multiple gestation
Open neural tube defects
Congenital nephrotic syndrome
Bladder neck obstruction
Upper gastrointestinal atresia
Omphalocele
Gastroschisis
Sacrococcygeal teratoma
Pilonidal sinus
Turner syndrome (monosomy X)
Fetal death
Fetal hemorrhage into amniotic fluid
Fetomaternal hemorrhage
Fetal growth retardation

examination or amniocentesis. If the elevated MSAFP remains unexplained (e.g., by fetal death, twins, incorrect gestational age, or definite anomaly), amniocentesis for measurement of amniotic fluid AFP is usually offered. Recent studies have suggested that improvements in the accuracy of ultrasound diagnosis may make it possible to detect neural tube and ventral wall defects with high sensitivity, thus possibly alleviating the need for amniocentesis in the presence of a normal ultrasound examination.

As experience accrued with MSAFP, it became apparent that patients with values at the low end of the normal distribution have an increased risk of fetal Down syndrome. These women have been offered amniocentesis for karyotyping. Only about 1 in 40 women with low MSAFP (after ultrasound elimination of those with inaccurate dating of the gestation) is found to have a chromosomally abnormal fetus, and the use of AFP alone identifies only about 20 percent of cases of Down syndrome. The accuracy of risk assessment can be greatly improved by using three maternal serum markers: AFP, human chorionic gonadotropin (hCG), and estriol (see Fig. 15-2). In normal pregnancies, estriol levels increase with increasing gestational age, while hCG levels decline. Measurements of these three serum markers, together with maternal age, enable the determination of a specific risk of Down syndrome for each pregnancy. It is now possible to detect over 60 percent of fetuses with Down syndrome with this approach, and the false-positive rate is an acceptable 5 percent. This means that there is now a safe, low-cost, sensitive, accurate way to detect Down syndrome in mothers younger than 35 years old who bear 80 percent of Down syndrome fetuses, and to reduce the number of mothers in the over-35 group who require amniocentesis because of their increased risk of nondisjunction.

It should be apparent from the above considerations that there is more to using MSAFP for prenatal diagnosis than buying a test kit. Performance of the test requires rigorous quality control, accurate dating of gestation, availability of ultrasound and cytogenetic diagnostic expertise, and genetic counselling resources to assist patients to understand the data so that they are able to make informed choices. The main drawback of MSAFP testing at the present time is that it has been done only in the second trimester, and results are not available before 17 weeks' gestation. Earlier diagnosis and termination, if elected, would be desirable for both psychologic and safety reasons.

Amniocentesis

Following the pioneer work of Riis and Fuchs, it rapidly became clear that many fetal pathophysiologic states are reflected by changes in the biochemical makeup of the amniotic fluid and that amniocytes could serve as representative samples of fetal genetic and metabolic events. Second-trimester amniocentesis has now been in clinical use for over 25 years, and has become the standard against which newer procedures are evaluated. The technique is relatively simple: the placenta is localized (and avoided) with ultrasound examination; a needle is inserted transabdominally into the amniotic sac, avoiding the fetus; and a 20-cc sample of fluid is aspirated (Fig. 15-3). The procedure is usually carried out at 16 to 17 weeks after the last menstrual period. The fluid may be subjected to a number of tests, depending on the clinical question posed. Earliest applications involved the use of amniotic fluid bilirubin levels to follow the course of hemolytic

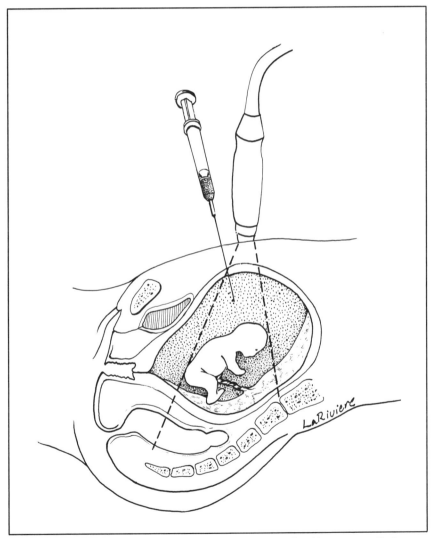

Fig. 15-3.   Technique for amniocentesis. Under ultrasound guidance, a needle is inserted into the amniotic sac. The fetus and placenta are avoided, and about 30 ml of amniotic fluid is withdrawn.

disease, usually Rh incompatibility. Amniotic fluid lecithin-sphingomyelin ratio and phosphatidyl glycerol levels are used to assess fetal lung maturity in situations such as maternal diabetes and abnormal antepartum biophysical testing when elective preterm delivery may increase the fetus's likelihood of survival. In cases of abnormal MSAFP, measurements of amniotic fluid AFP and acetylcholinesterase levels may clarify the fetal problem. Acetylcholinesterase (AChE), like AFP, leaks into the amniotic fluid in pregnancies complicated by neural tube defects, but AChE does not vary with gestational age, and it is not elevated by contamination with fetal blood.

More recently, applications of immunologic and molecular genetic techniques have been utilized to demonstrate intrauterine infection.

Early genetic applications of amniocentesis were limited to detection of karyotypic anomalies and metabolic conditions in which the abnormal enzyme or its metabolic product had been characterized and was known to be expressed in amniocytes (Fig. 15-4). The diagnosis of other conditions in which the metabolic defect was unknown, or expressed only in selected fetal tissues, was either completely impossible or required other invasive techniques to sample the involved tissue. Diagnosis of hemoglobinopathies, for example, could be carried out only by fetoscopy to sample fetal blood. The breakthroughs of the last decade in molecular genetic techniques have largely obviated the need to sample other fetal tissues, because the entire genome is potentially available for study in all diploid fetal cells, including amniocytes. Extraordinary progress has been made in understanding the genetic basis of human diseases. The genes responsible for hundreds of metabolic disorders have been isolated and cloned. The use of restriction endonuclease cleavage of the genome followed by hybridization with specific oligonucleotide probes makes it possible to detect single-base substitutions, deletions, recombinations, and translocations. Minute specimens containing a few copies of the gene in question may be amplified by polymerase chain reaction so that a very tiny number of cells can provide a definitive diagnosis. Examples of conditions in which the abnormal locus may be directly inspected in fetal cells include sickle-cell disease, the thalassemias, Duchenne's muscular dystrophy, and hemophilia. In diseases in which the exact gene is unknown, it is still possible to detect carriers and affected fetuses by looking at genetic polymorphisms that are known to be so closely linked to the locus in question that the rate of recombination is very small. This indirect way of looking at genes by the company they consistently keep is called restriction fragment-length polymorphism analysis; it is used for prenatal diagnosis in cystic fibrosis and autosomal-dominant ("adult type") polycystic kidney disease.

In practice, not all genetic diseases can be detected and prevented in this way. For one thing, these techniques are complicated, expensive, and require fastidious attention to quality control and avoidance of specimen contamination. They are not suitable for screening for multiple diseases, since each gene must be looked for individually. However, in a population

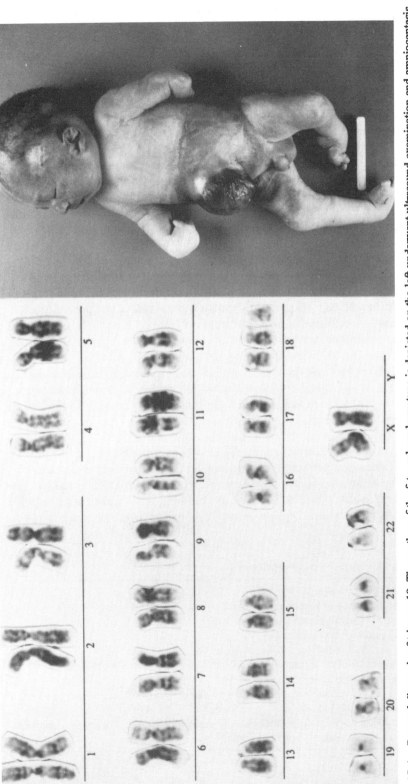

Fig. 15-4. Prenatal diagnosis of trisomy 18. The mother of the fetus whose karyotype is depicted on the left underwent ultrasound examination and amniocentesis after maternal serum alpha fetoprotein was found to be elevated. Cytogenetic analysis of amniocytes revealed an extra chromosome 18. The infant on the right has many features of this condition, including a dysmorphic face, low-set ears, limb deformities, and omphalocele. Affected infants are severely retarded; most die in the neonatal period. (Karyotype courtesy of Dr. Hon Fong Mark, Rhode Island Hospital, Department of Pathology.)

at known high risk for a specific defect like sickle cell anemia, screening is both feasible and desirable. Another problem arises from the fact that a single metabolic abnormality may be caused by several (or even hundreds of) different mutations, not all of which may be known. In many single-gene disorders, each family has a different "private" mutation; beta-thalassemia and hemophilia A are examples of conditions that are extremely heterogeneous at the molecular level. Sickle-cell disease, however, is always T > A at codon 6 of the beta-globin gene.

Amniocentesis, therefore, is useful only in the context of a specific clinical question. As imaging techniques continue to improve, and means are devised to obtain diagnostic fetal specimens by less invasive means, its use may be expected to decline. At the present time the majority of amniocenteses are performed to exclude Down syndrome. The current indications for amniocentesis are summarized in Table 15-3.

Several large collaborative studies have demonstrated that second-trimester amniocentesis is both safe and accurate. The fetal loss rate of less than 0.5 percent is not significantly increased over controls, and diagnostic accuracy exceeds 99 percent. In assessing the risk of any procedure, it is important to realize that the "background" rate of spontaneous abortion in fetuses of documented viability at 10 weeks is over 2 percent, and this risk increases with increasing maternal age.

The risks of second-trimester amniocentesis include trauma to the fetus, placenta, or umbilical cord (much diminished by ultrasound), infection, and abortion and premature labor. Isoimmunization due to fetomaternal hemorrhage is a risk, and amniocentesis is an indication for administration of Rh immune globulin in the Rh-negative mother.

The main problem with second-trimester amniocentesis is the timing; by 16 weeks, the pregnancy is obvious, family and friends are aware, and parental attachments may have formed. The time available for elective termination is short, and the risk to the mother of abortion increases with increasing gestational age. Recent trials of earlier amniocentesis, between

Table 15-3. Indications for amniocentesis

Advanced maternal age (>35 years)
Maternal serum alpha fetoprotein elevated or low
Previous child with a chromosomal abnormality
Parental chromosomal abnormality
Parents at risk for a known and detectable inborn error
Maternal carrier of an X-linked disorder
Previous child with neural tube defect
Previous child with major malformation but without cytogenetic diagnosis
Habitual abortion
Fetus at risk for condition in which elective preterm delivery or intrauterine intervention may be indicated

13 and 16 weeks, suggest that the accuracy, risk, and complications of the earlier procedure are acceptable in comparison to traditional amniocentesis and CVS. Studies of the safety and accuracy of amniocentesis between 9 and 13 weeks are in progress.

Chorionic Villus Sampling (CVS)

The psychosocial problems arising from postponing prenatal diagnosis until relatively late in gestation have been mentioned. Further anxiety may result from the delay necessitated by the fact that amniocytes must in most cases be established in tissue cultures before testing can be carried out. The risk to the mother of terminating a pregnancy increases with gestational age. These considerations have provided the impetus for development of safe and accurate diagnostic procedures applicable early in gestation. Successful direct sampling of the chorionic villi in the first trimester (CVS) was described in 1983 and has been in use since 1984. The first approach utilized was transcervical; a small plastic catheter is passed through the cervix into the uterus under ultrasound guidance, and a biopsy of the placenta is performed (Fig. 15-5). The specimen obtained can in many cases be analyzed directly, without the delay imposed by tissue culture, so that cytogenetic diagnosis is available in a few hours. Many controlled studies in many centers have confirmed that first-trimester CVS is a reasonably safe and accurate means of prenatal diagnosis. A transabdominal approach has theoretical advantages of lower infection rates and greater ease of performance because it is so similar to amniocentesis, but controlled studies have not demonstrated any advantage of either the transcervical or transabdominal route. In general, the indications, risks, and complications of CVS are similar to those of amniocentesis with certain exceptions.

Worrisome recent reports from the United Kingdom and Italy have called attention to an apparent association between oral and limb reduction defects and CVS, and in the United States fetal hemorrhagic lesions have been documented following CVS. These lesions were not seen in the large collaborative United States and Canadian studies, and it has been suggested that the European patients underwent CVS somewhat earlier in gestation than the North Americans. These observations, although unconfirmed by rigorously controlled studies, have raised concern over the safety of CVS.

CVS is slightly less successful than amniocentesis in obtaining cells, but if a diagnostic specimen is obtained, the accuracy of diagnosis is comparable.

A major problem with CVS not usually encountered in amniocentesis is mosaicism; rarely, fetus and placenta do not have the same karyotype. This comes about because the karyotypic abnormality arises after embryonic and extraembryonic cells have differentiated, resulting in placental but not fetal genetic abnormality or the reverse. Contamination of fetal cells with maternal cells is also a source of error. For this reason, certain abnormal CVS results will continue to have to be confirmed by amniocentesis.

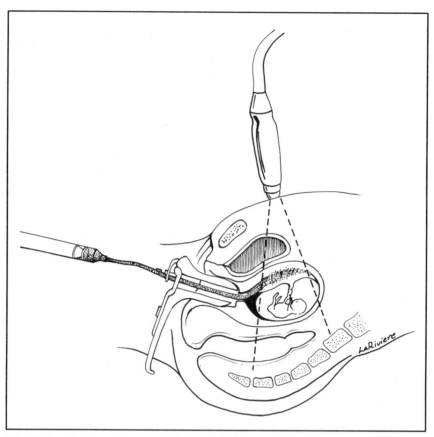

Fig. 15-5. Technique for transcervical chorionic villi sampling. A catheter containing a biopsy forceps is introduced into the placental bed and a small biopsy specimen of placental tissue is taken. The chorionic villi are fetal tissue and can be utilized for genetic or metabolic studies to detect genetic and metabolic disease.

In general, the primary utility of first-trimester CVS or amniocentesis is rapid diagnosis of cytogenetic abnormalities.

Fetoscopy and Embryoscopy

Direct endoscopic observation of the fetus has been feasible since 1954, but the procedure carries a high risk of fetal loss. Its main use has been to obtain fetal blood by cordocentesis for diagnosis of hemoglobinopathies in high-risk populations, but these diagnoses can now be made at the DNA level by amniocentesis, a much less risky procedure, and so fetoscopy is rarely employed. For those few conditions in which fetal blood sampling is still indicated, cord blood can be sampled by PUBS under ultrasound guidance.

Embryoscopy as a means of early first-trimester structural diagnosis or as a route of access to the fetal circulation in the first trimester is being explored but is currently limited to use as a research tool. Potential applications include verification of sonographic findings and access to the embryo for biopsy, surgery, or gene therapy.

Obtaining Fetal Blood and Tissue

The necessity for PUBS and fetal biopsy diminishes in inverse proportion to increasing sensitivity and accuracy of imaging modalities and molecular genetic methods. However, at the present time, fetal blood sampling is useful in clarifying cytogenetic questions raised by mosaicism, in certain (rare) immune deficiencies or hematologic disorders in which direct study of lymphocytes, platelets, or coagulation is necessary, and in establishing fetal infection in cases of maternal disease that may or may not have been transmitted to the fetus.

Fetal blood sampling is performed under ultrasound guidance using a technique similar to amniocentesis. A needle is inserted percutaneously into the amniotic sac and then into an umbilical vessel, usually at the insertion of the cord into the placenta, where movement of the umbilical cord is minimized. Percutaneous umbilical blood sampling has a low complication rate, and the main problems are related to contamination by maternal blood. Such contamination is readily identified using a Kleihauer-Betke test for fetal hemoglobin or by identification of the i antigen, found only on adult erythrocytes.

Biopsy of fetal tissues has been useful in dermatologic disorders. This group is also shrinking, but at present includes such things as epidermolysis bullosa, oculocutaneous albinism, and Harlequin syndrome. Fetal liver biopsy has historically been useful in diagnosis of metabolic disorders expressed only in hepatocytes (urea cycle defects, primarily), but these conditions are now amenable to direct DNA diagnosis.

In sum, ultrasound and its refinements (echocardiography, Doppler flow analysis, color mapping) are not known to carry any risk to mother or fetus. They provide detailed information as to the structural and physiologic integrity of the fetus. Invasive methods (early and late amniocentesis, CVS, PUBS) can provide accurate genetic and metabolic diagnoses, but none are entirely risk-free. What is needed is a test that is as easy and safe as MSAFP, as sensitive and accurate as second-trimester amniocentesis, and can be done well within the first trimester. This type of test may be a reality in the near future. Mueller and Hawes have demonstrated that fetal villous trophoblastic cells may be identified and isolated from maternal peripheral blood using monoclonal antibodies to trophoblast cytoplasmic membrane proteins and cell-sorting technology. This test is well within the realm of experimental medicine at the moment, but the possibilities are exciting and the promise is great.

Intervening on Behalf of the Fetus:
The New Obstetrics

We have thus far emphasized the diagnostic aspects of fetal medicine, concentrating on the detection, at a relatively late date, of anomalies that in the main either are not compatible with life or are productive of crippling mental or physical deformity. Many of these conditions, particularly malformations and malformation sequences resulting from genetic disorders, will not in the foreseeable future be amenable to any therapeutic intervention save termination of pregnancy. However, as has been shown in our discussion of teratogenesis, many congenital defects result from disruptions and deformities that are of known etiology or pathogenesis, which develop in a sequential, cumulative, and predictable fashion, and which are capable of being interrupted at some period in their development. This group of birth defects is clearly preventable, or at least capable of amelioration.

The most obvious strategy is to control or eliminate the underlying cause of the defect by treating the mother. The almost complete elimination of congenital rubella syndrome is an example of the successful application of this approach. There is no question that the incidence of malformation ascribable to maternal diseases like diabetes and PKU can be much reduced by appropriate metabolic control of the mother. The effects of intrauterine syphilis are greatly reduced by prompt treatment of the mother with antibiotics, and there is evidence that prenatal diagnosis and treatment of fetal toxoplasmosis may ameliorate the fetal disease. Not all exogenously produced problems will be solvable by the usual obstetric approaches; fetal alcohol effects and crack infants are going to require a broader societal approach for effective prevention.

Direct interventions on behalf of an individual fetus are of two types: those that basically aim at getting a compromised fetus out of the uterus before the condition gets worse, and those aimed at changing the course of intrauterine development. For the former group, management consists largely of elective preterm delivery; this is applicable for some infants of diabetic mothers, in cases of premature membrane rupture with infection, and for other conditions associated with increased risk of asphyxia or fetal death near term. For some infants, it may be advantageous to choose a time and place of delivery that will ensure immediate access to neonatal intensive care or prompt surgical intervention. Bowel obstruction and diaphragmatic hernia are examples of the latter group. Finally, the choice of route of delivery is frequently dictated by the prenatal diagnostic evaluation.

Fetal surgery in utero has been attempted in a few centers, but except for intrauterine transfusion, it has not clearly been demonstrated to be of benefit. Most surgical approaches have involved various types of shunt procedures to relieve disruptive damage to tissues caused by obstructive lesions. Fetal bladder shunts can at least theoretically prevent ongoing destruction or dysplasia of the kidneys in fetuses with lower urinary tract obstruction.

CSF shunts may alleviate neuronal loss due to increased intracranial pressure in obstructive hydrocephalus. Pleural effusions leading to pulmonary hypoplasia may be treated by intrauterine chest tubes. All of these procedures are invasive, carry a risk of infection, and may pose significant maternal risk. None is of proven benefit at the present time.

Recommended Reading

Benacerraf, B. (ed.). Fetal ultrasound. *Radiol. Clin. N. Amer.* 28:1, 1990.

Chambers, S. Prenatal Diagnosis by Ultrasound. In G. B. Reed, A. E. Claireaux, and A. D. Bain (eds.), *Diseases of the Fetus and Newborn: Pathology, Radiology, and Genetics.* St. Louis: Mosby, 1989. Pp. 573–595.

Firth, H. V., et al. Severe limb abnormalities after chorion villus sampling at 56–66 days gestation. *Lancet* 337:762–763, 1991.

Graham, J. M., and Otto, C. Clinical approach to prenatal detection of human structural defects. *Clin. Perinatol.* 17:513–546, 1990.

Haddow, J. E., et al. Prenatal screening for Down's syndrome with use of maternal serum markers. *N. Engl. J. Med.* 327:588–593, 1992.

Platt, L. D., and Carlson, D. E. Prenatal diagnosis—when and how? *N. Engl. J. Med.* 327:636–638, 1992.

Rhoades, G. G., et al. The safety and efficacy of chorionic villus sampling for early prenatal diagnosis of cytogenetic abnormalities. *N. Engl. J. Med.* 320:609–617, 1989.

Simoni, G., and Brambati, B. Fetal Karyotype Diagnosis by First Trimester Chorionic Villus Sampling. In G. B. Reed, A. E. Claireaux, and A. D. Bain (eds.), *Diseases of the Fetus and Newborn: Pathology, Radiology, and Genetics.* St. Louis: Mosby, 1989. Pp. 627–639.

Simpson, J. L., and Elias, S. Prenatal Diagnosis of Genetic Disorders. In R. K. Creasy, and R. Resnik (eds.), *Maternal-Fetal Medicine.* Philadelphia: Saunders, 1989. Pp. 78–107.

Smith, C. V. Amniotic fluid assessment. *Obstet. Gynecol. Clin. North Am.* 17:187–200, 1990.

Valenti, C., and Musenga, M. Mid Trimester Diagnostic Amniocentesis. In G. B. Reed, A. E. Claireaux, and A. D. Bain (eds.), *Diseases of the Fetus and Newborn: Pathology, Radiology, and Genetics.* St. Louis: Mosby, 1989. Pp. 641–660.

Viscarello, R. R., Gollin, Y. G., and Hobbins, J. C. Alternate methods of first trimester diagnosis. *Obstet. Gynecol. Clin. North Am.* 18:875–890, 1991.

16

Fetal Assessment

Donald R. Coustan

The fetus is our most inaccessible patient. We cannot observe, palpate, auscultate, or percuss the fetus as we would any other patient. We cannot take a history, and the fetus cannot tell us if he or she is uncomfortable. Fortunately, nature has designed the fetolplacental unit, and the mother, to maintain the very best conditions for safety, growth, and development under most circumstances. Because no system is perfect, and some pregnancies develop medical or obstetric problems, or both, a number of approaches have been developed to allow us to assess fetal status. All fetuses are monitored in some way during labor, and some require assessment at various times prior to the onset of labor.

Biophysical Fetal Monitoring in Labor

Labor is a time during which normal physiologic events predispose the mother and fetus to pathologic occurrences. Labor is a natural event that is experienced, under ordinary circumstances, by the mother of every member of the human race. However, it is also a potentially stressful event for the fetus. Each uterine contraction is accompanied by a decrease in maternal blood flow through the intervillous space, potentially diminishing the availability of oxygen and nutrients for transport to the fetus. Although the healthy fetus will tolerate such intermittent hypoxic episodes with no adverse effects, preexisting fetal compromise may diminish the fetoplacental reserve, the ability to maintain homeostasis under suboptimal conditions. Excessively strong or frequent contractions, brought about by events such as abruptio placentae or excessive oxytocin stimulation, may have an adverse impact even on a fetus with normal reserve. Various unpredictable mechanical events may complicate labor. Umbilical cord prolapse or compression against the bony pelvis may diminish blood flow between the placenta and fetus, decreasing the availability of oxygen and nutrients. Abruptio placentae may involve a large enough proportion of the placental surface area to compromise maternal-fetal gas exchange. Diminished uterine blood flow from aortic compression or maternal hypotension from diminished venous return due to the supine position may similarly compromise the fetus. Any or all of the above conditions can arise suddenly and unpredictably, so that the fetal condition may change rapidly.

Because stillbirths and depressed neonates often occur without warning, obstetricians for many years have attempted to evaluate fetal well-being. Fetal auscultation was investigated by Kergaradec in Paris in the 1820s. With a stethoscope, fetal heartbeats were counted over a time interval, generally a minute, and the average heart rate (in beats per minute [bpm]) was expressed. A normal range of 120 to 160 bpm was described; this is still considered to be the normal range. Uterine contractions were first recorded by Schatz in Rostock, Germany, in the 1870s. A mercury-filled bag was inserted into the uterus during labor, and the bag was connected to a manometer that inscribed intrauterine pressure levels on a rotating drum. These observations were of little practical value, since there was no way to treat the fetus if a problem was suspected. The focus of obstetric care at the time was the survival of the mother, with the offspring afforded secondary consideration.

Advances in anesthesia, surgical technique, blood transfusions, and antibiotics during the first half of the twentieth century provided obstetricians the luxury of performing a cesarean section with relative safety for the mother, and allowed more attention to be paid to the fetus. It became routine for obstetricians and obstetric nurses to listen to the fetal heart beat and calculate a rate that was an average of all the beats heard during the 30- or 60-second listening interval. It became clear that fetuses whose heart rates were slow (less than 100–120 bpm), or fast (greater than 160–180 bpm), or erratic were more likely to be stillborn or depressed at birth. These changes in average fetal heart rates became important factors in determining whether to perform an emergency cesarean section or rapid instrumental delivery out of concern for fetal jeopardy.

The 1950s and 1960s saw the development of methods for directly recording intrauterine pressure by means of an intraamniotic catheter, and for recording the fetal ECG by a clip electrode attached to the fetal scalp (Fig. 16-1). The electronic signals were fed into a computer that measured the interval between each two beats and used this interval to calculate a rate instantaneously after each pair of beats. The instantaneous fetal heart rate was then displayed on a cathode ray tube screen and on a permanent paper strip record. This electronic fetal monitor (EFM) design has been improved on in various ways, but still forms the basis for fetal monitoring

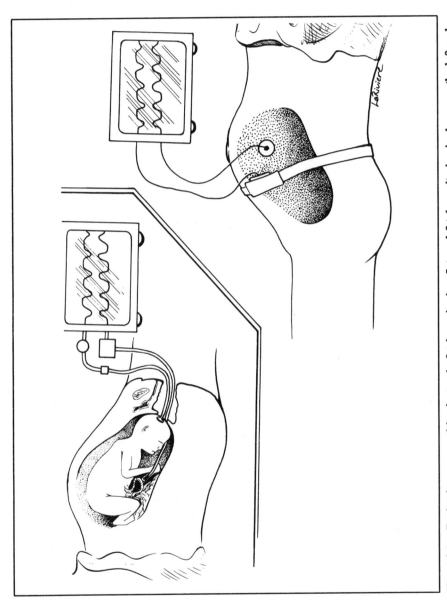

Fig. 16-1. Basic elements used in electronic fetal monitoring. Internal fetal monitoring is shown on the left and external fetal monitoring is depicted on the right.

in most of the obstetric units in the United States. Its main features are simultaneous recording of uterine contractions and instantaneous fetal heart rate, displayed together on a continuous record, so that short- and long-term changes in heart rate and their association with contractions can be appreciated. The use of instantaneous heart rates, rather than averaging over many beats, avoids the loss of potentially important details in heart-rate adjustments of the fetus.

The original method of direct fetal monitoring required the membranes to be ruptured in order to place an electrode on the fetal scalp. During the late 1960s an ultrasonic signal of low power was used to detect the movement of the walls of the fetal heart. Sound reflected from a moving surface returns to the transducer at a higher or lower frequency than when it was emitted, depending on whether the surface is moving toward or away from the transducer. The use of such Doppler transducers allowed the monitoring of the fetal heart prior to rupture of the membranes, and indeed prior to the onset of labor if desired (Fig. 16-1). The development of the abdominal pressure transducer, similar in principle to a tonometer used to measure intraorbital pressure in the eye, likewise allows the recording of the timing of contractions despite intact membranes, although contraction intensity and baseline resting tone cannot be measured accurately with this device.

Interpretation of the fetal monitor strip is performed in a systematic manner. The contraction pattern and heart rate pattern are each evaluated, and their relationship is assessed. Baseline fetal heart rate is normally in the range of 120 to 160 bpm. Mild *tachycardia* is 161 to 180 bpm, and marked baseline tachycardia is >180 bpm, persisting for at least 10 minutes. Tachycardia may be transient, and is associated with fetal movement or alertness. However, when there is baseline tachycardia the possibility of maternal fever, fetal hypoxemia, fetal infection, or fetal thyrotoxicosis should be considered. In the case of maternal fever, the fetus attempts to dissipate excess heat by increasing blood flow to the skin. Because this process is ineffective while the fetus is in utero, it leads to tachycardia as the fetus increases cardiac output to provide even more peripheral blood flow. When fetal hypoxemia occurs, tachycardia may develop over time. Tachycardia alone is not a reliable sign of fetal hypoxemia; other suggestive heart rate changes are generally present. A number of drugs administered to the mother may also be associated with fetal tachycardia, including sympathomimetics and parasympatholytics.

Baseline fetal *bradycardia* is mild at 100 to 119 bpm, moderate at 80 to 99 bpm, and severe at < 80 bpm, lasting at least 10 minutes. Moderate and severe baseline bradycardias are considered "nonreassuring" fetal heart rates, and may be associated with hypoxemia. Nevertheless, mild and moderate bradycardias may be benign or associated with fetal head compression, and even severe bradycardia may be secondary to fetal heart block. The baseline fetal heart rate is only one attribute of fetal tracing, and should be interpreted in the context of associated findings.

One of the most important elements of fetal heart rate tracing is baseline "beat-to-beat" *variability*. Normally heart rate is under the control of both cardioinhibitory and cardioaccelerator centers of the autonomic nervous system. The baseline rate is maintained by successive adjustments. When an internal scalp electrode is used, and each R-R interval is used as the basis for calculating instantaneous fetal heart rate, the continuous tracing can be seen to "jiggle" up and down around the baseline rate (Fig. 16-2). The changes about the baseline are described as "short-term" and "long-term." The usual short-term variability (STV) is approximately 3 to 7 bpm

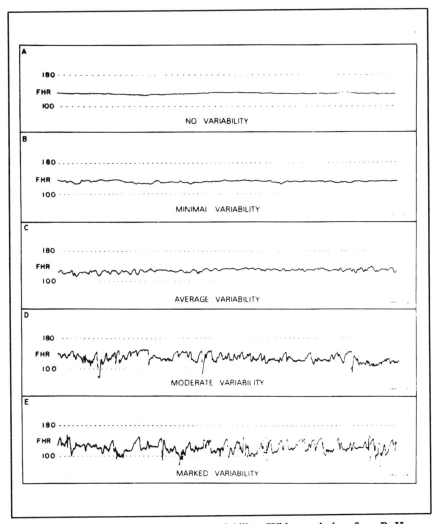

Fig. 16-2. Examples of fetal heart rate variability. (With permission, from R. H. Paul, et al. Clinical fetal monitoring. *Am. J. Obstet. Gynecol.* 123:207, 1975.)

on each side of the baseline. Long-term variability (LTV) generally has a fluctuation of 3 to 5 cycles per minute. The presence of normal short-term and long-term variability is extremely reassuring of fetal well-being, regardless of other aspects of the tracing. However, with external fetal heart rate monitors using Doppler systems to count heart beats, it is possible to induce "false" short-term variability as the changes in the distance from heart to transducer caused by fetal movement, fetal breathing, and maternal abdominal wall movement may be interpreted by the equipment as changes in fetal heart rate. Most current equipment incorporates computer logic to minimize this problem, but the only way to be absolutely sure that STV is present is with internal monitoring. When there is less than 3 bpm of short-term variability and less than 2 cycles per minute of long-term variability, diminished or absent variability is diagnosed. Diminished variability may be due to benign causes such as fetal sleep state or the use of drugs such as parasympatholytics or depressants. However, it may be indicative of long-term fetal neurologic dysfunction, or shorter-term decreased autonomic function secondary to acidemia. The absence of beat-to-beat variability is probably meaningful even with external fetal monitoring techniques, as random movements are unlikely to induce greater apparent regularity to the fetal heart rate.

Accelerations of the fetal heart rate, generally present in response to fetal movement, are another sign of fetal well-being. To be counted these accelerations should reach a peak of at least 15 bpm above baseline, and last for at least 15 seconds.

Periodic decelerations of the fetal heart rate are classified as early, late, and variable, depending on their relationship to contractions and the slope of their fall and return to baseline. Early and late decelerations are generally recognizable only with electronic fetal monitoring, while some variable decelerations may be appreciated by auscultation as well (Fig. 16-3).

Early decelerations are symmetric patterns that are "mirror images" of the contraction tracing. They begin with the onset of the contraction, end with the end of the contraction, and do not outlast it (Fig. 16-4). These early decelerations are believed to represent a fetal response to compression of the head against the bony pelvis during labor, and are mediated via the vagus nerve. They can be eradicated with parasympatholytic drugs such as atropine. Early decelerations are believed to be entirely benign, and their presence does not imply any compromise of the fetal condition.

Late decelerations are similar in form to early decelerations, with a gradual and smooth downslope and recovery. However, the timing of the onset and recovery, with respect to contractions, is different. Late decelerations begin well after the onset of each contraction. They reach their nadir after the peak of the contraction, and they do not recover completely to baseline until after the contraction is over; hence the name, "late" deceleration. Late decelerations are not significant when they occur as isolated events; they must be repetitive. A term formerly used to describe this pattern is

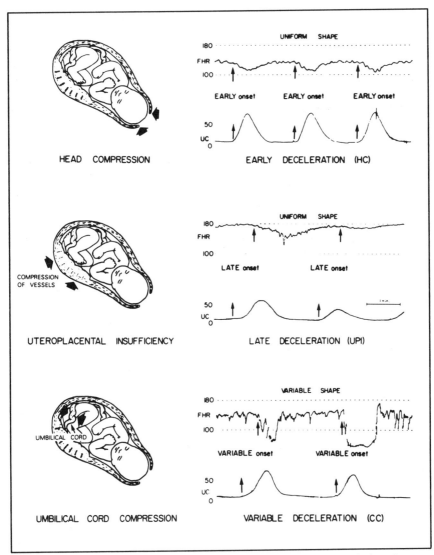

Fig. 16-3. Three different types of periodic decelerations. (With permission, from E. Hon. *An Introduction to Fetal Heart Rate Monitoring.* Los Angeles: University of Southern California, 1973.)

uteroplacental insufficiency (UPI). This name refers to the presumed patho-physiology of the genesis of late decelerations. As the uterus contracts, maternal blood flow to the intervillous space diminishes, ceasing altogether when the pressure within the uterus exceeds that in the spiral arteries. As the contraction persists, the concentration of oxygen in the maternal blood of the intervillous blood diminishes because umbilical blood flow from

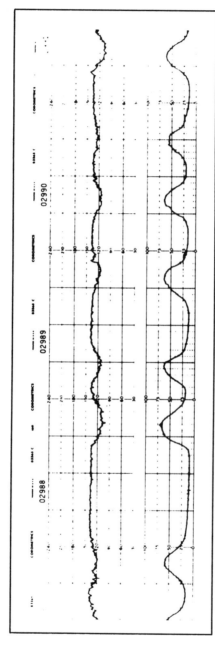

Fig. 16-4. Fetal monitor tracing showing early decelerations (top line). Note that decelerations are mirror images of the contractions (bottom line). (Top) line indicates fetal heart rate and (bottom) line indicates contractions. (Reproduced, with permission, from T. P. Barden. *Intrapartum Fetal Monitoring* [revised 2nd ed.]. American College of Obstetricians and Gynecologists. Intrapartum Fetal Monitoring. ACOG Self Learning Package, Program 2, 2nd ed. Washingon, DC: ACOG, 1985.)

the fetal villous circulation continues to carry away oxygen. As relative hypoxemia develops in the fetus, chemoreceptors respond by triggering an arterial pressure, which then stimulates baroreceptors to send a vagal signal, slowing the fetal heart rate. The onset of the deceleration is late, and occurs after the onset of the contraction, because of the time needed to deplete the intervillous blood of oxygen. The nadir of the deceleration occurs after the peak of the contraction because of the time needed for intervillous maternal blood flow to resume and replenish the oxygen supply.

Initially, late decelerations are mediated via the vagus nerve, and are reflexive in nature. With continued hypoxemia and the development of acidemia, direct myocardial depression may supervene. This ominous development is unlikely when the fetal heart rate tracing shows normal variability (Fig. 16-5), but should be suspected when variability is absent or markedly diminished in the presence of late decelerations (Fig. 16-6).

The causes of late decelerations may be maternal, such as hypoxemia, hypotension, severe anemia, or ketoacidosis; placental, such as abruptio placentae or placental insufficiency; or fetoplacental, such as dysmaturity. Excessively strong uterine contractions, whether spontaneous or oxytocin-induced, may cause late decelerations.

The form of *variable* decelerations is very different from those of early and late decelerations. The fall and rise in fetal heart rate are not smooth and gradual as in the latter conditions, but rather are abrupt and often "sawtoothed." In particular, the return to baseline occurs at an acute angle, rather than being rounded and smooth. The timing of variable decelerations does not have a particular characteristic except that it is variable. Variable decelerations may occur before, during, or after contractions (Fig. 16-7). When their timing is similar to that of late decelerations, the only way to distinguish them is by their form. Variable decelerations are caused by umbilical cord compression. Even mild impingement on the umbilical cord, without interruption of flow, causes arterial vasospasm. This vasospasm leads to increased peripheral resistance in the fetus, which elicits a baroreceptor response. Vagal stimulation then results in a variable deceleration. When cord impingement ceases there is a rapid fall in fetal peripheral resistance, cessation of baroreceptor firing, and return to baseline of the heart rate. Variable decelerations are often categorized as "mild" (lasting less than 30 seconds), "moderate" (lasting between 30 and 60 seconds and reaching a nadir below 60 bpm, or lasting more than 60 seconds with a nadir of 70–80 bpm), and "severe" (longer than 60 seconds, less than 70 bpm).

Variable decelerations are present in the majority of labors, and usually are innocuous. However, when variable decelerations are persistent and severe, hypercarbia may develop. This condition may be apparent from an "overshoot" in the fetal heart rate after a variable deceleration has recovered, when the fetal nervous system attempts to "blow off" the hypercarbia by means of a transient fetal tachycardia. The fetal bradycardia occurring

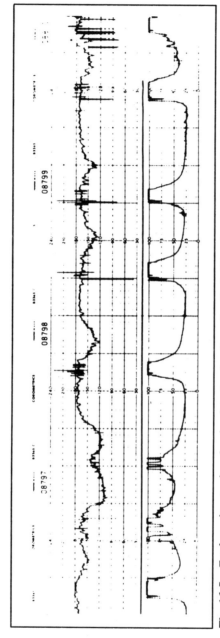

Fig. 16-5. Fetal monitor tracing showing late decelerations (top line). Note that the decelerations begin after the onset of contractions (bottom line), and outlast the contractions. The presence of beat-to-beat variability is somewhat reassuring. (Reproduced, with permission, from T. P. Barden. *Intrapartum Fetal Monitoring* [revised 2nd ed.]. American College of Obstetricians and Gynecologists. Intrapartum Fetal Monitoring. ACOG Self Learning Package, Program 2, 2nd ed. Washington, DC: ACOG, 1985.)

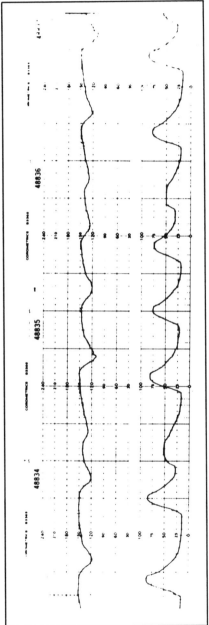

Fig. 16-6. Fetal monitor tracing late decelerations (top line; bottom line indicates contractions). Variability is now minimal or absent. This is a much more worrisome tracing than Fig. 16-5. (Reproduced, with permission, from T. P. Barden. *Intrapartum Fetal Monitoring* [revised 2nd ed.]. American College of Obstetricians and Gynecologists. Intrapartum Fetal Monitoring. ACOG Self Learning Package, Program 2, 2nd ed. Washington, DC: ACOG, 1985.)

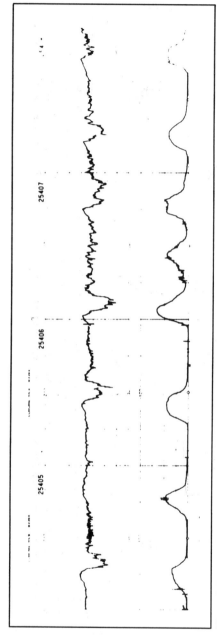

Fig. 16-7. Mild variable decelerations (top line indicates fetal heart rate; bottom line indicates contractions). Note the rapid falls and abrupt rises in heart rate. (Reproduced with permission from T. P. Barden. *Intrapartum Fetal Monitoring* [revised 2nd ed.]. American College of Obstetricians and Gynecologists. Intrapartum Fetal Monitoring. ACOG Self Learning Package, Program 2, 2nd ed. Washington, DC: ACOG, 1985.)

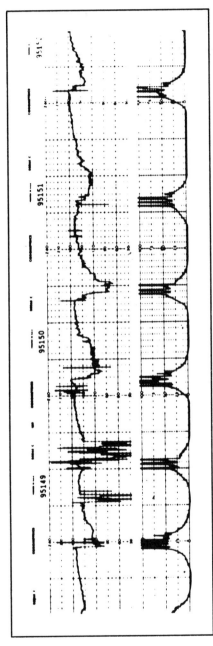

Fig. 16-8. Severe atypical variable decelerations (top line indicates fetal heart rate; bottom line indicates contractions). Note the slow return to baseline at the end of the decelerations. This tracing is clearly worrisome. (Reproduced, with permission, from T. P. Barden. *Intrapartum Fetal Monitoring* [revised 2nd ed.]. American College of Obstetricians and Gynecologists. Intrapartum Fetal Monitoring. ACOG Self Learning Package, Program 2, 2nd ed. Washington, DC: ACOG, 1985.)

during a variable deceleration may also cause decreased tissue perfusion by limiting cardiac output, resulting in metabolic acidemia. When this happens it is typical to see a slow return to baseline at the ends of successive variable decelerations, often called *atypical variable* decelerations or a *mixed pattern*. Such patterns have a similar significance to repetitive late decelerations, and are particularly nonreassuring when accompanied by diminished or absent variability (Fig. 16-8).

The response to a nonreassuring EFM tracing is not limited to immediate delivery. Very often other measures can be taken to improve fetal oxygenation. Maternal hypovolemia may decrease placental perfusion, which may be improved by rapidly increasing intravenous hydration. When the mother labors in the supine position the uterus may impinge on the maternal vena cava, interfering with venous return to the right side of the heart and decreasing cardiac output. Alternatively the uterus may compress the abdominal aorta, causing a decrease in local blood flow to the uterus. Either mechanism may be responsible for a nonreassuring EFM tracing, and may be alleviated by moving the patient from the supine to the lateral position. Finally, as described in Chap. 9, increasing the ambient oxygen concentration in the air inhaled by the mother can result in significant increases in fetal blood oxygen content, even though partial pressure of oxygen increases only minimally. Women with nonreassuring tracings are generally given nasal or face mask oxygen and are turned to their sides as a first response, and these measures are often effective.

When EFM was first explored, the particular patterns were delineated by studies on animal models, primarily sheep. Subsequently the interpretations were validated by measurement of acid-base values in scalp and cord blood of human pregnancies. In these studies pH was unaffected by mild variable (called "cord compression" at the time) decelerations and early (called "head compression") decelerations. However, as variable decelerations became more severe and as late decelerations (UPI) appeared, average fetal pH values fell (Fig. 16-9). Subsequent studies showed that for a given fetal heart rate pattern, the pH was likely to be lower if beat-to-beat variability was absent (Fig. 16-10).

After EFM was introduced clinically, a number of retrospective studies demonstrated decreases in perinatal mortality rates that were attributed to monitoring. Intrapartum fetal deaths all but disappeared in centers that used EFM on a regular basis. In some large centers, perinatal mortality rates were lower among "high-risk" patients whose labors were monitored electronically than among "low-risk" unmonitored patients. EFM was widely assumed to be effective at preventing perinatal mortality, and it was taken for granted that its widespread use would significantly reduce the prevalence of cerebral palsy and other neurologic problems in the offspring, since early signs of "asphyxia" would allow immediate delivery by cesarean section or other means, preventing permanent damage from occurring. Unfortunately, this expectation was not realized when perinatal mortality

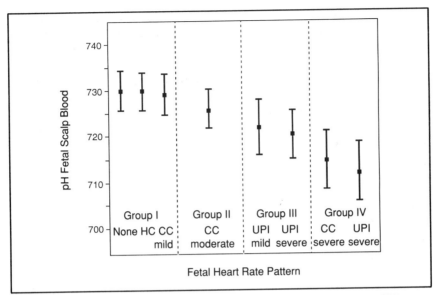

Fig. 16-9. Correlation between FHR patterns and fetal scalp blood pH. NONE = no decelerations. HC = head compression (early deceleration). CC = cord compression (variable deceleration). UPI = uteroplacental insufficiency (late deceleration). (With permission, from F. W. Kubli, et al. "Observations on heart rate and pH in the human fetus during labor." *Am. J. Obstet. Gynecol.* 104:1190, 1969.)

rates were evaluated in randomized trials; EFM was not associated with decreases in mortality or morbidity, although one trial showed a decrease in neonatal seizures, which are considered to be a marker for perinatal asphyxia. In addition, a number of these studies demonstrated higher cesarean section rates in monitored patients, without apparent benefit.

There are many possible explanations for the lack of demonstrable advantages when outcomes research was applied to EFM. Perinatal mortality is such a rare event that many pregnancies would have to be studied to detect differences. The studies published as of this writing have been large enough, in aggregate, that clinically significant differences would have been expected to emerge, if present. Another possibility is that monitor tracings were not evaluated appropriately, or that clinical responses were inappropriate; this might explain the increase in cesarean section rates in some studies. Although it is possible that our understanding of the meaning of fetal heart rate patterns is simply wrong, this seems unlikely since correlations between nonreassuring patterns and lower pH values are widely reported. The most likely explanation is that we have overestimated the contribution of labor events to perinatal mortality and neurologic damage.

Many studies have demonstrated that perinatal events account for only a small proportion of cases of cerebral palsy. Prematurity in particular, but also antepartum infections and congenital anomalies, and postnatal events,

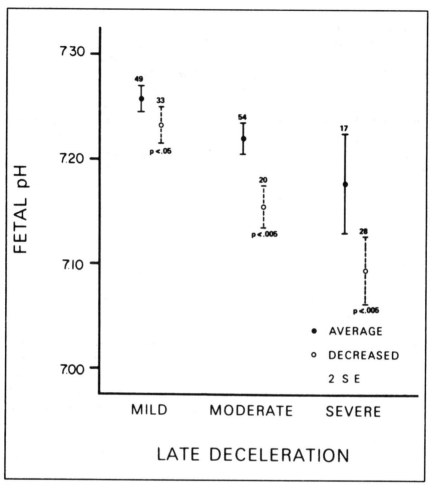

Fig. 16-10. As late decelerations become more marked, the mean pH falls. However, when FHR variability is present in association with late deceleration patterns, the mean pH is consistently higher than when it is absent. (With permission, from R. H. Paul, et al. Clinical fetal monitoring. *Am. J. Obstet. Gynecol.* 123:207, 1975.)

appear to be more frequent precursors of neurologic damage. Furthermore, abnormal fetal heart rate tracings may be the result of, rather than the cause of, neurologic dysfunction. Most abnormal fetal heart rate tracings are associated with benign outcomes, just as most infants with low Apgar scores survive and are developmentally intact. The EFM is very accurate at telling us that the fetus is tolerating labor well. However, when we interpret the tracing as showing that there is a problem, we are usually wrong. Another way to express this is that the predictive value of a normal tracing for the absence of acute hypoxemia and acidemia is extremely high, in the range of 99 percent, whereas the predictive value of an "abnormal" tracing for the presence of these conditions is fairly low, perhaps only 25 percent. Thus we have probably expected too much of EFM.

One largely semantic problem that has arisen with widespread utilization of EFM is the use of the term *fetal distress*. Tracings showing recurrent late decelerations, with decreased variability, or severe variable decelerations, are often labelled as diagnostic of fetal distress, and operative delivery is recommended as the treatment. More often than not, cesarean section produces a very healthy baby with no evidence of acidemia or hypoxemia. The term fetal distress is certainly inappropriate for such a patient, and fails to convey the high false-positive rate of EFM. This problem is compounded by the fact that most cases of neurologic dysfunction, such as cerebral palsy, are not related to intrapartum events. Nevertheless, when the above-described child, with good Apgar scores and an uncomplicated neonatal course, later manifests developmental delay for one of a score of reasons unrelated to birth, the diagnosis of fetal distress in the medical record may be a tempting target for assigning blame to the obstetrician. It is well established that "perinatal asphyxia" is not present when the child has an uncomplicated neonatal course. The combination of low Apgar scores, neonatal seizures, and other evidence of ischemic damage must be present before this diagnosis can be made. It has now become standard to refer to worrisome fetal monitoring patterns as "nonreassuring." This term conveys the lack of reassurance that would be provided by a perfectly normal tracing while not implying that the fetus is necessarily in danger. It is the most reasonable approximation of the meaning of such tracings. Obviously a tracing with no variability and recurrent late decelerations is more "nonreassuring" than a tracing with good variability and moderate variable decelerations.

In the controversies that continue to surround EFM, it must be remembered that the monitor is an inanimate object, incapable of making a decision or performing an unnecessary cesarean section. It can provide information to the health care team, but it is up to the obstetrician or midwife to interpret that information and decide how the patient's labor should be managed. We should not blame fetal monitoring for the increases in cesarean section rates during recent years; we should blame ourselves. Having more information about our hidden patient cannot be a bad thing; our use of the data is the issue.

Because of the absence of data to support universal EFM, the American College of Obstetricians and Gynecologists recommends that monitoring during labor be either continuous EFM or intermittent auscultation. For high-risk patients, it is recommended that if intermittent auscultation is used, it be performed and the results recorded, preferably following a uterine contraction, at least every 15 minutes during the first stage of labor and every 5 minutes during the second stage. For low-risk patients maximum intervals of 30 minutes during the first stage and 15 minutes during the second stage are advised. In practical terms, intermittent auscultation requires a nurse for each patient in labor. This is quite expensive, particularly when the number of laboring patients on a particular unit may fluctuate markedly so that the number of nurses required is difficult to predict. For this reason, many units continue to use EFM as the routine approach to assessment of fetal well-being during labor. Most patients find the monitoring process reassuring. However, a "low-risk" patient who prefers not to have EFM should not be made to feel that she is placing her fetus at increased risk, since the available data do not support that concept.

Fetal and Neonatal Acid-Base Analysis

The significance of particular EFM patterns was derived from their correlation with fetal blood-gas measurements, particularly pH. Blood gas analysis is a much more precise and accurate way to evaluate the fetal-neonatal condition than is the EFM tracing or the Apgar scores, because factors other than hypoxia, such as congenital malformations, drugs, and prematurity may be associated with low Apgar scores.

Under normal circumstances, during labor, the fetus has a PO_2 in the range of 17 to 24 mm Hg, and a PCO_2 of 33 to 55 mm Hg. The pH is in the range of 7.3 to 7.4. If maternal-fetal gas exchange is impaired, PCO_2 increases. As carbon dioxide tension rises, carbonic acid is produced and the pH tends to fall; this is a respiratory acidemia. As gas exchange is further impaired, the fetus may receive inadequate oxygen to carry out aerobic metabolism, or poor tissue perfusion may limit delivery of oxygen to the periphery. Anaerobic metabolism then assumes greater prominence. Whereas aerobic metabolism produces primarily carbonic acid, which can be dissipated as carbon dioxide, anaerobic metabolism produces lactic acid and ketone bodies, which are not so easily disposed of. As acids accumulate, the pH is maintained by a system of buffer bases in the blood. These include hemoglobin and bicarbonate as well as other bases. Although the buffers maintain the physiologic pH despite increased acid production, they can become depleted. The depletion of buffer bases is called *base deficit* or, in some centers, *negative base excess*. The presence of a base deficit suggests a metabolic acidemia. Blood gas analyzers measure pH, PO_2, and PCO_2. The bicarbonate level and base deficit are then derived. When acidemia is present (low pH), a respiratory source is indicated by a high PCO_2 and normal bicarbonate and buffer base level. A metabolic cause is present if there is a normal PCO_2 and a high base deficit or the bicarbonate is low, or both. Many cases will be mixed.

Although the normal range of umbilical artery pH at birth is usually given as 7.20 to 7.39, definitions of clinically significant acidemia vary widely. Many authors report that there is no increase in the likelihood of adverse outcome unless the umbilical cord pH is < 7.0, and others point out that two standard deviations below the mean is approximately 7.15. Most infants whose pH is above 7.0 do well.

It cord blood-gas determinations are needed, at the time of birth a segment of umbilical cord can be isolated with clamps, and a blood sample can be drawn from one of the two umbilical arteries. Umbilical venous blood can also be used, but arterial blood should more closely approximate the fetal condition, since venous blood is returning from the placenta. Heparin is used as the anticoagulant.

It is also possible to obtain fetal blood gas determinations during labor. This can be very useful in helping to decide whether a nonreassuring EFM tracing is associated with fetal acidemia. In some centers fetal scalp pH measurement is performed prior to any intervention for nonreassuring fetal heart rate patterns, in order to avoid unnecessary intervention. Scalp samples yield capillary blood and pH is usually considered low if < 7.20, with 7.20 to 7.25 being a "gray zone." Maternal acidemia or alkalemia can influence fetal blood gases, so simultaneous maternal blood gases (venous blood is acceptable) may be helpful when there is reason to suspect that maternal pH is high or low. Membranes must be ruptured and the cervix dilated to at least 2 to 3 cm in order to obtain a fetal scalp sample. In some circumstances it is necessary to obtain fetal blood prior to active labor. Percutaneous umbilical blood sampling is sometimes used for this purpose.

Antepartum Fetal Evaluation

Although labor is a time when the fetus may be exposed to increased risk, some pregnancies are at risk even prior to labor. For example, when the mother has poorly controlled type I diabetes, the likelihood of an "unexplained" antepartum fetal demise has been reported to be as high as 20 percent. Severely hypertensive pregnancies may be complicated by poor placental perfusion, fetal growth retardation, and fetal death. Prolonged pregnancies that are developing dysmaturity may show evidence of fetal compromise prior to labor. For these reasons many approaches have been developed to evaluate the fetus before labor and delivery. The principles of intrapartum EFM also have been applied prior to labor.

Antepartum Electronic Fetal Monitoring

Intrapartum EFM is based on the concept of uterine contractions being potential stressors for the fetus. It is logical, then, to apply this principle to the maternal-fetal pair not in labor by inducing uterine contractions with oxytocin and observing the fetal response. The *oxytocin challenge test* is carried out by using external EFM while an infusion of dilute oxytocin is administered intravenously. If consistent late decelerations are present, the test is considered "positive" and consideration is given to delivering the baby, usually but not always by cesarean section. A variation of this test is the *contraction stress test* (CST), which applies to testing during contractions that occur for any reason, not just those induced by oxytocin. Thus, a patient having spontaneous contractions but not actually in labor would have a CST. Contractions also may be induced by stimulation of the mother's nipples (usually with a washcloth), which then induces endogenous oxytocin release and contractions; this is called the *nipple stimulation test.*

Performing a CST may be time-consuming and relatively expensive. Another approach is to look for evidence of fetal well-being in the baseline fetal heart rate tracing, even in the absence of contractions. This approach is usually referred to as the *nonstress test* (NST), and the hoped-for evidence of fetal well-being is the acceleration of the fetal heart rate in response to fetal movement. In practice, the mother is given a button to push that makes a mark on the tracing when she perceives the fetus to have kicked. If, coincident with fetal movement, the heart rate increases by at least 15 bpm, and the acceleration lasts at least 15 seconds, a fetal heart rate acceleration has occurred. If two of these events occur during a 10-minute interval, or three occur during a 20-minute interval, the test is considered "reactive" (Fig. 16-11). In the absence of an acute intervening event, a reactive NST or a negative CST is considered reassuring of fetal survival for the ensuing week.

One important principle of antepartum fetal testing is the significance of *a priori* risk. Both NSTs and CSTs have a significant likelihood of false-positive results, i.e., the test suggests problems when the fetus is perfectly well. To simplify discussion of this issue, let us assume that the automatic response to a positive test is to deliver the fetus. Let us further assume that 5 percent of all tests of normal individuals give falsely positive results. Consider two populations of 100 patients each. One group is at very low risk, having a likelihood of fetal compromise of 1 percent. The other group is at high risk, with a likelihood of fetal jeopardy of 10 percent. Antepartum testing is then applied to all members of both groups (Table 16-1).

The low-risk group will have six positive tests (five false-positives plus one true positive). Of the positive tests, only 17 percent (1/6) are true positives. The high-risk group will manifest 15 positive tests (five false-positives plus 10 true positives), with 67 percent (10/15) being true positives. It is clear that an abnormal test in a patient with low *a priori* risk is much less worrisome than an abnormal test in a patient with high *a priori* risk. If the pregnancies were all at a gestational age when neonatal survival is only

Table 16-1. Predictive accuracy of antepartum testing

	N	True positive	False positive	Total positive
Low risk	100	1	5	6
High risk	100	10	5	15

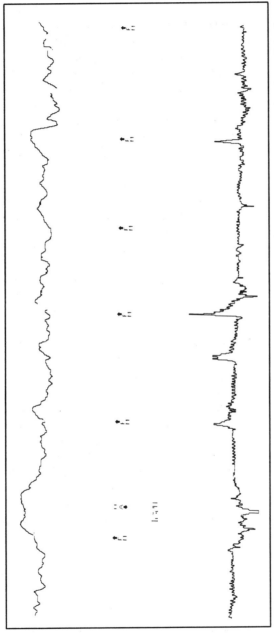

Fig. 16-11.   Reactive nonstress test. Arrows represent maternally perceived fetal movements. Note accelerations of fetal heart rate with most fetal movements. (Top line indicates fetal heart rate; bottom line indicates contraction.)

50 percent, it is clear that delivering the low-risk patient with a 17 percent likelihood of truly being in trouble makes much less sense than delivering the high-risk patient with a 67 percent likelihood of fetal death. The greater the risk associated with delivery, the greater the risk of testing a low-risk population. Thus there is no point in testing a normal pregnancy "just to find out if everything is OK" at 25 weeks' gestation, when delivery is likely to be disastrous. Even at term, since most abnormal results in low-risk patients will be false-positives, careful consideration must be given before indiscriminate testing is ordered. Another strategy used to lower the risk of false-positive results is to use one test as a "screening" test, and then perform a second test for confirmation before acting. Very often an NST is performed first, and if it is nonreactive a CST is carried out.

Biophysical Profile

The use of ultrasound to diagnose congenital anomalies is discussed in Chap. 15. Another application of ultrasound is to determine fetal well-being. The *biophysical profile* (BPP) is comprised of four elements determined by ultrasound plus an NST. The four elements are (1) fetal tone (active extension with return to flexion); (2) fetal movement (at least 30 seconds of movement during a 30-minute observation); (3) fetal breathing (at least 30 seconds of breathing during a 30-minute observation); and (4) amniotic fluid volume (at least one pocket measuring $\geq$ 2 cm x 2 cm). By convention, each element is assigned a score of 0 if absent or 2 if present, so the maximum total score is 10. Scores of 8 or 10 are considered normal. A score of 4 or 6 is suspicious, and a score of 2–3 is extremely suspicious. A score of 0–1 is ominous. The various elements of the BPP reflect different aspects of fetal well-being. Fetal breathing movements are normally observed during the second half of pregnancy, and are believed to be "practice" for extrauterine respiration. A fetus who is hypoxemic and acidemic will stop breathing. However, breathing may be absent for totally innocuous reasons such as fetal sleep or maternal medications or cigarette smoking. Fetal movements and tone are also lost when the fetus is hypoxemic and acidemic. Amniotic fluid volume diminishes with chronic fetal compromise, as renal blood flow is diminished by hypotension and reflex vasoconstriction. The BPP, by evaluating a number of different markers, does not rely on a single indicator of fetal compromise.

Because the BPP is more time-consuming than the NST, many centers use the NST as a screening test and the BPP as a confirmatory test of fetal jeopardy. In addition, a number of investigators have found that the use of two elements of the BPP, the NST plus amniotic fluid volume, is particularly useful in evaluating prolonged pregnancies. When either or both of these is worrisome, the remainder of the BPP can be completed.

Another ultrasound technique being explored as a means of assessing fetal well-being is *Doppler velocimetry*. Special ultrasound equipment utilizes the Doppler principle to detect the flow of blood through fetal or maternal vessels, or both, most commonly the umbilical artery. Some fetuses will manifest reversal of diastolic flow, which suggests hypoperfusion and vaso-constriction. If it can be demonstrated that assessment of blood flow offers a significant benefit in diagnosing fetal compromise, Doppler velocimetry may someday become a part of our armamentarium for antepartum fetal assessment.

Fetal Activity Determinations

A pregnant woman perceives most of the fetus's gross body movements. A fetus whose condition is deteriorating will frequently become less active for some time prior to death. It is common for mothers whose fetuses die to report that days of fetal inactivity were present before the death. Many studies have utilized maternal counting of movements as an "early warning system" for fetal compromise. Typically mothers are instructed to keep a diary of the number of hours it takes to experience 10 fetal movements each day. If more than 12 hours elapse, or there is a significant decrease in movements from the established pattern, the mother is instructed to come in for more formal antepartum testing by NST, CST, or BPP. Other approaches include the counting of fetal movements for an hour each day, with further testing if a considerable reduction is noted. Using historic controls, one study of maternal "kick counting" demonstrated a significantly lower rate of stillbirths. Two randomized trials reported conflicting results regarding the value of fetal movement determinations. The approach costs nothing except for the additional testing generated, and most studies demonstrate that 5 percent or fewer patients require further testing. At the very least, fetal activity determinations offer relatively inexpensive reassurance that the fetus is in good condition. Many obstetricians recommend daily kick counting for all pregnant women, but the benefits of such a recommendation are not yet clear.

Biochemical Determinations

Prior to the widespread availability of the above-described biophysical means of antepartum testing, a number of substances were measured in an attempt to detect existing or impending fetal compromise. The measurement of serum or urinary estriol levels on a daily basis is described in Chap. 9, and has now been abandoned because of its high expense and poor predictive value. Measurements of human placental lactogen have likewise not proven useful. At one time the measurement of heat-stable alkaline phosphatase, originating in the placenta, was also investigated and found to have inadequate discriminatory value. Currently there are no biochemical tests of fetal well-being that are considered useful except under very unusual circumstances, such as estrogen measurements to diagnose placental sulfatase deficiency (see Chap. 9).

Assessing Fetal Lung Maturity

Most of the major complications associated with premature birth are related to the *respiratory distress syndrome* (RDS). For this reason it is axiomatic that pregnancies should be allowed to progress to term, and elective premature delivery is not practiced. However, some pregnancies are complicated and the obstetrician is faced with weighing the alternatives of premature delivery with possible RDS as opposed to continuing the pregnancy with the possibility of continuing maternal or fetal compromise and deterioration. In such circumstances it may be useful to estimate the likelihood of RDS developing if the pregnancy is delivered. This syndrome is believed to be due to a deficiency of surfactant, a group of chemicals that stabilize the alveoli so that they do not completely collapse after each exhalation. Surfactant production by lung cells called *type II pneumocytes* increases in a maturational process. The timing of this process is such that RDS becomes less and less likely until approximately 35 to 36 weeks' gestation, when most fetuses produce adequate amounts of surfactant. Although the recent development of artificial surfactants, which can be administered to the neonate at risk for prematurity, has diminished the danger of RDS to a certain extent, it is better not to deliver a baby at high risk for RDS if possible.

Many tests for chemicals and objects in the amniotic fluid have been developed to help assess the likelihood of RDS. Lecithin, a major component of surfactant, is quantified by measuring its ratio to sphingomyelin; this is the *L-S ratio*. Sphingomyelin is present in relatively constant amounts, and the use of a ratio allows the lecithin measurement to be standardized for varying amniotic fluid volumes that would cause dilution or concentration. If the L-S ratio in amniotic fluid is ≥ 2, the chance of RDS is less than 2 percent. However, the fetus whose L-S ratio is "mature" may still develop RDS if hypoxia or acidemia, or both, occur during the perinatal period. It is only after the appearance of phosphatidylglycerol (PG) in the amniotic fluid that surfactant production is stabilized against intervening insults. Thus, in many centers, PG is measured in the amniotic fluid when maturity testing is needed. Immunologic test kits are widely available for this determination. Respiratory distress syndrome is quite unlikely when the L-S ratio is mature and PG is absent, unless the fetus or neonate is challenged by "asphyxia." Other tests of fetal lung maturity rely on the physical properties of surfactant. Thus the "shake test" and "foam stability index" make use of the fact that when an ethanol solution is mixed with amniotic fluid and shaken, the small bubbles that form will not break down rapidly if surfactant is present in adequate amounts to prevent RDS.

Recommended Reading

American College of Obstetricians and Gynecologists. Intrapartum fetal monitoring. *ACOG Technical Bulletin.* No. 132, Sept., 1989.

Freeman, R. K., Garite, T. J., and Nageotte, M. P. *Fetal Heart Rate Monitoring* (2nd ed.). Baltimore: Williams & Wilkins, 1991.

Gabbe, S. G. Antepartum Fetal Evaluation. In S. G. Gabbe, J. R. Niebyl, and J. L. Simpson (eds.), *Obstetrics: Normal and Problem Pregnancies* (2nd ed.). New York: Churchill-Livingstone, 1991. Pp. 377–424.

Petrie, R. H. Intrapartum Fetal Evaluation. In S. G. Gabbe, J. R. Niebyl, and J. L. Simpson (eds.), *Obstetrics: Normal and Problem Pregnancies* (2nd ed.). New York: Churchill-Livingstone, 1991. Pp. 457–491.

17

Labor: Normal and Dysfunctional

Carol A. Wheeler

Parturition, labor, and childbirth are all terms used to describe the complex process involved in the transition from intrauterine to extrauterine life. The anatomic and physiologic changes that occur in the human female for prevention, preparation, and occurrence of this event are not nearly as well understood as they are in various animal species. Timing of this process is critical in order to ensure survival of the newborn.

Pelvic Anatomy and Uterine Function

In order for delivery to be accomplished, the fetus must negotiate the bony and ligamentous walls of the maternal pelvis. During pregnancy, there is hormonally mediated relaxation of the ligaments and joints interconnecting these bones to allow for easier fetal passage.

Generally speaking, there are four types of female pelvic structures that have certain characteristics and diameters. The specific anatomic parts assessed in the clinical evaluation or clinical pelvimetry of the pelvis are the inlet, sacrum, sacrosciatic notch, sidewalls, ischial spines, and pubic arch. Although the current obstetric practice dictates a trial of labor regardless of the pelvic type or size, clinical pelvimetry is still performed as part of the initial obstetric examination. At that time a determination is made as to the type of pelvis and its adequacy for the passage of the fetus. Most female pelves are a combination of one or more of the types of pelves and can be described as such.

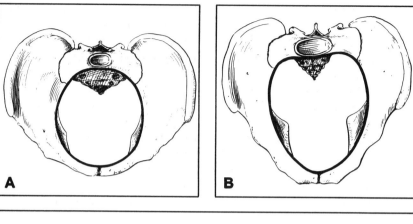

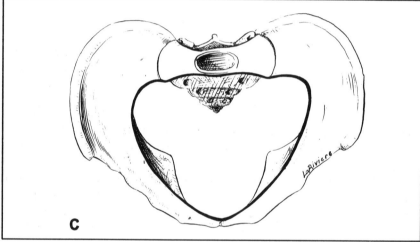

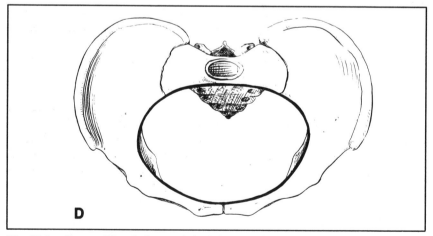

Fig. 17-1. Types of female bony pelvis. (A) Gynecoid. (B) Anthropoid. (C) Android. (D) Platypelloid.

The four types of female pelves are the gynecoid, anthropoid, android, and platypelloid (Fig. 17-1). The gynecoid pelvis is known as the true female pelvis and occurs in approximately 42 percent of the United States population. It is ideal for vaginal birth of an average-weight fetus. An anthropoid pelvis is more common in the nonwhite population. The shape of this pelvis allows for posterior positioning of the fetal head and can be adequate for a vaginal birth. The android pelvis is known as the male pelvis because it occurs more frequently in men than in women. Since the pelvic inlet is heart-shaped, the posterior sagittal diameter is short. This shape allows for very little room posteriorly for the fetal head. In addition, the pelvic sidewalls generally converge, creating a funnel shape. The platypelloid (flat) pelvis often is not adequate for a vaginal delivery. It has a very short anteroposterior diameter and a very wide transverse diameter. This pelvic type occurs in less than 3 percent of the population.

The uterus itself is composed of a corpus and a cervix. The corpus can be divided into three layers: serosa, myometrium, and endometrium (decidua). The myometrium and cervix play crucial roles in the labor process. The myometrium is composed of two-thirds smooth muscle cells in two spirals and one-third matrix of collagen and glycosaminoglycans. The uterus increases in size from a prepregnancy weight of 50 g to approximately 1000 g at term. This increase in size occurs primarily by cellular hypertrophy and to a lesser extent by cell division. Because of this extensive stretching and the tendency towards contraction by the smooth muscle, it is amazing that a pregnancy is maintained.

Cellular contact zones, or gap junctions, appear at the onset of labor and serve as a communication mechanism between adjacent cells (Fig. 17-2). Electrical and chemical signals transmitted through these gap junctions ensure an orderly and coordinated contraction. Formation of these gap junctions is promoted by estrogen and prostaglandins but is inhibited by progesterone. Gap junctions are found in the myometrium in both normal and preterm labor and inhibition of their synthesis may be important in preventing labor onset.

The actual uterine contraction involves the interaction of the proteins actin and myosin. This interaction is initiated by the phosphorylation of myosin light chain, which is regulated by a calcium-modulated protein kinase. Cyclic adenosine monophosphate (cAMP), which reduces calcium ion availability by stimulating Ca^{2+} uptake into cellular organelles and lowering free Ca^{2+}, leads to uterine relaxation. Therefore, drugs that stimulate cAMP production and lower Ca^{2+}, such as ß-adrenergic agonists, will cause uterine relaxation. Myosin light-chain kinase is inactivated by its own phosphorylation and this also leads to relaxation.

$$\text{Myosin light chain} \xrightarrow[\substack{\text{kinase} \\ (Ca^{2+} \text{ activated})}]{} \text{Phosphorylated myosin light chain} + \text{Actin}$$

$$\longrightarrow \text{Phosphorylated actomyosin}$$

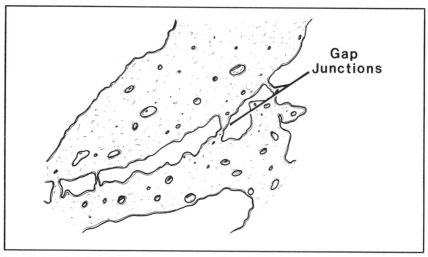

Fig. 17-2. Gap junctions between myometrial cells are utilized for intercellular communication.

The nerve supply to the uterus is controlled by the presacral ganglia that mediate pain, but the uterus also contains autonomous adrenergic ganglionic cells. This adrenergic innervation is increased by estrogen and decreases during pregnancy. The decidua is richly vascularized with spiral arteries and venous lakes. It provides a critical separation of the placenta and fetal membranes from the myometrium. The decidua also secretes prolactin, prostaglandins, and relaxin.

The cervix is composed of smooth muscle (6–25 percent) in a collagen and glycosaminoglycan matrix. Biochemical changes known as cervical ripening occur by gradual breaking and proteolysis of the collagen fibers. These changes lead to increased flexibility and stretchability of the cervix to permit dilatation. This process is promoted by relaxin, estrogen, and prostaglandins. Effacement of the cervix, which occurs prior to or in the early stages of labor, involves a shortening of the cervical length due to muscular action pulling cervical tissue up into the lower uterine segment (Fig. 17-3).

Endocrine Physiology of Labor

There are many factors leading to the onset of labor. Progesterone withdrawal leads to menstruation in humans, yet there is no solid evidence to link progesterone withdrawal with the onset of human labor. This lack of evidence for many years has frustrated researchers who have attempted to explain human labor by this mechanism. Other agents are therefore critical and must be explored. Oxytocin clearly stimulates labor; this may be

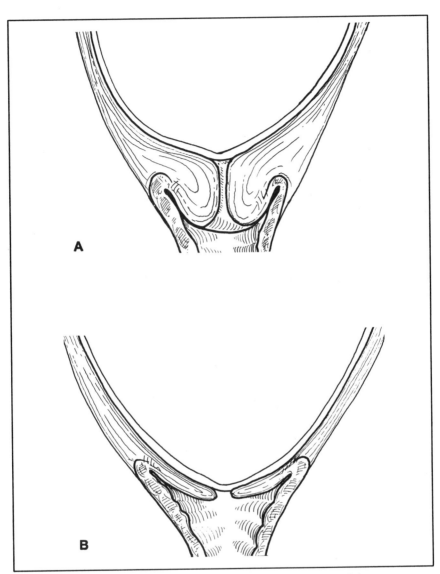

Fig. 17-3. Effacement of the cervix. (A) Noneffaced cervix prior to labor.
(B) Effaced cervix.

related to an 80-fold increase in myometrial oxytocin receptors without an
increase in endogenous secretion.

Oxytocin is secreted in spurts so that evaluation of its secretion rate is
difficult. The fetus secretes oxytocin as well (umbilical artery levels are
twice umbilical vein levels) and this secretion may play a part. It is unknown, however, if oxytocin is important in the initiation of labor or if it
acts in a secondary mechanism.

Prostaglandins are effective agents for the pharmacologic initiation of labor and may play an important physiologic role as well. Very small amounts of $PGF_{2-\alpha}$ are needed to induce labor and this amount is easily formed in myometrial tissue. The amnion and chorion secrete primarily PGE_2 while the decidua preferentially produces $PGF_{2-\alpha}$. Prostaglandin synthetase inhibitors such as indomethacin can delay the onset of labor and have been used to arrest preterm labor. Oxytocin and prostaglandins may work together, in that oxytocin may stimulate prostaglandin production by the decidua.

Two main groups of endogenous substances may act to cause uterine relaxation. Catecholamines (primarily epinephrine) and relaxin (an ovarian hormone also secreted by the decidua and placenta) may play a role in maintenance of the uterus in a resting state and prevention of preterm delivery.

Other hormones of possible importance in labor include estrogens, which stimulate the formation of gap junctions, oxytocin receptors, and beta-adrenergic receptors. Estrogens also increase prostaglandin synthesis. Cortisol plays a role in sheep with a rise just prior to labor, but this is not seen in humans. Glucocorticoids do, however, help mature the fetal lung in the human.

These considerations have led to the use of various agents for tocolysis (inhibition of labor). Magnesium sulfate inhibits calcium influx into myometrial cells and therefore prevents the action of myosin light-chain kinase. Beta-adrenergic agonists stimulate cAMP generation and lead to inactivation of the kinase enzyme as well as lowering intracellular free Ca^{2+}. Ethanol, although not used clinically any longer due to side effects, inhibits oxytocin release and may interfere with calcium transport. Prostaglandin synthetase inhibitors, as mentioned previously, decrease the production of prostaglandins as potent stimulators of contractions. Calcium channel blockers are potentially useful for tocolysis since they inhibit entry of calcium through the cell membrane, although their clinical use has been limited due to concerns over fetal effects (Table 17-1).

Course of Labor

Labor is defined as regular uterine contractions leading to progressive cervical change. This cervical change begins as ripening (softening of the cervix) and continues as effacement (shortening of the cervix) that is often simultaneous with dilatation. In addition to these changes, a process of fetal descent through the birth canal occurs, generally simultaneously.

These changes of labor have classically been divided into three stages. The first stage of labor begins from the time of onset of regular contractions to the time of complete cervical dilatation (corresponding to 10 cm). This stage is subdivided into a latent phase and an active phase. The active phase is further divided into an acceleration phase, a phase of maximum slope, and a deceleration phase.

Table 17-1.   Classes of tocolytics

Compound	Mechanism of action
Magnesium sulfate	Inhibits calcium influx
β-adrenergic agonists	Stimulate cyclic adenosine monophosphate generation
	Lower intracellular Ca^{2+}
Ethanol	Inhibits oxytocin release
Prostaglandin synthetase inhibitors	Decrease the production of prostaglandins
Calcium channel blockers	Inhibit Ca^{2+} entry into cells

The second stage of labor begins with complete cervical dilatation and ends with the expulsion of the entire fetus. The third stage begins after delivery of the baby ends with expulsion of the placenta and the membranes (Fig. 17-4).

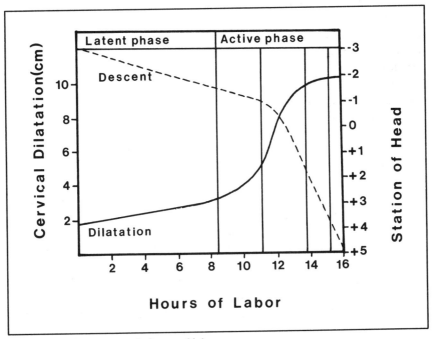

Fig. 17-4.   The stages and phases of labor.

During the first stage of labor, the latent phase, which averages 8 to 12 hours in nulliparas and 6 to 8 hours in multiparas, may normally last up to 20 hours and 14 hours, respectively. The latent phase is variable in length depending on many factors such as sedation and oxytocic agents. The cervix effaces and dilates up to approximately 3 cm during the latent phase. Active-phase labor generally begins at about 3 cm and consists of contractions usually every 3 to 5 minutes lasting approximately 1 minute. Once active phase has been reached, the cervix should dilate at least 1.2 cm per hour in the primigravida and 1.5 cm per hour in the multigravida.

Concomitant with cervical dilatation is descent of the fetus. Prior to labor the presenting part may be floating, that is, at or above the pelvic inlet, especially in multiparas. Station, or position of the presenting part (generally the head) is defined by its relationship to the ischial spines. *Engagement* is when the biparietal diameter of the fetal head has passed the pelvic inlet, which occurs when the presenting part is at the level of the spines, or at 0 station. The pelvis then can be divided by centimeters above and below the spines, such that at above 0 station the head is unengaged and at +5 station the presenting part is at the perineum. These are important clinical criteria based on serial vaginal examinations used to evaluate labor progress (Fig. 17-5).

Obviously, not all fetuses enter the delivery process in the same manner. The fetal "lie" is the relationship of the long axis of the fetus with the

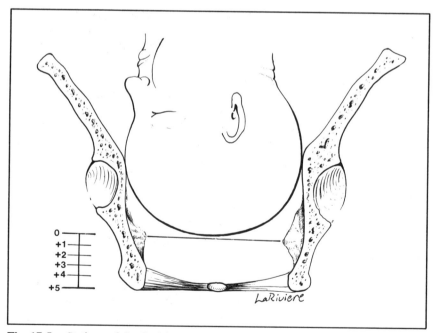

Fig. 17-5. Stations of the fetal head.

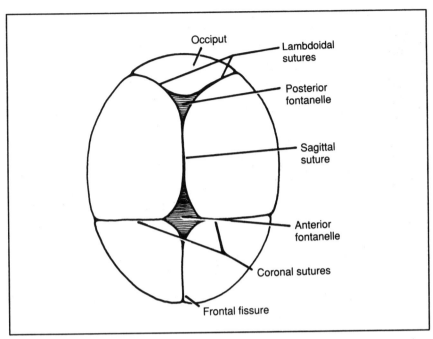

Fig. 17-6.   Diagram of the fetal head, superior view, indicating the major landmarks.

mother; it is either longitudinal, transverse, or oblique. A transverse lie may be further described as the fetal back being up—toward the maternal head in the uterine fundus—or back down at the pelvic brim. Both transverse and oblique lies are considered abnormal lies in labor.

The *presentation* is the part of the fetal body that is first in the birth canal and is generally felt on vaginal examination. Presentation, in order of decreasing frequency, may be fetal vertex (occiput), breech (buttocks), face, shoulder, compound (an extremity along with the presenting part), or brow. Breeches are further subdivided into frank (buttocks only); full, or complete (buttocks and feet); and footling (single or double).

The *position* of the presenting part is defined in relationship to the maternal pelvis. The sutures and fontanelles of the fetal skull are palpated and used as landmarks to describe the position in the occiput presentation. The saggital suture runs in an anterior-posterior direction and serves to guide the examiner to the fontanelles. The junction of the occipital to the parietal bones is at the posterior fontanelle. This is the smaller and more triangular of the two fontanelles and is used as the landmark for position. The larger, anterior fontanelle is diamond shaped (Fig. 17-6). Positions are labelled left occiput anterior (the occiput is in the left anterior portion of the maternal pelvis); left occiput posterior; left occiput transverse; right occiput anterior, etc.

The cardinal movements of labor are the positional changes that a fetus must accomplish in order to be born. *Engagement* usually occurs with the sagittal suture directed transversely or obliquely and occurs prior to labor in most primigravidas. *Descent* of the fetus occurs because of fundal pressure on the breech due to contraction of the abdominal muscles and straightening of the fetal body. When the descending head encounters resistance on the pelvic floor, it begins to flex so that the chin is brought closer to the thorax and the head presents to a smaller diameter for passage through the pelvis.

If *flexion* fails to occur, the fetus may have difficulty negotiating the pelvis. The position of the head in this situation is called *military position* or in extreme cases of failed flexion, hyperextension (Fig. 17-7). *Internal rotation* involves turning of the fetal head to a position with the occiput located anteriorly or posteriorly. Following internal rotation, the head reaches the perineum and *extends* to permit passage through the vulva. Following delivery of the head, it *restitutes,* or *externally rotates,* to return to the transverse position, probably because the shoulders assume an anterior-posterior orientation in the pelvis. Soon thereafter, expulsion of the fetal body occurs, completing the second stage of labor. Thus, the cardinal movements of labor are descent, flexion, internal rotation, extension, and restitution, or external rotation (Fig. 17-8).

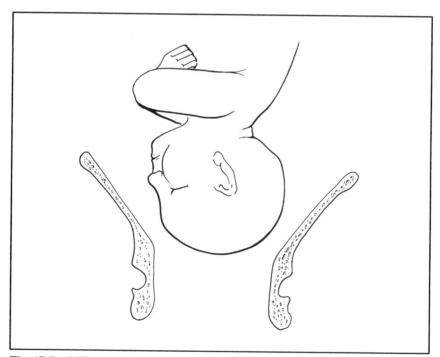

Fig. 17-7. Military position of the fetal head.

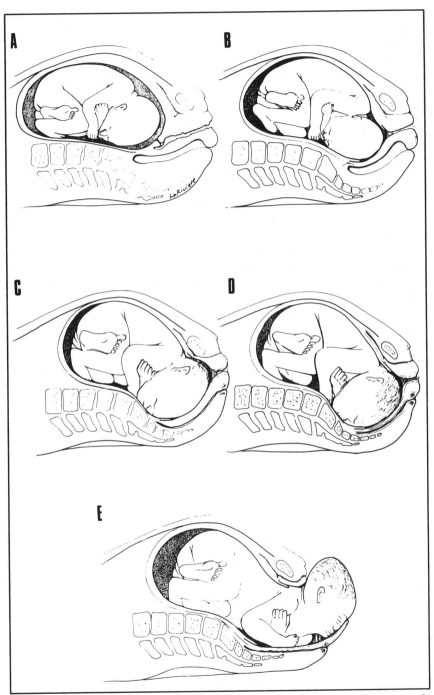

Fig. 17-8. The cardinal movements of labor. (A) Floating head prior to the onset of labor. (B) Descent. (C) Flexion. (D) Internal rotation. (E) Extension.   *(Continued)*

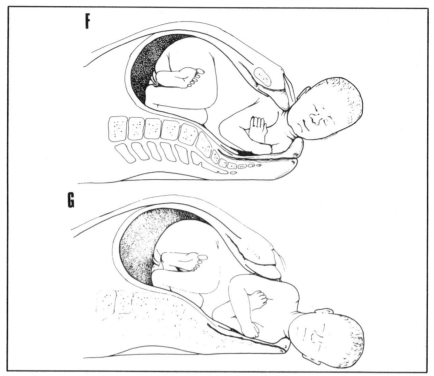

Fig. 17-8. *(Continued)* (F) External rotation. (G) Expulsion.

Dystocia, difficult or abnormal labor, occurs when there is a problem with the "powers, the passenger, or the pelvis." Problems with the "powers," or contractions, exist when the contractions are of inadequate duration, frequency, or strength for cervical dilatation or descent. These problems may occur for a number of reasons, but some of these include overdistention of the uterus from twins, excess amniotic fluid, or a multiparous uterus. The second group of dystocias relate to the "passenger," or fetus. Abnormalities such as breech presentation, transverse lie, persistent occiput transverse position, or an excessively large (macrosomic) or anomalous fetus may all interfere with the normal progress of labor. Lastly, maternal pelvic contracture may prevent the normal progress of the mechanisms of labor. This type of contracture may be due to genetics, pelvic injury, or, years ago, to childhood rickets.

One method of evaluating labor progress is by plotting a graph of the patient's progress, or a labor curve (Fig. 17-9). This graph depicts both cervical dilatation and fetal descent and may be compared to population averages. One of the most common causes of dystocia is a prolonged latent phase, greater than 20 hours in a primigravida or greater than 14 hours in a multipara; this may in fact represent false labor or be related to excess analgesia or anesthesia. The woman may be treated with narcotic sedation to permit a 6- to 10-hour rest. If this has been false labor, it will resolve. A majority of patients will awaken in the active phase. Prolonged latent phase does not necessarily signify that vaginal delivery will be difficult, and is not an indication for cesarean section.

During the active phase one can see protraction and arrest disorders. Protraction of dilatation occurs when the slope of cervical dilatation is less than 1.2 cm per hour in the nullipara or less than 1.5 cm per hour in the parous patient. Protraction of descent occurs when descent is < 1 cm per hour in the nullipara or < 2 cm per hour in the parous patient during the second stage.

As long as contractions are adequate and slow progress continues, no intervention should occur in a protraction disorder. A secondary arrest of dilatation exists when there is no cervical change over a period of 1 hour, although many clinicians will wait a second hour for confirmation. A secondary arrest of dilatation may be due to cephalopelvic disproportion and, if so, should be treated by cesarean section. A similar picture exists with arrest of descent, where despite adequate contractions and complete cervical dilatation, there is failure of the presenting part to progress through the birth canal. In either arrest disorder, if contractions are not adequate in frequency or strength, oxytocin administration may lead to progress. Excess analgesia or anesthesia may interfere with maternal expulsive efforts and may lead to arrest of descent. Allowing excess anesthesia to wear off may allow for progress. If these measures fail to lead to progress, cesarean section will be necessary.

Precipitate labor is when labor is excessively rapid. Precipitate dilatation is greater than 5 cm per hour in a primigravida or greater than 10 cm per

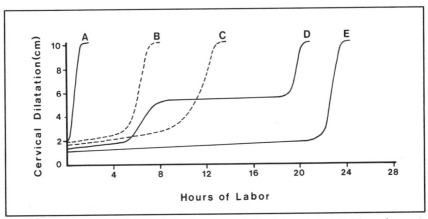

Fig. 17-9.   Normal and abnormal labor curves. *A.* Precipitate labor. *B.* Normal multiparous labor. *C.* Normal primigravida labor. *D.* Secondary arrest of dilatation. *E.* Prolonged latent phase.

hour in a multipara. It may also be defined as total labor of less than 3 hours. No treatment is generally necessary but the physician must be aware that the patient is at increased risk for postpartum excessive bleeding.

Rupture of the fetal membranes may happen at any time prior to or during the course of labor and delivery. Rupture is accompanied by a sudden gush of generally clear and colorless liquid of variable amounts. Fluid that is dark or greenish in color may indicate the presence of meconium stool passage by the fetus and may be a sign of fetal stress or distress. Meconium passage is fairly common, particularly in term and postterm pregnancies, and does not always indicate a problem. Artificial rupture of the membranes may be performed by the caregiver and will allow placement of internal monitoring devices of the fetal heart rate and contractions. Premature rupture of the membranes occurs anytime prior to the onset of labor and preterm rupture of the membranes occurs prior to 37 completed weeks' gestation. Rupture of the membranes more than 24 hours before delivery is called *prolonged rupture of the membranes* and is of concern because of the increased risk of infection.

Electronic fetal monitoring became generally accepted in the 1970s as a way to evaluate the fetus during labor. It may be performed externally by placing gauges and small ultrasound devices on the maternal abdomen, or internally by using a small electrode attached to the fetal head and a catheter inside the uterus to measure contractions. It is unclear whether electronic monitoring has actually improved fetal or maternal outcome over careful monitoring by a trained individual performing intermittent auscultation. For low-risk patients, an alternative approach is auscultation of the fetal heart rate during, and for 30 seconds after, a contraction at least every 30 minutes during the first stage of labor and every 15 minutes during the second stage. More frequent intervals are recommended for high-risk patients. Most labor and delivery suites are unable to provide one-on-one attendants, however, and therefore electronic fetal monitoring is practical and useful. All data from these monitor strips should be carefully evaluated and interpreted by an individual who is knowledgeable in their use.

Patient Care in Labor

Management of the patient in labor should have two main goals—comfort and safety. A low-risk mother and fetus may be followed with minimal intervention if labor is progressing normally. An initial evaluation of medical and prenatal history should be obtained. Vital signs and a brief physical examination including a vaginal examination should be performed. An assessment of the status of the fetal membranes should be made based on the history and examination. If the patient is experiencing bleeding that is heavy, a placenta previa should be ruled out before a vaginal examination is performed.

The vaginal examination should include a rapid clinical evaluation of the adequacy of the pelvis, as well as the presentation, position (if possible), dilatation, effacement, and station. This examination is performed in an aseptic manner by inserting two gloved examining fingers into the vagina and advancing toward the fetal presenting part. If any problems arise in this initial evaluation, further procedures such as ultrasound may be indicated. The fetal heart should be auscultated, preferably during and after a contraction, and auscultation should be repeated at intervals if no electronic monitoring will be employed. An assessment of uterine contractions should be made either by palpation or electronic monitoring. Frequency, duration, and strength of contractions should all be noted.

During the early stages of labor, the mother may remain ambulatory if everything is progressing normally. She may have small amounts of clear liquids but should avoid solid foods because of concern over aspiration if vomiting occurs. An intravenous line may be started if the patient needs hydration or will receive analgesia or anesthesia.

Repeat auscultation or evaluation of the fetal heart rate should be performed approximately every 15 minutes. The vaginal examination interval will vary depending on the stage of labor. Examinations may be as frequent as hourly in the active phase and second stage in order to accurately assess progress. Too frequent examinations, however, may lead to an increased risk of infection and may be uncomfortable for the patient.

Anesthesia and analgesia should be provided as the patient requests. Maternal response to labor can have an impact on the progress of labor. It is believed that the greater the mother's anxiety, the greater the amount of catecholamine release, which then may impede the progress of labor. Analgesia or anesthesia may help block catecholamine release and may be indicated during labor for some patients. Emotional support from family and close friends may be all that is necessary in other situations. The goal when labor is progressing normally is to avoid excess interference in this personal and intimate experience.

Recommended Reading

American College of Obstetrics and Gynecology. Intrapartum fetal heart rate monitoring. *ACOG Technical Bulletin*. No. 132, Sept., 1989.

Cunningham, F. G., MacDonald, P. C., Gant, N. F., Leveno, K. J., and Gilstrap, L. C. III. *Williams Obstetrics* (19th ed.). Norwalk: Appleton & Lange, 1993. Pp. 363–394.

Friedman, E. A. *Labor: Clinical Evaluation and Management* (2nd ed.). New York: Appleton, 1978.

Gabbe, S. G., Niebyl, J. R., and Simpson, J. L. (eds.). *Obstetrics: Normal and Problem Pregnancies* (2nd ed.). New York: Churchill-Livingstone, 1991. Pp. 147–174. Pp. 427–456.

18

Birth

Cydney I. Afriat and Donald R. Coustan

The culmination of labor, a process described in Chapter 17, is the birth of the fetus and placenta. The cardinal movements of the fetal head are descent, flexion, internal rotation, extension, and restitution/external rotation. This chapter describes the mechanisms and methods by which vaginal delivery and cesarean section are accomplished.

Much attention has been focused in recent years on the increasing cesarean section rate in the United States. Thirty years ago typical cesarean section rates were 5 percent or less, whereas currently more than 20 percent of American babies are delivered abdominally. The reasons usually given for this rising cesarean rate are numerous, and include the improved safety of abdominal surgery, increasing prevalence of the diagnosis of "dystocia" (usually taken to mean lack of vaginal delivery after an abnormal labor), and a prevailing view that difficult forceps deliveries and breech deliveries under all but ideal circumstances should be avoided. The widespread use of electronic fetal monitoring also has been linked to increasing cesarean section rates. This connection has not been proven unequivocally, since it is also likely that cesarean sections previously performed for ausculted fetal bradycardia may be avoided by continuous observation of fetal heart rate patterns. The desire to avoid professional liability for adverse fetal outcomes also has been cited frequently, as well as the widespread misperception that obstetricians receive higher fees for cesarean than vaginal deliveries. In fact, most third-party payors compensate similarly for either type of delivery. Nevertheless, it is true that the amount of time and anxiety required to manage labor with vaginal deliveries is greater than that involved in performing a cesarean. Finally, the increasing rate of primary cesarean sections has led inevitably to an increase in the number of repeat cesarean sections, particularly when the dictum "once a cesarean, always a cesarean" is followed.

It appears that cesarean section rates in the United States have leveled off in the low– to mid–20 percent range. Professional organizations such as the American College of Obstetricians and Gynecologists have strongly recommended attempted vaginal birth after cesarean section, and hospital quality assurance efforts have focused increased attention on cesarean deliveries. Patients are becoming more aware of these issues, and with increased education has come a willingness to try for vaginal birth after a previous cesarean. It is to be hoped that patients will also be educated to view a cesarean section not as an "easy way out," but as an operation that is appropriate only under specific circumstances. No "ideal" cesarean section rate has yet been established, but an achievable goal would be that each cesarean section be clinically indicated.

Hand Maneuvers for Birth

Despite the controversy noted above, most babies are born vaginally. The beginning medical student or house officer is bound to be insecure as to how to "perform" his or her first few deliveries. Specific movements of the hands for the birth of the infant are described to help the reader to provide a safe, atraumatic birth for the mother and infant. These maneuvers are designed to facilitate and occur in synchrony with the cardinal movements, and to provide security in handling the baby. Variations of these hand maneuvers exist and most are very effective. An example of the sequence of hand maneuvers is shown in Figs. 1 through 9.

As the presenting part of the baby is crowning in the occiput anterior (OA) position (Fig. 18-1), the birth attendant may be standing to one side or the other. The pads of the fingers of one hand of the birth attendant are placed on the anterior aspect of the presenting vertex, to assist the fetus in flexion. The fingertips should not slip inside the vagina, as this may cause lacerations. As more of the fetal head appears, the fingers spread to encompass the head. Controlled pressure should be exerted, but not so much that it impedes the birth process (Fig. 18-2).

Many clinicians believe the perineum must be "supported" simultaneously with the birth of the head in order to prevent perineal tears or extension of the episiotomy. If necessary, the clinician's remaining hand is covered by a sterile towel to prevent the hand from being contaminated by fecal matter and then it is placed against the perineum. The thumb is placed in the crease of the groin on one side and the middle finger is placed on the opposite groin. Pressure is applied downward and inward toward the perineal body. Throughout this process, the perineum is closely observed for signs of tearing.

As the head is delivering, the birth attendant's hand on the fetal head assists it in extending (Fig. 18-3) in order to bring the baby's face and chin

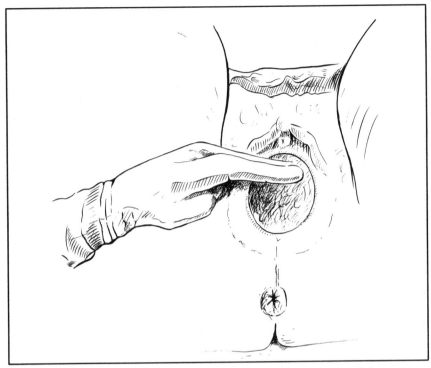

Fig. 18-1.   Hand maneuvers. The baby's head is beginning to crown and the attendant's hand is used to assist the vertex in flexion.

across the curve of Carus, an imaginary line defining the curvature of the birth canal. At this point, the towel is dropped and the birth attendant's fingertips examine the baby's neck for evidence of a nuchal loop of umbilical cord. If one is present and tight, it is clamped with two clamps and then cut between them (Fig. 18-4). If it is a loose nuchal cord, it can be lifted gently over the fetal head. Then the child's nose and mouth are suctioned with a bulb syringe. If meconium is present in the amniotic fluid, a De Lee suction apparatus connected to a mechanical or wall suction device is used to aspirate the fluid from the baby's alimentary canal in order to lessen the likelihood of meconium aspiration.

While waiting for the next contraction, it is instructive to watch the baby's head restitute/externally rotate to realign with the shoulders. The clinician then should adjust to either the mother's right (if the fetus rotated to right occiput transverse [ROA-ROT]0 or left side (if the fetus rotated left occiput anterior–left occiput transverse [LOA-LOT]). One of the clinician's hands is placed on each side of the baby's head, with the fingers pointed toward the baby's nose and the palmar surfaces over the ears (Fig. 18-5).

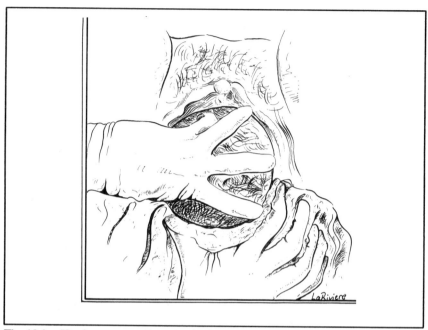

Fig. 18-2. Hand maneuvers. Crowning is almost completed. Attendant's left hand is controlling extension of the fetal head, while the right hand is supporting the perineum.

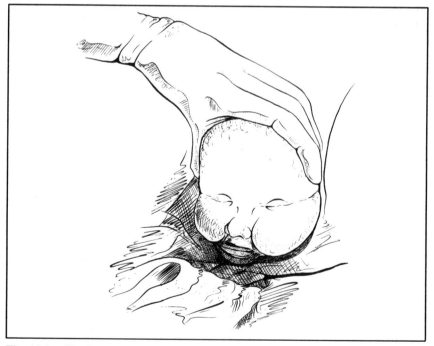

Fig. 18-3. Hand maneuvers. The head has delivered, and restitution has not yet occurred.

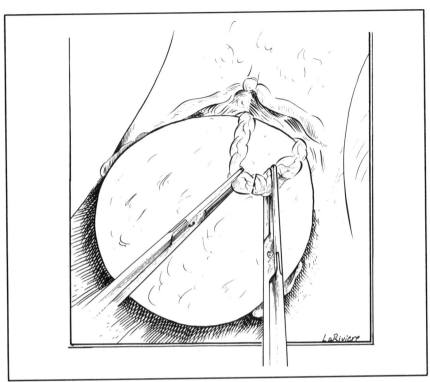

Fig. 18-4. Hand maneuvers. A tight nuchal cord was identified, so the birth attendant has placed two clamps and is about to cut the cord.

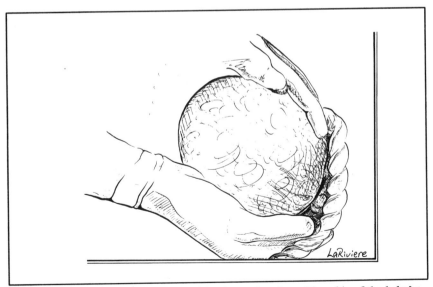

Fig. 18-5. Hand maneuvers. One hand has been placed on either side of the baby's head, and gentle downward traction is being applied.

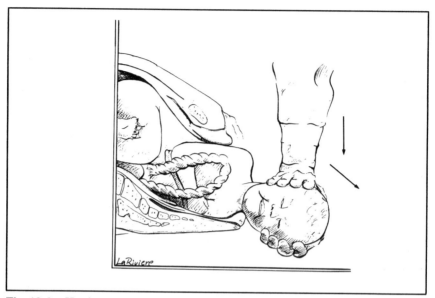

Fig. 18-6. Hand maneuvers. The anterior shoulder is born.

Care must be taken not to allow the hands to drift down to the infant's neck. Gentle downward pressure is then exerted until the anterior shoulder is born (Fig. 18-6). Then upward and outward pressure is placed on the side of the baby's head until the posterior shoulder is visible (Fig. 18-7).

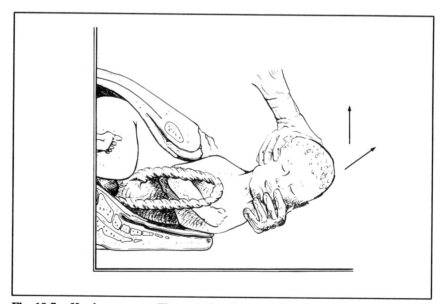

Fig. 18-7. Hand maneuvers. The posterior shoulder is born.

The movement actually lifts the baby's head towards the ceiling while the clinician watches the perineum. The birth attendant's bottom hand then slides down the baby's neck to the shoulder and elbow as they are born, in order to keep them from causing tears in the vagina and perineum. At this point the baby's upper torso is in the deliverer's bottom hand, the thumb of which is on the baby's back, while the rest of his or her fingers press the baby's arm to the body and the fingertips embrace the baby's chest (Fig. 18-8).

The clinician's top hand then slides down the baby's back and with the middle finger between the baby's legs, the legs are grasped as the entire infant is moved to a secure "football," or safety hold, leaving one hand free to clamp and cut the umbilical cord (Fig. 18-9). The baby's head is kept in a dependent position so that secretions can drain and further suctioning of secretion is accomplished.

One variation of these hand maneuvers involves standing in the middle facing the mother's head and placing the hands on either side of the baby's head with the fingertips directed at his or her neck. Caution must be used with this technique so as not to encircle the baby's neck, as this direct pressure can cause trauma to the child. A second variation is to place the infant directly on the mother's abdomen after birth by lateral flexion rather than placing the infant in a safety hold.

The speed of the birth is dependent on two factors: maternal effort and uterine contractions. In some situations, particularly with multiparous women, it is possible to slow the delivery process by coaching the woman to refrain from pushing with contractions and allowing the contraction

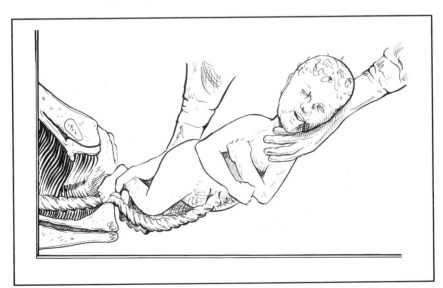

Fig. 18-8. Hand maneuvers. The birth attendant's left hand cradles the baby's shoulder, while the right hand slips down to the legs.

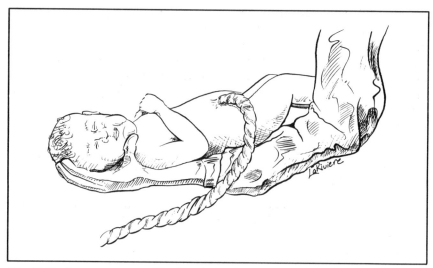

Fig. 18-9. Hand maneuvers. The "football hold."

itself to "expel" the infant or by having the woman push between contractions, which also will decrease the force of the expulsion. By diminishing the force behind the birth, greater control over the delivery can be effected, thus decreasing the chance of vaginal and perineal lacerations or extension of the episiotomy.

Delivery of the Placenta

The third stage of labor begins with the completed birth of the baby and ends with the birth of the placenta and membranes, which occurs in two phases. First is placental separation, followed by placental expulsion. The average length of time for the third stage of labor is 5 to 10 minutes. However, it can last as long as 30 minutes without necessitating intervention.

A combination of the dramatic decrease in the size of the uterine cavity and sustained uterine contractions cause placental separation following a brief respite after the birth of the baby. The decrease in uterine size causes the area of placental attachment to also decrease, with the placenta thus buckling and separating and descending into the lower uterine segment. The placenta then continues through the cervix and along the curve of Carus (the curvature of the pelvis) to complete expulsion.

The four traditional signs of placental separation include a sudden rush of blood, lengthening of the umbilical cord at the introitus, a change in the shape of the uterus from discoid to globular, and elevation of the uterus in the abdominal cavity. Maternal symptoms of placental separation may include cramping and contracting of the uterus and an urge to push.

The Brandt-Andrews maneuver, along with maternal effort, is used to deliver the placenta (Fig. 18-10). For this maneuver one of the birth attendant's hands is placed on a sterile drape suprapubically and pressure is exerted on the mother's lower uterine segment, not the fundus. The other hand then places gentle traction on the umbilical cord clamp in a downward fashion until the base of the placenta is visualized. Then gentle upward pressure is applied to the lower uterus by the hand on the abdomen. When the bulk of the placenta is seen, the hand on the abdomen moves under the placenta to catch it and gradually lower it into the placenta basin, enduring that all membranes are delivered as well.

The above described Brandt-Andrews technique is used to prevent inadvertent inversion of the uterus should the placenta still be partially attached to the uterine wall, For this reason, vigorous suprafundal pressure should be avoided. If, after 30 minutes, the placenta has not separated, a manual removal of the placenta may be required. If the fetal side of the placenta presents first it is called a *Schultz presentation*. If the maternal side of the placenta presents, it is referred to as a *Duncan presentation*. Most medical students learn the mnemonics "shiny Schultz" and "dirty Duncan."

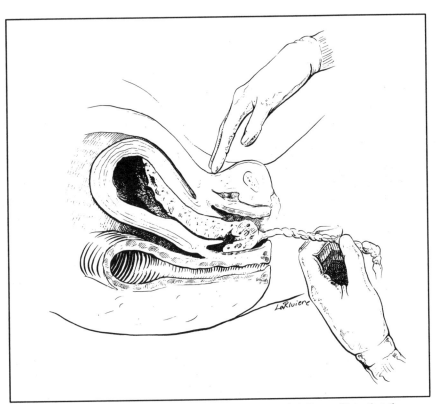

Fig. 18-10. The Brandt-Andrews maneuver for placental delivery. Note that the abdominal hand exerts upward pressure on the lower uterine segment, rather than suprafundal pressure.

Following its delivery, both maternal and fetal sides of the placenta, the membranes, and the cord are inspected to ensure that they are intact and complete. The uterus then will continue to contract, diminishing blood loss from the site of placental implantation. These "afterbirth pains," or cramps, can be more severe in multiparous women and often require analgesia during the postpartum recovery period.

Episiotomy

An epitiotomy is a surgical incision into the perineum to enlarge the vaginal orifice for the birth of the fetus. It is the most common operation in obstetrics and the subject of some controversy. Since births have moved from the home to the hospital, with a concomitant increase in episiotomies, the incidence of symptomatic cystocele, rectocele, uterine prolapse, and stress incontinence have apparently decreased. However, this decrease has not been statistically substantiated and has frequently been disputed by researchers. A few of the proposed reasons for performing an episiotomy in all parturients are that a clean surgical incision is easier to repair than a jagged laceration, it shortens the second stage of labor, it spares the fetal head from excessive pressure during the second stage, and it may spare the pelvic floor musculature. Arguments opposing routine episiotomy include maternal discomfort and the potential for later dyspareunia, extension to third- and fourth-degree lacerations, and that the depth of the episiotomy will most likely be greater than that of a spontaneous laceration.

An episiotomy is usually cut when the fetal head is crowning approximately 3 to 4 cm in diameter. At that point, the perineum is thinned sufficiently to tamponade small bleeding vessels. If the perineum is still thick, excessive bleeding could occur. The incision is made under local or some other form of anesthesia.

Two of the birth attendant's fingers are placed inside the mother's vagina with the knuckles against the fetal head and the front of the fingers facing the perineum (Fig. 18-11); this protects the fetus from inadvertent harm. With the clinician's fingers in place, a scissors is used to cut straight down toward the mother's rectum. One smooth cut is preferable to several snips, as they may cause a jagged edge. This is called a midline or median episiotomy and it cuts into the central tendinous point of the perineum, separating the two sides of the bulbocavernosus and superficial transverse perineal muscles.

A mediolateral episiotomy may be performed instead if concern exists that the midline episiotomy may extend into the rectum, for example in a woman who has a short perineum. The mediolateral episiotomy begins at the central tendinous point of the perineum, then extends laterally through the bulbocavernosus and the superficial and deep transverse perineal muscles, and into the pubococcygeus muscle. Lacerations or extensions into the rectum are highly unlikely with this type of episiotomy. However,

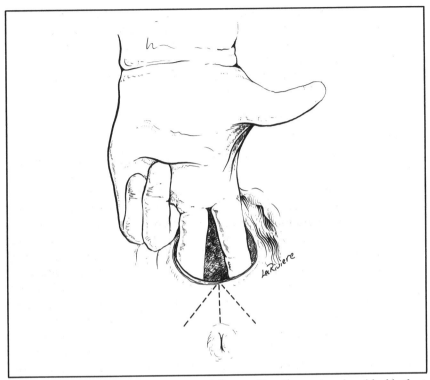

Fig. 18-11.   Preparation for cutting an episiotomy. Two fingers are placed inside the perineum to protect the fetal head. Middle dotted line shows placement of median episiotomy. Outside dotted lines depict paths of right mediolateral and left mediolateral episiotomy.

the potential exists for extention into the fatty tissue of the ischiorectal fossa, with a greater likelihood of significant bleeding and even hematoma or abscess formation. Generally, the healing process for this type of episiotomy presents more maternal discomfort and the potential for long-terms dyspareunia. Repair of the midline episiotomy is depicted in Fig. 18-12.

Lacerations of the birth canal are classified by their degree or depth. A first-degree laceration involves the fourchette, the perineal skin, and the vaginal mucous membranes. A second-degree laceration involves the above plus the fascia and muscles of the perineal body. A third-degree laceration extends into the anal sphincter. A fourth-degree laceration extends through the rectal mucosa to expose the lumen of the rectum.

Operative Delivery
Although the mechanisms of spontaneous delivery described above are applicable in most cases, situations arise from time to time wherein spon-

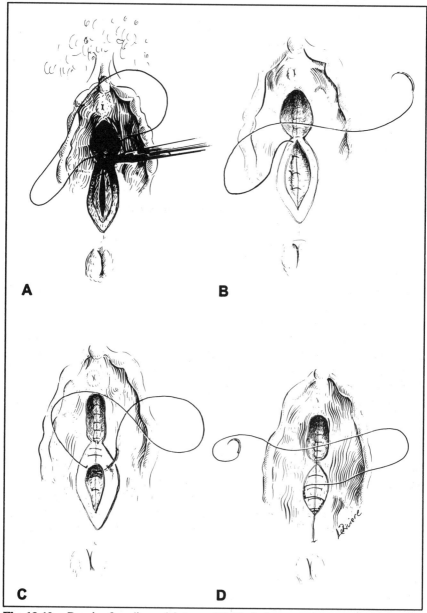

Fig. 18-12. Repair of median episiotomy. (A) Vaginal mucosa is sutured with a running, locking technique down to the hymeneal ring. (B) Interrupted stitches are used to approximate deep muscles of the perineum. (C) Running suture is used to close the perineal subcutaneous tissue. (D) Running subcuticular suture is used to close the perineal skin. When the suture is tightened the skin edges will approximate and no suture material will be visible.

taneous delivery is not possible or not desirable. In such situations obstetricians may find it necessary to perform an *operative vaginal delivery* (an *instrumental delivery* with obstetric forceps or vacuum extractor), or an *abdominal*, or *cesarean delivery*.

Operative Vaginal Delivery

Certain prerequisites are necessary before an instrumental vaginal delivery is performed. The presenting part of the fetus must be engaged in the maternal pelvis, the mother's cervix must be fully dilated, the membranes must have ruptured, the position of the fetal head must be known, there must be adequate analgesia, and the operator must be experienced, or be supervised by someone who is experienced. Obstetric forceps deliveries are classified according to the station of the fetal head when the instruments are applied. If the head is not engaged in the maternal pelvis, i.e., the presenting part is above 0 station (see Chap. 17 for a discussion of station of the presenting part), such an operation would be classified as a *high forceps* delivery and is considered absolutely contraindicated because under such circumstances it is impossible to predict whether the fetal head will fit through the mother's pelvis, and because the chance of injury to the fetus or mother is quite high.

If the head is engaged but the station is above +2 cm, the procedure is called a *midforceps* delivery. Midforceps are used only under unusual circumstances such as sudden severe fetal or maternal compromise; simultaneous preparations should be made for cesarean section in case the procedure is not successful.

Low forceps deliveries involve application of the forceps to a fetal head that is at least at +2 cm station but not all the way down to the pelvic floor. Low forceps deliveries are divided into those in which more than 45 degrees of rotation are required as opposed to those in which less than 45 degrees of rotation occur. Low forceps may be applied when spontaneous vaginal delivery has not occurred after an appropriately managed second stage. The American College of Obstetricians and Gynecologists suggests that consideration be given to low forceps delivery when the second stage has exceeded 2 hours in a nulliparous patient and 1 hour in a parous patient, in the absence of regional anesthesia. When regional anesthesia has been administered, an additional hour is generally added to the waiting time because of the belief that the anesthesia may decrease the urge to push and thus slow the descent of the fetal head. These are general guidelines, and certainly do not mandate the application of forceps after a given period of time. Other appropriate indications for low forceps delivery include "presumed fetal jeopardy," i.e., a nonreassuring fetal heart rate tracing, and the occasional situation in which maternal indications exist. Examples would include the necessity to avoid the Valsalva maneuver in patients with certain cardiovascular or cerebrovascular problems.

Finally, *outlet forceps* deliveries are those in which the fetal head is on the perineum with caput, or fetal scalp, showing at the introitus without the operator having to spread the labia apart. To be classified as an outlet forceps application, the fetal head must be in the direct OA or OP, or LOA or ROA position, so that forceps rotation of the head does not exceed 45 degrees. In addition to the same indications described for low forceps, outlet forceps may be applied electively in order to shorten the second stage of labor, since such forceps deliveries have been shown to result in no greater fetal morbidity than is attributable to spontaneous delivery.

Forceps come in over 600 shapes and sizes, but most are variations on a common theme. The "classic" forceps are of two general designs, Simpson's and Elliot. Elliot forceps have a more rounded cephalic curve (the portion of the forceps designed to fit around the baby's head), and thus are considered most appropriate in situations in which little *molding* (the change in fetal head configuration from round to oblong due to compression within the maternal pelvis) has taken place. Simpson's forceps, on the other hand, have a more oblong cephalic curve, and are generally employed when the head has been molded (Fig. 18-13). Countless variations on these two designs were introduced during the first half of this century, when the "art" of obstetrics centered around the physician's skill at instrumental deliveries. "Special" forceps deviate widely from the "classic" designs, and were intended for particular situations, such as the Barton forceps for deep transverse arrest of the fetal head and the Piper forceps for delivering the aftercoming head when the baby presents as a breech.

The *vacuum extractor* is another category of instrument used to effect vaginal delivery. Both metal and plastic cups, which fit over the occiput of the fetal head, are available (Fig. 18-14). A vacuum is generated, causing adherence of the cup to the head, and downward traction is exerted to advance the station. In many parts of the world the vacuum extractor has replaced forceps for instrumental vaginal deliveries. The same precautions and classifications are appropriate to both approaches.

Cesarean Section Delivery

Cesarean section is the removal of the fetus through an incision in the abdominal wall and uterus. The usual *lower uterine segment transverse* approach involves a horizontal incision, made in the lower uterine segment, which was part of the cervix prior to effacement (Fig. 18-15). The advantages of such an incision include the likelihood that in subsequent pregnancies the old scar will be part of the cervix and lower uterus until very late in gestation or until labor, and thus will be protected from the tension exerted by the growing conceptus. Such scars are highly unlikely to rupture prior to labor in future pregnancies.

Occasionally a *classical incision* in the uterus becomes necessary. Such an incision is made in the upper portion of the uterus, and stretches vertically between the round ligament insertions (Fig. 18-16).

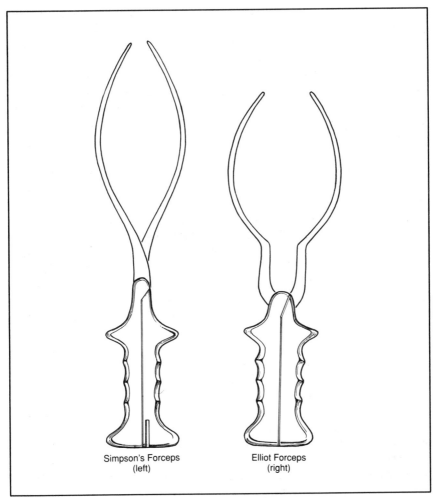

Simpson's Forceps
(left)

Elliot Forceps
(right)

Fig. 18-13. The classic forceps. Simpson's forceps, on the right, are used for delivery of a molded head. It has a more oblong cephalic curve than the Elliot forceps on the left. Note the separated shanks of Simpson's forceps and the overlapping shanks of the Elliot forceps.

An intermediate approach is called a *low segment vertical incision.* Here the operator attempts to make the incision in the lower uterine segment after peeling back the bladder flap of peritoneum as in a low transverse incision, but the incision is oriented vertically (Fig. 18-17). Theoretically some of the risk of rupture associated with a classic incision should be avoided, since the incision is still in an area that will be part of the cervix during subsequent pregnancies, but this is dependent on the amount of cervical effacement that has occurred prior to the operation, and on the success of the operator in confining the incision to the lower segment.

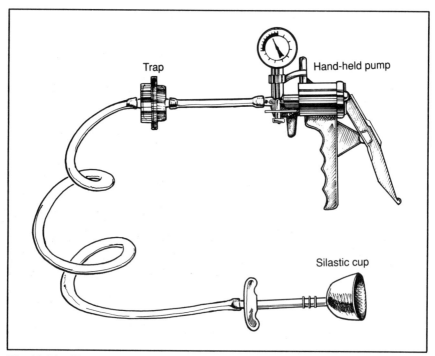

Fig. 18-14. Vacuum extractor. This particular model employs a hand-held pump and Silastic cup.

Currently, classical and low vertical incisions are rarely utilized, except for patients with anterior placenta previa and transverse lie for whom an approach to the upper uterus is preferable; and some breech presentations when the lower segment has not been effaced and widened sufficiently by labor to allow for atraumatic delivery through a transverse incision.

The likelihood of dehiscence of a previous cesarean section scar during subsequent pregnancies is in the range of 1 percent. These dehiscences are just as likely to be discovered at the time of repeat cesarean section as they are to manifest themselves during a trial of labor. In most cases the dehiscence of a transverse lower uterine segment scar is relatively benign, although on occasion hemorrhage may be life-threatening to the mother or fetus. Extrusion of the fetus into the abdominal cavity may be catastrophic, but is rare with transverse scars because the lower uterine segment is generally separated from the peritoneal cavity by the overlying bladder. When a classical cesarean section is performed, the incision involves the uterine musculature. During subsequent pregnancies, the potentially weak scar is exposed to increasing intrauterine pressure, and rupture may occur prior to active labor. Furthermore, the location of the scar means that extrusion of the fetus into the abdominal cavity is considerably

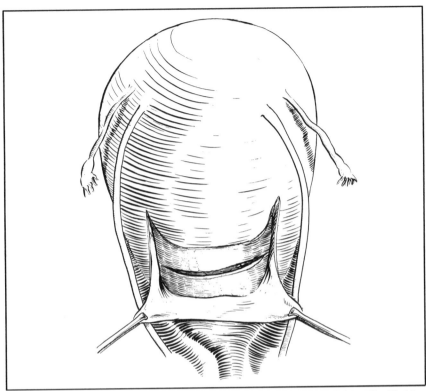

Fig. 18-15. Lower uterine segment transverse cesarean section incision. The bladder flap peritoneum has been opened and dissected downward and an incision has been made into the myometrium of the lower uterus.

more likely than with the low transverse scar. For this reason, patients with previous classic cesarean sections are generally advised to undergo planned repeat cesarean section without lbor.

Breech Delivery

When the presenting part of the fetus is the buttocks (breech), or the feet (footling breech), the risk of vaginal delivery is increased. Because the head of the fetus presents the widest diameter to the pelvis, it is possible that the body will delivery normally but the head be unable to fit through the bony pelvis. If this were to happen, the baby would likely be deprived of nutrients and oxygen as the umbilical cord is compressed between the head and the bony pelvis, and intact delivery would be highly unlikely.

When the feet present first the situation is theoretically even worse. The feet do not make a very good "dilating wedge" for the cervix, so that it is difficult to achieve full dilation before the head must be delivered rapidly.

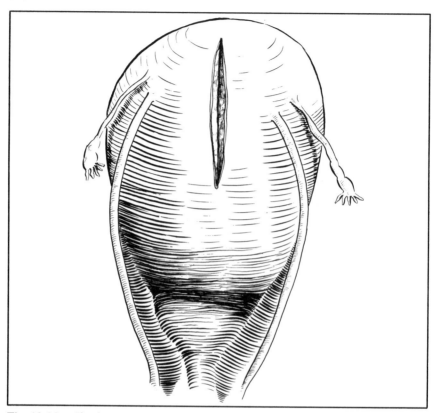

Fig. 18-16. Classic cesarean section incision. The incision is made in the upper portion of the uterus. The bladder flap is not dissected.

Furthermore, as the feet descend there is a good deal of room around them, with no head or breech to "plug" the cervix. Umbilical cord is more likely to prolapse with or ahead of the feet, again causing decreased availability of oxygen and nutrients as the cord vessels go into spasm when exposed to the lower temperature and drying of the outside air, or as the cord is compressed against the bony pelvis.

A number of case series' have demonstrated lower intellectual performance for breech-presenting babies delivered vaginally than for babies delivered headfirst. These studies are confounded by the fact that babies in certain high-risk situations are more likely to present as breech, and it may be the underlying problems rather than the presentation that are responsible for the poor performance on mental and motor function testing. For example, approximately 11 to 20 percent of babies delivered at 30 weeks' gestation present as breech, whereas only 2 to 3 percent are breech at term. Since prematurity is one of the highest risk situations for neuro-

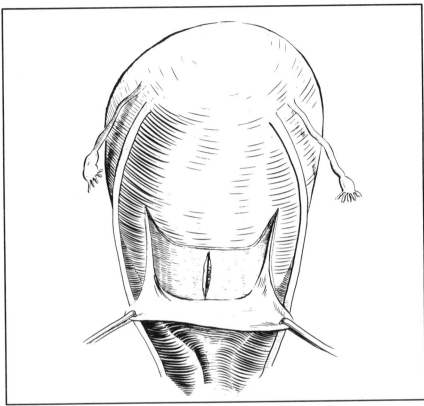

Fig. 18-17. Lower uterine segment vertical cesarean section incision. As in a low segment transverse incision, the bladder flap has been dissected downward.

logic impairment, delivery as breech may not be the most important problem. The fetus with oligohydramnios is more likely to present as breech, as are fetuses with underlying neurologic abnormalities. It is believed that these two situations make breech more likely because these fetuses cannot move around as easily, either because of very little amniotic fluid or because of an underlying motor disorder.

Vaginal breech delivery has become increasingly unusual in recent years, probably because of concern about adverse outcomes and because obstetricians in training are less likely to gain experience in the appropriate techniques for breech delivery. Nevertheless, vaginal breech delivery is considered an appropriate alternative to cesarean section in situations in which the bony pelvis can be shown to be large (by x-ray or CT pelvimetry), the baby is not overly large and is at or near term, and the labor progresses normally.

Recommended Reading

American College of Obstetricians and Gynecologists. Operative vaginal delivery. *ACOG Technical Bulletin.* No. 196, 1994.

Carpenter, M. W. Safety of Forceps Vaginal Delivery and Principles of Application. In D. H. Nichols (ed.), *Gynecologic and Obstetric Surgery.* St. Louis: Mosby-Year Book, 1993. Pp. 1061–1066.

Dennen, P. C. *Dennen's Forceps Deliveries* (3rd ed.). Philadelphia: F. A. Davis, 1989.

Depp, R. Cesarean Delivery and Other Surgical Procedures. In S. G. Gabbe, J. R. Niebyl, and J. L. Simpson (eds.), *Obstetrics: Normal and Problem Pregnancies* (2nd ed.). New York: Churchill-Livingstone, 1991. Pp. 635–693.

Oxorn, H. (ed.). *Oxorn-Foote Human Labor and Birth* (5th ed.). Norwalk: Appleton-Century-Crofts, 1986.

Varney, H. *Nurse Midwifery.* Boston: Blackwell, 1987.

19

Obstetric Analgesia and Anesthesia

Donald R. Coustan

Childbirth can be a painful process. How that pain is perceived differs markedly from one individual to another. The word *anesthesia* has come to mean the loss of pain perception, whereas *analgesia* denotes a reduction of the sensation of pain with maintenance of consciousness. *Regional anesthesia* completely blocks the transmission of pain along the spinal cord, while leaving the patient conscious. *General anesthesia* renders the patient unconscious and decreases the body's response to painful stimuli.

The goal of obstetric anesthesia and analgesia is to provide a safe and more comfortable childbirth experience for the parturient. This goal must always be balanced against the well-being of both mother and fetus. In the past, pharmacologic anesthesia was the leading cause of maternal mortality. Such deaths were primarily caused by the use of general anesthesia that eliminated the gag reflex and permitted aspiration of gastric contents into the pulmonary tree, particularly in laboring patients whose gastric contents are quite acidic and whose gastric emptying time is prolonged. Today maternal mortality due to anesthesia is rare, primarily due to improvements in our understanding of the physiology of the mother-infant unit, but also to the introduction of new agents and methods of pain relief. Furthermore, in recent years there has been an increased acceptance on the part of patients and caregivers alike that they must function as a team, and that no medical procedure such as anesthesia is totally risk-free; this acceptance has led to joint responsibility for decision making. This chapter describes the physiology of pain and stress; childbirth education as a form of analgesia; and analgesia for labor, for delivery, and for cesarean section.

Placental Physiology

Most of the analgesic and anesthetic techniques currently available involve the administration of a pharmacologic agent to the mother. Virtually all substances ingested by the mother cross the placenta and reach the fetal circulation. Most critical in determining the risk-benefit ratio of a given compound is the amount that reaches the fetus and the presence or absence of adverse fetal effects attributable to the agent. Factors that predispose to transplacental passage of a drug include low molecular weight, lipid-solubility, relative lack of ionic charge, slow metabolism by the mother, and a high ratio of free-to-bound drug in the maternal circulation. Drugs may be metabolized by the fetus to active compounds that, due to relative lack of the properties listed above, do not cross the placenta freely and ay accumulate in the fetal circulation.

Physiology of Pain and Stress

Although pain and stress are subjective experiences, it is possible to measure their effects on the mother by changes in vital signs such as heart rate, blood pressure, and respiratory rate. Women in labor have been reported to manifest increased blood levels of glucocorticoids, catecholamines, ß-endorphins, and enkephalins; these are responses similar to those seen in other types of pain and stress. Catecholamines, in particular, are capable of inducing constriction in the uterine vasculature, decreasing uterine blood flow, and in some circumstances reducing oxygen delivery to the fetus. Although these changes are not always detectable by cursory clinical examination, anxious patients with subjectively reported severe pain presumably are more prone to such adverse effects. Thus, the routine use of pharmacologic analgesia even in the absence of apparent pain and anxiety does not seem warranted. Furthermore, most pharmacologic agents administered to the mother make their way to the fetal circulation, and some have the potential for adversely affecting fetal well-being. These potential fetal side effects are discussed with the various approaches to analgesia and anesthesia.

The pain experienced by laboring women stems from uterine contractions, cervical dilation, and stretching of the pelvic floor and perineum. During the first stage of labor, uterine and cervical pain are mediated by sympathetic afferent neurons that enter the spinal cord at the lower thoracic and upper lumbar segments. Additional second-stage pain, from stretching related to descent of the fetus, travels via sensory fibers in the pudendal nerve to enter the spinal cord at sacral levels 2 to 4 (Fig. 19-1). For this reason, modes of anesthesia in which specific nerve roots are

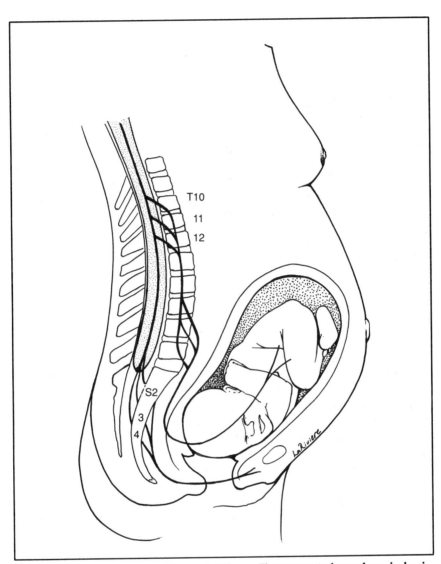

Fig. 19-1.   Pain pathways for labor and delivery. First-stage uterine and cervical pain is mediated by sympathetic afferent neurons entering the spinal cord in the lower thoracic and upper lumbar segments. Pelvic pain from descent of the fetus and stretching of the perineum is mediated by sensory fibers that travel via the pudendal nerve to enter the spinal cord at S2–4.

targeted may require modification depending on the stage of labor in which they are administered.

Preparation for Childbirth (Psychoprophylaxis)

A number of approaches to nonmedicated childbirth have been espoused over the years. One of the more popular of these is the Lamaze method, in which the patient and her support person learn techniques of positive conditioning such as specific breathing patterns, the refocusing of attention during contractions, and relaxation exercises. All such methods have in common education about the physiology of labor and childbirth, and the involvement of a support person. They are effective for many couples, and provide a sense of control and participation in the face of a medical care delivery system that may be perceived as sterile and disease-oriented.

The evolution of childbirth education has brought about many changes in obstetrics, mostly for the better. The widespread acceptance of family-centered childbirth with fathers present throughout labor and delivery, the emergence of the labor-delivery-recovery room paradigm, and the overall brightening of the environment for childbirth all have origins in the childbirth education movement. Routine use of pharmacologic agents has now disappeared from most maternity centers.

Psychoprophylaxis is not effective for all individuals. Operative births generally require analgesia or anesthesia, regardless of the preparation that has occurred. Some patients experience pain and stress during labor and birth despite the best of preparation, and request pain relief. It is important that childbirth preparation courses not set couples up in a "win-lose" situation, where the use of analgesia is looked on as a defeat. As mentioned earlier, there is evidence that maternal stress and pain can reduce uterine perfusion, potentially reducing oxygen delivery to the fetus. Thus various types of analgesia may be beneficial to both mother and child in particular circumstances. The remainder of the chapter is devoted to these options, but it should be borne in mind that, as for medicine in general, no intervention should be applied if it is not needed.

Analgesia During Labor

Narcotic Analgesics

Provision of *narcotic analgesics* is the most commonly used pharmacologic approach to pain relief during labor. They act centrally, decreasing the patient's perception of pain. Meperidine, a synthetic opioid, is the prototype drug for labor. It is given either intravenously (25–50 mg) or intramuscularly (50–75 mg). When injected intramuscularly the onset of analgesia generally occurs within 20 minutes and lasts for 2 to 3 hours. Intravenous meperidine has a more rapid onset of action and a duration of approximately 2 hours. Common side effects include nausea, vomiting, and lightheadedness. The use of any intravenous analgesic agent will, to a certain extent, change the mother's perception of her surroundings. Maternal respiratory depression may also occur, particularly with larger doses, because of depressed sensitivity of the respiratory center to carbon dioxide. Like other narcotics, meperidine crosses the placenta and enters the fetal circulation, with fetal blood levels rapidly reaching approximately 80 percent of maternal levels. Administration of meperidine to the mother between 1 and 4 hours prior to delivery has been associated with neonatal respiratory depression and measurably lower neonatal psychophysiologic test scores.

These fetal and neonatal effects are relatively short-lived, and may be due to the accumulation in the fetus of normeperidine, an active metabolite that may be trapped on the fetal side of the placenta. Repeated doses of meperidine appear to cause the greatest amount of respiratory depression. This problem can generally be reversed in the neonate by the administration of a narcotic antagonist such as naloxone (0.1 mg/kg). Administering the narcotic antagonist to the mother in order to decrease the effect of meperidine on the fetus is not logical, since the drug will reverse the analgesic effect of meperidine as well as the respiratory depressant effect.

Another potential side effect of meperidine, and most other narcotic analgesics, is the loss of fetal heart beat-to-beat variability and, in rare cases, the emergence of an unusual "sinusoidal" fetal heart rate pattern, which is described in Chap. 16. Although the sinusoidal pattern induced by meperidine is likely benign, it must be differentiated from the sinusoidal pattern related to fetal anemia, which is ominous. Although virtually all analgesic drugs can be addicting, this is not a realistic consideration in labor because of the transient nature of the need for analgesia.

Morphine, the prototype natural opioid, was formerly a common analgesic during labor. However, because of its later onset of action and longer duration of action, and probable greater propensity to cause nausea and vomiting, it has largely been abandoned except during prodromal labor as a way of "resting" the patient. Morphine also has been reported to cause greater neonatal respiratory depression than some of the other opioids.

Butorphanol is a more rapidly acting synthetic opioid than is meperidine or morphine. It is an agonist-antagonist, which suggests that respiratory depression does not increase as the dose rises, and that there is little cumulative neonatal effect of repeated maternal doses. Although butorphanol is absorbed after intramuscular or intravenous administration, there is considerable hepatic first-pass metabolism, which makes the intravenous route preferable. A dose of 1 to 2 mg intravenously provides analgesia quite rapidly; the effect lasts from 3 to 4 hours. Nalbuphine, another agonist-antagonist, has properties similar to those of butorphanol. Its analgesic potency is similar to that of morphine; the usual dose is 10 mg.

A relatively innovative approach to analgesia during labor is patient-controlled administration of an opioid by intravenous pump. Within certain limits preset to avoid overdosing, patients are able to determine when an additional intravenous dose is given. This approach provides greater patient autonomy and may be the most rational approach to delivering only that amount of medication that is desired by the patient.

Tranquilizers and Sedatives

Tranquilizers and sedatives may be administered to laboring patients to reduce anxiety or to decrease the nausea and vomiting associated with opioid analgesics. Although barbiturates were often utilized in the past, their potential respiratory depressive effect on the mother and neonate and their lack of analgesic activity have led to their abandonment except in early latent-phase labor, when administration of a drug such as secobarbital (100 mg) may allow the patient to rest more comfortably until active labor supervenes.

Phenothiazine tranquilizers are often used in combination with opioid analgesics to potentiate the analgesic effect and decrease side effects such as nausea and vomiting. Promethazine (25–75 mg intramuscularly or intravenously) and hydroxyzine (25–100 mg intramuscularly) are the most commonly used agents. These drugs may decrease fetal heart rate beat-to-beat variability, and in high doses may cause maternal hypotension or neonatal depression. Benzodiazepine tranquilizers are not commonly used during labor because of many potential adverse effects. They may cause a significant reduction in fetal heart rate beat-to-beat variability that would make interpretation of electronic fetal heart rate monitoring difficult. Impaired thermoregulation by the neonate has also been reported with diazepam. Other related agents such as lorazepam and midazolam have such potent amnestic properties that the mother may not recall labor or delivery; these agents have not been evaluated for use in labor.

Anticholinergic Agents

Anticholinergic agents such as scopolamine were once used widely during labor. They were generally combined with an opioid and a phenothiazine to form a "cocktail," the results of which were often referred to as "twilight sleep." The main function of the anticholinergic agent was to induce amnesia for the events surrounding labor and delivery. Unfortunately, the use of this drug was often associated with bizarre behavior and delirium. Because of its inhibition of vagal nerve activity, scopolamine also suppressed fetal heart rate beat-to-beat variability and rendered electronic fetal heart rate tracings difficult to interpret. Its use during labor has been abandoned.

Paracervical Block

As mentioned above, first-stage labor pain is mediated primarily by sympathetic fibers from the uterus and cervix that travel to the lower thoracic and upper lumbar spinal segments. Because these fibers coalesce in Frankenhäuser's ganglion, lateral to the cervix, it is possible to block the transmission of nerve impulses by anesthetizing these areas. An anesthetic solution is injected just lateral to the cervix, just below the mucosa, at the 3 and 9 o'clock positions (or the 4 and 8 o'clock positions). Although this technique is effective for first-stage labor pain, it has lost favor and is currently only occasionally used.

The major problem encountered with the paracervical block has been fetal bradycardia that occurs a few minutes after the injections. In some cases this problem has been of major clinical significance. Its frequent occurrence, which has been alternatively ascribed to fetal drug toxicity or uterine vasoconstriction, is alarming and has led to the infrequent use of the paracervical block in recent years.

Epidural Block
Epidural anesthesia is a popular form of pharmacologic analgesia for labor in the United States. Its administration involves the injection of a local anesthetic solution or narcotic, or both, into the epidural space, a potential space between the ligamentum flavum and the dura surrounding the spinal cord (Fig. 19-2).

One advantage of epidural anesthesia is its versatility; it can provide analgesia during labor, anesthesia for vaginal delivery, or surgical anesthesia for cesarean section. The Touhy needle, a blunt needle with an eccentric aperture, is inserted into the epidural space at the interspace between lumbar vertebrae 2 and 3, 3 and 4, or 4 and 5. A teflon catheter is inserted through the needle 2 to 3 cm into the epidural space. For pain relief during the first stage of labor, small doses of local anesthetic solution (0.25% bupivacaine, 2% 2-chloroprocaine, 1% lidocaine) and in many centers a narcotic (fentanyl) are injected through the catheter, which causes analgesia in the distribution of the lower thoracic and upper lumbar segments. Although traditionally the analgesia was "reinforced" from time to time with further doses of local anesthesia, it has now become common to utilize continuous infusion pumps to administer the anesthetic solution, thus maintaining a constant anesthetic level without episodes of "wearing off."

A number of different local anesthetic compounds are available, and the differences among them can be confusing. Based on molecular structure, they are divided into two broad categories: ester-linked agents and amide-linked agents. The two types have specific properties that determine their action and toxicity. Ester-linked drugs, such as procaine, tetracaine, and 2-chloroprocaine, are metabolized by pseudocholinesterase that circulates in the plasma. They differ with respect to the speed with which they are catabolized, with 2-chloroprocaine being the fastest and tetracaine the slowest. As a result, 2-chloroprocaine has a very rapid onset of action but short duration, and lasts only 30 to 60 minutes, whereas tetracaine's effects last for many hours. A drug that is broken down rapidly is less likely to

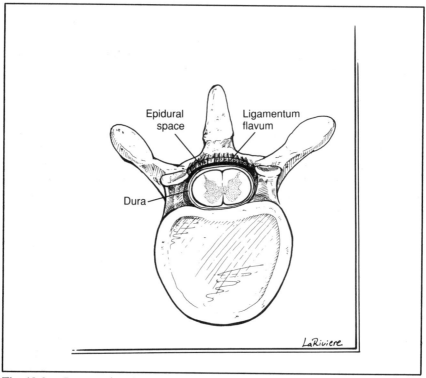

Fig. 19-2. Cross section through the spine at the lumbar level. The epidural anesthesia needle and catheter are placed through the ligamentum flavum into the potential space between that ligament and the dura surrounding the spinal cord.

have adverse effects on the fetus, since much of it is gone from the circulation before it can cross the placenta. However, the brief action of such a drug requires more frequently repeated injections. One drawback of ester-linked agents is their potential prolonged activity in patients with a deficiency of the pseudocholinesterase enzyme.

Amide-linked local anesthetic agents are, in general, catabolized in the liver and tend to have longer half-lives than ester-linked agents. Typical amide-linked drugs include bupivacaine, lidocaine, and mepivacaine. Placental transfer of these drugs is favored by their low molecular weight, lipid-solubility, the degree to which they are present in a nonionized form, and the degree to which they circulate in the free rather than protein-bound state. Because bupivacaine is more highly ionized and protein-bound, it does not cross the placenta as freely as the other two agents. Bupivacaine is currently the most popular agent for epidural anesthesia in the United States. This agent is advantageous because it provides more of a sensory blockade and less of a motor blockade than many other local anesthetic agents. Another variation currently popular in the United States is the addition of an opioid such as fetanyl, which binds to specific spinal opioid receptors and improves the sensory anesthesia without a marked effect on motor nerve function. The use of this adjunctive narcotic also results in a lower total dosage of local anesthetic.

Adverse effects of epidural anesthesia are related to maternal and fetal toxicity of the drugs used as well as to the physiologic effects of the block induced. The latter effects are generally more important, and relate primarily to maternal hypotension due to the sympathetic blockade that commonly accompanies the sensory blockade. Decreased sympathetic tone results in vasodilation and pooling of blood, with decreased venous return leading to decreased cardiac output. In practice, this hypotension is usually prevented by the administration of a fluid preload, typically 500 to 1000 ml of crystalloid, prior to induction of epidural anesthesia. Dextrose-containing solutions should be avoided for these rapid infusions, since maternal hyperglycemia is rapidly transmitted to the fetus and may be associated with fetal acidemia. Furthermore, avoidance of the supine position during labor with concomitant vena cava compression and decreased venous return is an important principle regardless of the type of anesthesia administered.

When hypotension occurs despite these preventive measures, the administration of oxygen and increased intravenous fluids is appropriate. Ephedrine, which has both alpha- and beta-adrenergic properties, may be administered intravenously in doses of 5 to 20 mg to increase blood pressure without significantly decreasing uterine perfusion. This drug acts both by direct stimulation of adrenergic receptors and by causing the release of stored norepinephrine.

Epidural anesthesia may be associated with systemic toxicity of the agent used, particularly if intravascular injection occurs. Primary toxic effects are to the cardiovascular and central nervous systems. CNS toxic effects develop at a lower maternal blood level than cardiotoxicity; they are first manifest as tinnitus, a metallic taste in the mouth, or anxiety. These symptoms can progress to generalized seizures with hypoxia and acidosis. Cardiac toxicity usually involves arrhythmias, transient hypertension, and generalized cardiovascular collapse.

There is a good deal of controversy as to the likelihood of epidural anesthesia prolonging labor and predisposing to the need for instrumental delivery. Various studies support each side of the controversy, but most are not ideally designed. Current techniques with lower concentrations of anesthetic agents are less likely to have clinically significant effects on labor than are older techniques. Nevertheless, most obstetricians avoid the induction of epidural anesthesia prior to the active phase of labor. Although not all experts agree on the presence of a tocolytic (labor-slowing) effect of epidural anesthesia, some patients require oxytocin augmentation after the analgesia has taken effect.

Analgesia and Anesthesia for Vaginal Delivery

Local Anesthesia

Local anesthesia for vaginal delivery consists of perineal infiltration with a local anesthetic agent in preparation for episiotomy or for repair of a perineal laceration. Although local anesthetic agents can be transferred to the fetus relatively rapidly after local infiltration in the maternal perineum, little morbidity has been reported.

Pudendal Block

Pudendal block consists of the injection of local anesthetic into the pudendal nerves, which carry sensory fibers from the perineum to the spinal cord. Blocking this nerve relieves perineal pain, but not the pain of uterine contractions. Therefore, pudendal block is most useful for spontaneous deliveries or some outlet forceps deliveries. The pudendal nerve block is administered via a long needle of approximately 20 g that is inserted into the nerve just posterior and inferior to the ischial spine in the region of the sacrospinous ligament. A long tubular needle guard, called an "Iowa trumpet," is used to guide the needle tip to the appropriate spot on each side (Fig. 19-3). Pudendal block often suffices for an outlet forceps delivery, but in some cases additional local infiltration in the perineum is required if an episiotomy is necessary.

Epidural Anesthesia

Epidural anesthesia, if already in place during labor, is commonly employed to relieve the discomfort associated with spontaneous or operative vaginal delivery. Because the pain associated with delivery is mediated by neurons entering the spinal cord at sacral segments 2, 3, and 4, the blockade must include these segments in order to be effective. This lower blockade may be induced by administering an increased dose of local anesthetic agent through the epidural catheter, often while the patient is in a sitting position.

An effective epidural anesthesia blocks the sensation of bearing down experienced by parturients during the descent of the fetal head. In fact, that is one of the functions of the epidural anesthetic. Although many woman will "push" effectively and expel the baby while the epidural anesthesia is functioning, some are less able to push because of the lack of proprioception. If such individuals experience a prolonged second stage with lack of descent, it is reasonable to allow the epidural anesthetic to wear off in order to restore sensation and improve the patient's expulsive efforts. However, the discomfort associated with this maneuver may be more psychologically unsettling to the parturient than had she never received the epidural anesthesia. There is also some evidence, albeit controversial, that epidural anesthesia for delivery is associated with a higher likelihood of obstetric forceps utilization. The upper limit of normal second-stage duration should be extended by 1 hour when epidural anesthesia is used.

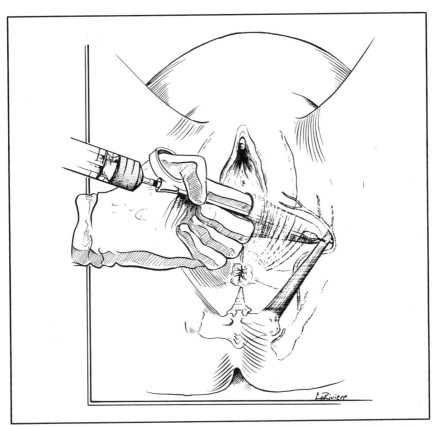

Fig. 19-3.   Administration of a pudendal nerve block. An "Iowa trumpet" is used to guide the needle to a point 1 cm inferior to and 1 cm medial to the ischial spine, where the pudendal nerve and blood vessels are located.

Spinal Anesthesia

Spinal anesthesia, often called "saddle block" because the area anesthetized is approximately that which would be in contact with the saddle during horseback riding, is particularly useful when an operative delivery is to be performed for a patient who does not have a preexisting epidural in place. Similar to an epidural anesthetic, a spinal anesthetic is administered through the intervertebral interspace at L2–3, 3–4, or 4–5. However, a small-gauge sharp needle is used and the dura is punctured so that the needle enters the subarachnoid space, caudal to the termination of the spinal cord itself. A small volume of hyperbaric (dense) solution is injected into the subarachnoid space while the patient is sitting. It settles down into the lower portion of the space, anesthetizing the appropriate region. Spinal anesthesia has a rapid onset and profound effect, which make it suitable for urgent operative manipulations. It has the same complications as epidural blockade, including hypotension due to sympathectomy. In addition, postspinal headache may result from leakage of fluid out through the puncture hole in the dura, decreasing the buoyant medium in which the brain floats. The use of very small-caliber needles has diminished the likelihood of headache considerably. In fact, postspinal headache also complicates epidural anesthesia, particularly when the large needle used for the introduction of an epidural catheter punctures the dura.

General Anesthesia

General anesthesia was at one time quite commonly used for vaginal delivery, but many considerations have combined to make this form of pain relief extremely rare. At one time the leading cause of maternal mortality was anesthesia, primarily aspiration due to vomiting of gastric contents when the gag reflex was suppressed. Because laboring women have delayed gastric emptying it became clear that if general anesthesia was to be used, rapid sequence techniques including immediate endotracheal intubation were necessary. In addition, as women expressed their wish to be awake for delivery, general anesthesia became less desirable. General anesthesia occasionally becomes necessary for manipulative deliveries such as a breech or difficult forceps, particularly when conduction anesthesia is unavailable or ineffective. However, inhalation analgesia with mixtures of nitrous oxide and oxygen is still in common usage. Although the patient is not asleep and still experiences her delivery, pain seems to be tolerated with greater equanimity. The gas mixture is administered via a mask that may be hand-held by the patient. Nitrous oxide and oxygen are premixed in the proper ratio to avoid hypoxia.

Anesthesia for Cesarean Section

Because cesarean section is a major surgical procedure, anesthesia is always necessary. Although in some unusual circumstances local infiltration of the abdominal wall (accompanied by intravenous sedation) may be used, the overwhelming majority of cesarean sections are performed under either general or conduction anesthesia.

General Anesthesia

General anesthesia may be accomplished with a variety of agents and is preferred by some patients because they would rather not be awake for the procedure. Anesthetic agents are chosen to minimize the likelihood of adverse fetal effects, and techniques are used to minimize the likelihood of maternal aspiration of gastric contents. Typically a liquid nonparticulate antacid is administered orally prior to induction of anesthesia in order to raise the pH of the gastric contents, decreasing the risk of chemical pneumonitis if aspiration should occur. Because the supine position used for abdominal surgery causes the uterus to compress the vena cava, diminishing venous return, and also the aorta, diminishing uterine and lower extremity perfusion, an object such as a rolled up blanket is placed under the mother's right hip to achieve left uterine displacement.

The patient breathes 100 percent oxygen through a face mask for a few minutes, and the unconscious state is then induced with intravenous thiopental or ketamine. A muscle relaxant is then administered and endotracheal intubation is performed immediately. Prior to intubation an assistant exerts gentle pressure on the cricoid cartilage to close off the esophagus and lessen the likelihood of regurgitation and aspiration. Once the tube is in place, a mixture of nitrous oxide and oxygen is administered to provide analgesia. Other agents are sometimes added to provide deeper anesthesia and amnesia. These include isoflurane and enflurane, among others. Although high concentrations of these agents may cause uterine relaxation and increased intraoperative bleeding, such problems are not likely to be associated with the low concentrations usually employed for cesarean section. Such combinations of anesthetic agents are often referred to as *balanced anesthesia*. They are intended to minimize the depressive effect of general anesthesia on the fetus. Once delivery has occurred, more profound analgesia may be provided by intravenous opioids or greater concentrations of nitrous oxide.

Conduction Anesthesia

Conduction anesthesia, which includes regional techniques such as spinal and epidural blocks, is used more commonly than general anesthesia for cesarean section. Most parturients wish to remain awake for the delivery, and to have the father of the baby present, and conduction anesthesia allows for this. Furthermore, intubation is not necessary. Risks of conduction anesthesia during delivery are similar to those described for its use during labor, such as hypotension and anesthetic drug toxicity. If an epidural anesthetic is already in place for labor when cesarean section is decided on, it may be reinforced with a greater concentration of drug and the level may be brought up to a surgical plane. Epidural anesthesia may be placed specifically for cesarean section, but this requires that the indication for the procedure be nonemergent in order to allow enough time for the block to solidify. Spinal anesthesia can be administered rapidly, and tends to provide a more reliable and solid anesthetic block than does epidural. The personal preference of the anesthesiologist is also a consideration. With either type of conduction anesthesia there may be some discomfort associated with intraabdominal manipulations and peritoneal "tugging," so it is common to supplement with an intravenous opioid analgesic once the baby has been delivered. Occasionally the conduction anesthetic does not provide a solid block and general anesthesia is required in addition.

In summary, a number of different techniques are available for pain relief during labor and delivery. The guiding principle to be followed should be the use of only those pain relievers that are indicated. The well-prepared mother who is tolerating her labor well does not require pharmacologic anesthesia, but the mother who is in pain and who is highly anxious should not be denied it.

Recommended Reading

Chestnut, D. H., and Gibbs, C. P. Obstetric Anesthesia. In S. G. Gabbe, J. R. Niebyl, and J. S. Simpson (eds.), *Obstetrics: Normal and Problem Pregnancies* (2nd ed.). New York: Churchill-Livingstone, 1991. Pp. 493–538.

Steude, G. M., and de Rosayro, M. Analgesia and Anesthesia for Delivery. In P. V. Dilts, Jr., and J. J. Sciarra (eds.), *Gynecology and Obstetrics* (Vol. 2). Philadelphia: Lippincott, 1992. Pp. 1–9.

The Puerperium

Donald R. Coustan and Diane J. Angelini

The alterations in maternal physiology described in Chap. 10 are no longer adaptive once the baby has delivered, and the *puerperium*, which is the 6- to 7-week period during which the uterus returns to its nonpregnant size and form, or *involutes*, is a time of dramatic change. During the first few minutes to hours after delivery of the placenta, when the intervillous space has ceased to exist, arterial inflow must stop lest the mother exsanguinate. The mother's cardiovascular system must maintain stability despite the sudden blood loss of ≥ 500 ml that takes place at delivery, and her endocrine system must adjust to the sudden fall in levels of estrogen, progesterone, human placental lactogen, and other hormones that accompany the delivery of the placenta. Lactation must be initiated and maintained. A stable attachment between mother (and father) and newborn, known as *bonding*, is necessary to ensure that the helpless and demanding neonate will have its needs met and will not be abandoned. Finally, the mother must adjust to the tremendous emotional and life-style changes brought about by the introduction of the child into her life and that of her family. This chapter will consider each of these requirements, and discuss the underlying physiology when appropriate.

Normal Physiologic Changes

Uterine Involution

The process by which organs return to their prepregnant state is defined as *involution* (Table 20-1). Following delivery, the uterus measures $15 \times 12 \times 7.5$ cm and weighs approximately 900 g. Four to 6 weeks after

Table 20-1. Involutional process

Postdelivery time	Location of fundus	Placental site diameter (cm)	Lochia	Uterine weight (g)	Cervix
Immediately postpartum	Halfway between the symphysis and pubis and the umbilicus	12.5	Lochia rubra (1–4 days)	900	Soft, flabby, admits 1–2 fingers
Postpartum day 1	At or below the umbilicus				
First week postpartum	7.5 cm above the symphysis pubis	7.5	Lochia serosa (5–9 days)	450	2 cm
Second week postpartum	Uterus not palpable as an abdominal organ	5.0	Lochia alba (10–15 days)	200	1 cm
Six weeks postpartum		2.5		60–100	Slit only

delivery, the uterus measures 7.5 × 5 × 2.5 cm and weighs somewhere between 60 and 100 g. Immediately postpartum, the uterine fundus reaches a little bit more than halfway between the symphysis and the umbilicus.

On the first day postpartum the uterine fundus is at or slightly below the umbilicus (Fig. 20-1). If the uterus rises above the umbilicus or is displaced to either side, consideration needs to be given to the possibility that the uterus is filling with clots or a distended bladder exists. Ultrasound can confirm whether an empty uterus exists, when clots are present, or when retained tissue may need to be evacuated.

By the first week postpartum, the uterine fundus is approximately 7.5 cm above the symphysis. The greatest reduction in uterine size occurs during the first postpartum week when the uterus diminishes by half. By approximately 12 to 14 days after delivery the uterus is usually not palpable as an abdominal organ.

This uterine involutional process is initiated by autolysis. The factor producing autolysis is thought to be a hormone or enzyme that causes protoplasm in the uterine muscles to break down, become absorbed, and then to be excreted in the vaginal discharge. Contraction and retraction of muscles compress the uterus, reduce uterine blood supply, and diminish

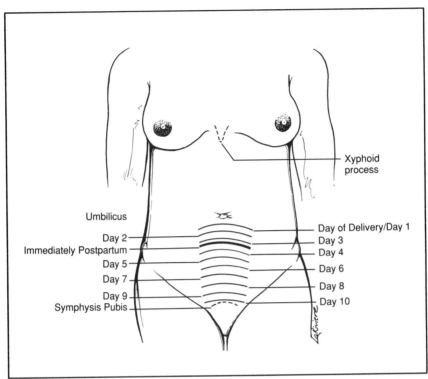

Fig. 20-1. Involutionary changes in the uterine fundus. (Redrawn with permission from H. Varney. *Nurse Midwifery* (2nd ed.). Boston: Blackwell, 1987.)

the overall uterine size and shape. The fibers of uterine muscles, which expanded exponentially during pregnancy, are now reduced in size to normal dimensions.

Placental Site Involution

It takes approximately 6 to 8 weeks after delivery for the placental site to be regenerated. The placental site is elevated and irregular after delivery and measures 12.5 cm in diameter. By the end of the first week postpartum, the placental site is 7.5 cm in diameter. It measures 5.0 cm at 2 weeks postpartum and 2.5 cm at 6 weeks postpartum. The process by which placental involution occurs leaves no scar at the site. Placental involution is often attributed to a process called *exfoliation*. Endometrial tissue develops from all sides and from beneath the placental site. By the eighth week postpartum, the placental site should be well healed.

Endometrial Involution

The shedding of the endometrium, or decidua, after delivery of the placenta occurs in two layers. The superficial layer sloughs off and is seen as lochia, or vaginal discharge, early in the postpartum process. The other layer is a more functional layer closer to the myometrium. This layer serves as the restored or rejuvenated endometrial lining. This process should be completed by about 3 weeks postpartum.

Lochia is the vaginal discharge from the sloughing off of the superficial layer of the endometrium. It begins as blood flow that changes in both appearance and color over the first 2 to 3 weeks of the postpartum course. The red, bloody discharge seen first is called *lochia rubra* and lasts approximately 1 to 4 days. It consists primarily of blood as well as some decidua and parts of chorion, amniotic fluid, fetal cells, vernix, lanugo, and meconium.

Lochia serosa, seen after lochia rubra, is more pinkish in color. It can be thicker and more mucoid in appearance. It is usually present between days 5 to 9 postpartum. This vaginal discharge is pinkish brown in color due to a decrease in the blood component and is composed mainly of serum, but also includes leukocytes and microorganisms.

The vaginal discharge then changes to *lochia alba,* which is yellow white or creamy green in color. It contains leukocytes, microorganisms, mucus, and debris from the uterine lining.

Lochia is normally alkaline and is a good culture medium for microorganisms to flourish as opposed to the normally acidic vaginal discharge. Lochia is usually heavier than menstrual flow in the first 5 days or so, and should not be malodorous. A foul odor may be an early sign of endometritis. Any shedding of blood and body fluids should be handled with universal precautions and lochia is no exception. Lochia is described as heavy, moderate, or scant as it changes from rubra to serosa to alba in appearance. It is not unusual for lochia to become heavier when women ambulate due to vaginal pooling when they are supine. Clots may be evident or an even heavier flow may occur in some women; this may occur between days 7 and 14 and is due to bleeding and sloughing at the placental site. This heavier flow is normal and women should be reassured. However, any steady increase in lochia rubra should be noted and the woman should be evaluated for postpartum hemorrhage from retained placental fragments.

Cervical Changes

Immediately following delivery, the cervix is soft, thick, and flabby. It contracts more slowly and can admit 1 to 2 fingers (2–3 cm) and is 3 to 6 cm long. The margins of the external os often are irregular, which gives the parous cervix its "fish mouth" configuration. Cervical lacerations at delivery are not unusual and very small tears that are not bleeding are often left unrepaired. The cervix can appear bluish black from bruising that occurs during the birth process, especially if the cervix was caught between the presenting part of the fetus and the vaginal outlet during pushing. The external os returns to its prepregnant state by the fourth week postpartum, and the cervical opening is seen as only a slit by 6 weeks postpartum.

Lower Uterine Segment and Ligaments

The thinned-out lower uterine segment also contracts and retracts. Over a 2-week postpartum period, it becomes a more dense structure, and eventually becomes the uterine isthmus. The round ligaments become lax during pregnancy, but by 4 to 6 weeks postpartum regain their prepregnant state.

Vagina, Perineum, and Rectum

Depending on the type of delivery, tissue friability, and repair of lacerations, if any, the vagina may be edematous, ecchymotic, and bruised. It goes through a fair amount of stretching as the vaginal floor accommodates the fetus during birth. The vaginal lining is smooth and has limited tone. The vagina eventually decreases in size but never fully returns to its prepregnant state. Rugae, which disappeared during birth, reappear by the third to fourth week postpartum. The hymen consists of irregular tissue tags called *myrtiform caruncles* in most women who have given birth.

The tone of the vagina usually increases by the end of the puerperium as it responds to vaginal tightening exercises. Kegel exercises, i.e., voluntary tightening of the relaxed vaginal floor, help to expedite this toning process. Loss of tone from overstretching may account for the later development of cystoceles and rectoceles, which are "hernias" of the urogenital diaphragm in which the bladder or rectum prolapse into the vagina.

The perineum may be intact or may have been sutured. The vulva may appear edematous after delivery due to tissue friability, the length of second-stage pushing efforts, trauma, or lacerations. Such vulvar edema is normal during the early puerperium and responds well to ice packs, especially in the first 12 hours after delivery. Cold and hot sitz baths further aid this process and help eliminate the edema.

Hemorrhoids often occur late in pregnancy and may worsen after labor and delivery. They may first appear or worsen during second-stage pushing due to the force of the fetal head that causes dilation of rectal veins. A third- or fourth-degree laceration may add to rectal discomfort and tenderness.

Abdominal Changes

The abdominal wall often remains soft and flabby due to stretching of the overlying muscles from the enlarged uterus. Improvement in abdominal wall tone takes several weeks. If muscles remain lax, a *diastasis recti,* or marked separation of the rectus muscles, may be detected on abdominal palpatation. If this diastasis persists, the muscle area fills in with peritoneum, fascia, and subcutaneous fat.

Striae, commonly seen as reddened stretch marks during pregnancy, change in appearance over the puerperium and eventually appear silvery white. They may fade but never totally disappear. The linea nigra of pregnancy fades. Facial petechiae are also seen early after delivery. They result from vigorous pushing and resolve without treatment.

Renal and Urinary Tract Changes

A decrease in bladder tone can result from trauma at birth or may be related to anesthesia. The bladder may be bruised and the urethra swollen and spasmodic due to trauma or lacerations. The edema seen at the urethra usually subsides in the first day postpartum. The bladder may be hypotonic from overdistention during labor. In addition, an increase in residual urine and incomplete emptying may result in urinary retention and stasis predisposing to the development of urinary tract infections. Stress incontinence may persist postpartum. Dilated ureters and renal pelves take from 2 to 8 weeks to return to their prepregnant states.

Diuresis is present in the first 48 hours and often up to 5 days postpartum. This is a normal physiologic process and is a response to the increase of extracellular fluid during pregnancy. Approximately 5 pounds are lost as a result of diuresis during the first week after delivery.

Gastrointestinal Changes

The decreased motility seen during pregnancy resolves quickly even in women who experience cesarean births. Occasional paralytic ileus can occur. Constipation may occur because of a decrease in solid food intake during labor, lack of exercise, dietary changes, and decreased fluid intake as well as hemorrhoids and rectal lacerations. Fear of tearing sutures or experiencing increased perineal discomfort often adds to difficulty with elimination.

Cardiopulmonary Changes

Immediately after delivery, the plasma volume decreases by 1000 ml due mainly to blood loss. There is a shift of extracellular fluid into the vascular space well into the third postpartum day. By the end of the first week postpartum, the blood volume has returned to prepregnant levels. Cardiac output remains elevated in the first 48 hours after delivery due to increased stroke volume. Once delivery occurs and the weight of the uterus against the diaphragm is removed, normal respiratory function returns.

Vital Signs and Hematology Changes

The mother's temperature should become normal during the first 24 hours after delivery. Dehydration may account for elevations in temperature during this interval. Fevers after this time require careful monitoring, workup, and possible treatment for puerperal infection. The blood pressure should be normal during the puerperium unless a predisposing problem exists such as chronic hypertension or pregnancy-induced hypertension. Hypotension may result from excessive blood loss and warrants careful monitoring. The pulse rate is usually normal unless there is excessive blood loss. Bradycardia can be seen in some women during the early postpartum period. The exact physiologic cause is unknown.

Hemoglobin and hematocrit levels may vary widely. Important factors include preexisting anemia and blood loss during labor. It often takes days for the hematocrit to equilibrate. If a woman has a low hematocrit but is asymptomatic, oral iron therapy is usually sufficient. Leukocytosis seen during labor extends into the postpartum period and can reach levels as high as 30,000 leukocytes; this is primarily an increase in granulocytes.

Return of Menses

Menses usually return within 6 to 8 weeks but may be delayed for up to 12 weeks postpartum for some women. Variations occur in the amount of bleeding and length of menses. Many of these early menstrual cycles are anovulatory, but since there is widespread variation, contraceptive counselling is important. For lactating women, menstruation can return anywhere from 2 months to 18 months or longer following delivery.

Resumption of sexual intercourse is dependent on many factors. Commonly, women are encouraged to return to sexual activity when they feel ready, when there is little perineal discomfort, and when contraception will be used. Return of muscle tone and healing time for episiotomy repair may take up to 4 weeks or longer for some women. Lack of vaginal lubrication is a common physiologic occurrence during the puerperium. The thinned and atrophic walls of the vagina do not lubricate well due to a decrease in estrogen. Breast-feeding may affect feelings of sexual responsiveness as well. Leaking breasts, sore nipples, and tenderness may add to discomfort and diminished sexuality. Body image concerns that encompass body functioning, appearance, and intactness are paramount during the postpartum period.

Bonding

There is evidence to suggest that the first few hours to days of life are an important time during which a loving, nurturing relationship is established between the parents, particularly the mother, and the neonate. When parents and their offspring have the opportunity for close interaction just after birth, a number of characteristic behaviors are observed. These include gazing at the infant with the parent's face in a plane parallel to that of the infant *(en face)*, cuddling and other forms of physical contact with the infant, and talking to the infant. Based largely on the writings of Klaus and Kennell, there has been considerable progress over the past 15 years toward enabling this kind of parent-infant bonding to take place in the hospital setting. Labor and delivery rooms are more home-like and comfortable, and mothers are encouraged to breast-feed their babies during the first few hours of life. Early breast-feeding also stimulates the release of oxytocin from the posterior pituitary gland of the mother, causing uterine contractions that decrease the amount of postpartum bleeding. Liberal visiting hours for fathers and siblings are helpful, as are instructions by the nursing staff regarding breast-feeding, child care, and other related issues. Although current trends toward early discharge after delivery may allow maternal-infant attachment to occur more readily at home, it is possible that the opposite effect will result because of lack of time for nursing observation and teaching in the hospital. This problem may be intensified by the evolution in our society away from the tradition of extended families being present in the home to help and support new mothers.

Postpartum Bleeding

Under ordinary circumstances immediate postpartum bleeding is stopped by uterine muscular contraction, which compresses the vessels, and arterial vasoconstriction. Occasionally these mechanisms fail to control the flow of blood through the placental attachment site, resulting in *immediate postpartum hemorrhage*. Under such circumstances the blood loss may greatly exceed the usual 500 to 600 ml associated with a normal vaginal delivery; life-threatening hemorrhage may be encountered. The most common cause of immediate postpartum hemorrhage is failure of the uterine muscle to contract adequately. This failure may be attributed to various causes, including retention of all or a portion of the placenta, which may prevent successful contractions, or lack of adequate contractile force. Predisposing factors to uterine relaxation include previous overdistention of the uterus by multiple gestation or a large fetus, the use of large doses of oxytocin during labor, infection, and the occasional use of anesthetic agents such as halothane, which have a uterine-relaxing effect. Other causes of immediate postpartum hemorrhage include bleeding from vaginal or cervical lacerations, and, very rarely, uterine rupture.

Immediate steps are necessary to control hemorrhage when it is present. In order to be certain that all placental fragments have been expelled, and that uterine rupture has not occurred, a *manual exploration* is performed. The fingers of the examining hand are introduced into the uterine cavity, usually with an opened gauze sponge wrapped around them. The uterine cavity is palpated and any placental fragments are removed. The examining hand is then withdrawn into the vagina, and bimanual uterine massage is begun. The fist in the vagina pushes upward while an open hand on the abdomen pushes downward, so that the uterus is compressed between them (Fig. 20-2).

In addition to bimanual uterine massage, *ecbolic agents* such as oxytocin should be administered. Because there is no longer a fetus present, hyperstimulation is no longer an issue and high doses may be given intravenously. A typical regimen would be 20 units of oxytocin in 1000 ml of normal (0.9%) saline solution, infused rapidly. Often the intravenous infusion is allowed to run "wide open" to achieve maximum effect. However, such a rapid flow rate is not necessary since maximal ecbolic effect will be reached at far lower doses. Furthermore, fluid overload is a potential problem when rapid infusion rates are used. Direct intravenous "push" infusions of pure oxytocin should be avoided, as transient hypotension may result.

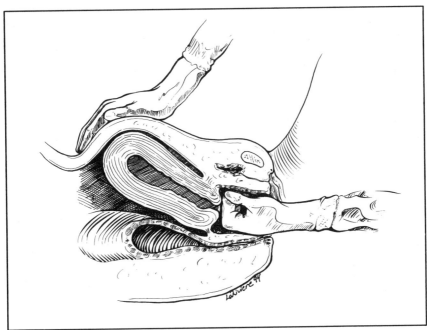

Fig. 20-2.   Bimanual massage of the uterus. The attendant's closed fist in the vagina pushes the uterus upward, compressing it against the open hand on the abdomen.

Other ecbolic agents such as ergot alkaloids and prostaglandins are commonly used as second- or third-line therapies. Ergonovine maleate is an ergot preparation which, while contraindicated during pregnancy because it causes prolonged tetanic contractions, may be quite useful once the baby has been born. It is usually given intramuscularly, because intravenous use may cause hypertension. A prostaglandin compound, 15-methyl prostaglandin $F_{2\text{-alpha}}$, is also used intramuscularly to promote uterine contractions. This drug may be given in any muscle, but some clinicians prefer to inject it directly into the myometrium through the abdominal wall.

If uterine massage and ecbolic agents are not rapidly successful in stopping postpartum hemorrhage, the vagina and cervix should be carefully inspected to identify and repair any lacerations that may be the source of bleeding. If all of the above measures are unsuccessful, abdominal surgical approaches such as ligation of the ascending branch of the uterine artery, hypogastric artery ligation, or hysterectomy may be required.

Delayed postpartum hemorrhage is that which occurs more than 24 hours after delivery. Commonly there is a transient episode of bleeding during the second week postpartum, representing the sloughing of the eschar at the placental implantation site. Delayed postpartum hemorrhage may occur at any time. The cause is often considered to be *subinvolution* of the placental implantation site, in which the uterus is larger than would be expected at a given interval since delivery. There may be retained fragments of placental tissue, and infection may also be present. Treatment is often unnecessary, but when bleeding is heavy and persistent the use of ecbolic agents, particularly ergot derivatives, is a good first step. Although curettage was traditionally performed for delayed postpartum hemorrhage, this may not be necessary and might make things worse, either by increasing the bleeding or by causing scarring of the endometrial cavity, which may lead to *Asherman's syndrome*, or intrauterine synechiae. It is useful to perform sonography to determine whether there is significant tissue remaining in the uterine cavity. If not, curettage is unlikely to be helpful.

Perineal Care

If an episiotomy has been performed, or a perineal laceration has occurred, the patient is often concerned about care of this incision or wound. Absorbable sutures are routinely used, and no special care is required. Patients are advised to bathe or shower as desired. If analgesia is required during the first few postpartum days, a nonsteroidal antiinflammatory agent, acetaminophen, or aspirin may be suggested. Cold or hot sitz baths may be helpful when there is more than the usual degree of discomfort. Some patients may have considerable pain, particularly if a mediolateral episiotomy was performed or a hematoma has formed in the subcutaneous tissues of the vulva and perineum. When patients complain of severe perineal pain it is important to examine the area and make certain that no treatable problem, such as hematoma or infection, is present. The perineum should be evaluated for redness, edema, ecchymosis, discharge, and skin approximation.

Although it was once routine to advise couples to avoid sexual intercourse until the 6-week postpartum visit, this advice was neither practical nor appropriate. There are many strains on a family as it adapts to the presence of a new baby without having to deal with 6 weeks of sexual abstinence. Because no data are available to support a particular recommendation, couples are now advised to resume sexual intercourse when it is comfortable for the woman. If a women has experienced a fourth-degree laceration, it is probably advisable for her not to resume intercourse until the 4- to 6-week postpartum checkup.

Lactation

The breast begins to develop in the fetus at about 35 days after conception when, along the mammary ridge from the axilla to the lower abdomen, a mammary bud invaginates from the surface epithelium. This bud will become the breast, and preparation for lactation begins during embryonic life. The nipple forms in the skin overlying the mammary bud. Between 15 and 25 milk ducts develop to carry milk from the glandular units of the

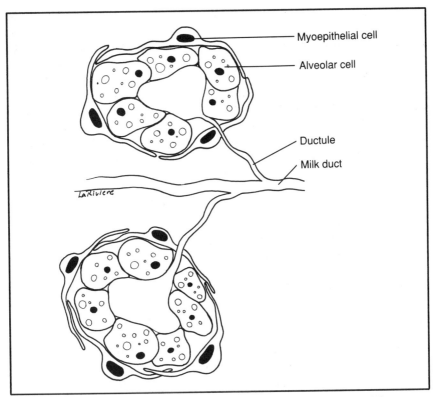

Fig. 20-3.   Functional unit of the breast. The myoepithelial cells surround the
alveolar cells, which secrete into a central opening. This fluid drains through a ductule
into a milk duct. (Adapted from D. H. Riddick. All about the human breast. *Contemp.
Ob/Gyn.* 19:103, 1982.)

breast to the nipple. Each glandular unit consists of alveolar cells that empty
into a central sinus, which in turn is drained by a ductule into a milk duct.
The alveolar cells are surrounded by myoepithelial cells that compress the
alveoli, squeezing milk into the ductules (Fig. 20-3).

At the time of birth, some infants lactate, presumably secondary to the
withdrawal of maternal estrogen. However, further development of the
breasts is necessary before lactation can support nutrition in a neonate.
Little happens during infancy and childhood, but at *thelarche,* which is the
development of the breasts at puberty, there are a series of stages that culminate in the mature breast. Prolactin stimulates the production of estrogen receptors in the mammary epithelial cells. Rising estrogen during the
menstrual cycle causes arborization of the milk ducts, while progesterone
promotes the growth of alveolar epithelium. Insulin, growth hormone, cortisol, and thyroxine are permissive but not rate-limiting for breast

development. The fatty tissue in the breasts serves as a matrix of support, and also as a source of steroidogenesis.

Once the individual begins to ovulate and menstruate, the breasts go through cyclic changes each month. During the proliferative phase of the menstrual cycle, estrogen leads to increased ductal proliferation, and during the secretory phase the combination of progesterone and estrogen enhances glandular development and water content.

Once pregnancy occurs, rising levels of prolactin, estrogen, and progesterone exaggerate these changes and the mature functional breast is ready to lactate by the third trimester. All that remains for *lactogenesis* (the initiation of milk production) to occur is the precipitous fall in maternal estrogen and progesterone levels, which is brought about by delivery of the placenta. As the inhibitory effects of estrogen and progesterone are released, lactose is produced and water is incorporated into the secretions of the glands. Prolactin and cortisol are permissive for this process. In addition, the surge in prolactin just before delivery increases the production of casein, the primary milk protein.

At one time breast-feeding was not fashionable, and many women wanted to prevent lactation, particularly the sometimes painful "engorgement" of the breasts when milk is produced but not removed by suckling. Large doses of estrogen, in depot form to prolong absorption, can delay lactogenesis by converting the sudden drop in estrogen to a gradual diminution. For many years this approach was used to prevent lactation. It was effective in delaying breast engorgement until the mother was home from the hospital. The many theoretical risks of high-dose estrogen combined with a trend toward breast-feeding have caused this approach to lose favor, and now there are no estrogen preparations approved by the Food and Drug Administration for lactation suppression.

Bromocriptine, a dopamine receptor agonist that inhibits the release of prolactin, is available for lactation inhibition. It is rather expensive, and must be taken over a 2-week interval, but is relatively effective. Side effects include nausea and vomiting, hypotension, and rarely cardiovascular manifestations such as hypertension, stroke, and myocardial infarction.

Because of these potential side effects, most women who do not wish to lactate are not given drugs, but are advised to avoid suckling, so as to avoid the stimulus for prolactin secretion as well as prevent milk removal. Breast engorgement is treated with mild analgesics and ice packs and usually abates within 24 to 48 hours. Patients who do not lactate after delivery may have *Sheehan's syndrome,* which is a rare condition also known as *pituitary apoplexy.* It is due to pituitary infarction secondary to hypotension, usually resulting from postpartum hemorrhage. Absence of lactation is the first sign of this complication.

During lactogenesis the presence of large amounts of prolactin is necessary, with serum levels averaging 200 ng/ml during the first week. There is a reflex in which suckling of the breast evokes an outpouring of pituitary prolactin. Once lactation is established, prolactin is not as critical. Levels are elevated during the first few months, and increase 10- to 20-fold during suckling, but by the fourth postpartum month prolactin levels are only slightly elevated and do not respond so briskly to suckling. Another important reflex that becomes established during lactation is the milk ejection response. Stimulation of the nipples at suckling leads to release of oxytocin from the posterior pituitary gland. The oxytocin causes the myoepithelial cells in the breasts to contract, causing the "milk let-down" reflex. The oxytocin also stimulates uterine contractions, decreasing postpartum bleeding. Eventually the reflex becomes generalized, so that even hearing the baby cry may cause a milk let-down.

The maintenance of milk production, called *galactopoiesis*, requires the removal of milk via breast-feeding, adequate nutrition, and the proper mental state. The latter is aided by a relaxed and unhurried environment. As the mother continues to nurse her baby, the high prolactin levels present during the first few months lead to continued low levels of gonadotropin-releasing hormones, and thus low levels of luteinizing hormone and follicle-stimulating hormone, so that ovulation is inhibited. Although nonlactating women usually ovulate by 2 months postpartum, those who lactate and breast-feed exclusively may not ovulate for considerably longer periods of time. Nevertheless, 5 percent of lactating women ovulate by 2 months postpartum and most do so by 10 months. Thus, "lactational infertility" may reduce the overall pregnancy rate, but it is not a very reliable approach for the individual who does not want to conceive. Other means of contraception should be made available to lactating mothers.

Emotional Changes

Major emotional adjustments are necessary with the birth of a baby, particularly the first baby. The woman must make the transition from being someone's daughter to being someone's mother. The couple must expand their relationship to include the mutual responsibility for, and intrusion of, a third individual who is helpless and unrelenting in his or her demands for attention and care. The pregnancy has been a time of high anticipation and excitement; once the child has been born there may be a sense of "letdown" because the eagerly awaited event has passed.

Most new mothers experience the "blues" for a few days during the week following childbirth. The cause has not been determined, but the symptoms are so universal that many clinicians assume that there is a hormonal or physiologic basis. The most common manifestations include crying for no apparent reason, or a reason that seems trivial to others, lability of mood, and confusion. These self-limited "blues" are not pathologic, and should not be mistaken for postpartum depression.

It has been estimated that upwards of 10 percent of women undergo clinically significant postpartum depression, usually characterized by somatic symptoms such as fatigue. It may be difficult to distinguish depression from normal postpartum symptoms, but the depressed patient continues to experience symptoms long after the average woman has returned to normal functioning. Postpartum depression often is not diagnosed until 4 to 6 months after delivery. Although many investigators have sought evidence of a hormonal relationship between pregnancy and depression, no such association has been adequately documented. Women who have had previous depressive episodes are at particular risk, and there is a 50 percent recurrence rate if a women experienced postpartum depression in her previous pregnancy. Because postpartum thyroiditis may evoke symptoms similar to those of depression, it is worthwhile to evaluate thyroid function in patients with depression. Although postpartum thyroiditis may have a hyperthyroid phase, the depressive symptoms are generally associated with hypothyroidism. This diagnosis is made by the presence of low thyroxine and high thyroid-stimulating hormone, and may be confirmed by the presence of antithyroid antibodies, usually measured as microsomal antibody. Postpartum psychosis is the most extreme form of emotional disturbance experienced after birth, but it is not clear that this is a specific form of psychosis. Psychosis is considerably more common during the weeks after delivery, and the prognosis for such patients is better than with psychosis at other times. The relationship with pregnancy has not been delineated.

Common Postpartum Discomforts

During the postpartum period, a number of discomforts are experienced by childbearing women. Most fall within the range of normal. Many postpartum women can benefit from health teaching about such complaints.

Breast Tenderness and Engorgement

Engorgement is swelling of the breasts. It is a normal physiologic condition that occurs 2 to 5 days following birth. Pain and tenderness are associated with fully engorged breasts that are hard and warm to the touch. For the nonlactating woman, wearing a tight-fitting bra, using ice on the breasts, taking analgesics, and not putting the infant to the breast (i.e., natural suppression) suppress milk production and diminish engorgement. For the lactating woman, placing the infant to the breast assists in the subsidence of engorgement by emptying the breasts. Nursing every 2 to 3 hours prevents milk from backing up and engorgement from occurring; this situation is especially likely to occur at night. Short, frequent feedings, applying moist heat to the breasts, using breast massage, and hand or pump expression help. Within a few days, the supply of milk is regulated by the demands of the infant and the engorgement lessens.

Fatigue and Weakness

Lethargy and fatigue are common complaints during the postpartum period. Exhausting or long labors coupled with the widespread requirements of insurance companies for early postpartum discharge (in order to lower cost by shortening the length of stay) often mean that women have very little time for recuperation early in the puerperium. Fatigue is often perceived as muscle soreness, especially in the upper arms, shoulders, and legs. Having someone to provide support at home can be helpful. Mothers tire easily due to the demands of infant care and feeding along with the need to provide restorative care for themselves. With increased availability of parental leave, more time is now set aside for parenting during this period. Daily naps and adequate sleep are necessary. Hot showers and slow advancement of activities help. Nothing is more tiring than having to deal with visitors at home. Allowing others to do laundry, shopping, cooking, and errands as well as taking the phone off the hook are all helpful ways for mothers to limit energy demands. Fatigue coupled with a body trying to heal may make driving uncomfortable. Stairs can be difficult for some women. Blood volume and hormonal changes can predispose the woman to dizziness. Prolonged fatigue that does not resolve may signal thyroid dysfunction.

Afterpains
Intermittent uterine contractions that occur after delivery are called *afterpains*. To most women they resemble severe menstrual cramps and can be the most discomforting symptom experienced during the puerperium. They often begin immediately after delivery of the placenta and can last until the uterus becomes a pelvic organ at around 2 to 3 weeks. Afterpains seem to be more intense after second and subsequent babies than after the first baby. Women who are breast-feeding also experience stronger afterpains, since suckling stimulates oxytocin production. Such cramps often signal that the uterus is contracting and beginning to involute. The discomfort of afterpains can be limited in a number of ways. During the early puerperium the nursing staff should ensure that the bladder is empty, and the woman may feel better when lying prone with a pillow under her lower abdomen. Various mild analgesic medications may also provide relief.

Stiffness and Cramps in the Lower Extremities
Muscle stiffness and cramps in the lower extremities are often attributed to a long labor during which muscles that have not been actively used in the past are suddenly called on. Hot showers and the slow progression to increased activity ease the discomfort. It is important to ensure that lower extremity discomfort is not due to superficial or deep vein thrombosis.

Abdominal Wall Relaxation
Many patients find that abdominal wall muscle tone is diminished after childbirth. This loss of tone is a result of overstretching due to enlargement of the uterus. The abdomen appears somewhat pendulous after delivery. Abdominal binders are not effective. Abdominal-strengthening exercises should be initiated as soon as possible after birth to improve abdominal muscle tone. If the delivery or birth has been uncomplicated,

abdominal-tightening exercises can be started immediately while the woman is in bed. Exercises that can be initiated early on are the pelvic tilt and modified leg lifts. Abdominal- and pelvic-tightening exercises (Kegels) can be started in the hospital as well. After cesarean birth women can benefit by initiating a few exercises early on, but the incision should be splinted to manage postoperative gas and coughing.

The resumption of active exercise should not be restricted after the first 2 weeks postpartum if vaginal bleeding is minimal and the woman is well rested. However, it often takes months to regain original abdominal tone. A longer period of time before initiation of an active program of exercise is advised after cesarean section, at least until the 4- to 6-week checkup.

Diuresis and Diaphoresis

Initially in the postpartum period, urinary frequency and perspiration are very evident. The body is managing to rid itself of extra fluid. Some women experience night sweats even to the point of having to change clothing. The diaphoresis is just an additional route for the body to rid itself of increased extracellular fluid accumulated during pregnancy. If women are told about this problem, they can anticipate it. The excessive fluid loss adds to the overall weight loss most women experience after delivery.

Diet and Appetite Changes

Women are often hungry following labor since they may have eaten very little prior to labor and are without solids during labor. Many are ready for a meal soon after the birth experience. Appetite swings are not unusual during the entire postpartum period. Women are often too tired to cook or prepare food and this may affect eating habits. Puerperal women need foods high in iron and protein to prevent anemia and to aid in tissue healing. If a women is breast-feeding, an increase in caloric intake of 500 additional calories per day is required.

Difficulty Voiding

Several factors may affect the ability to void after birth. Anesthesia, perineal swelling, and bladder overdistention can affect bladder sensation, and urethral discomfort may inhibit voiding. Edema of the vulva from periurethral lacerations or vigorous pushing during second-stage labor may increase perineal swelling. Women should be encouraged to void as soon as possible after delivery. Intake and output are monitored carefully during this time to detect and prevent urinary retention. Bladder catheterization may be necessary, and sometimes an indwelling catheter is used if the problem does not resolve.

Constipation and Hemorrhoids

Constipation and hemorrhoids are common discomforts during the postpartum period. Contributing factors include decreased abdominal wall tone, third- or fourth-degree lacerations, constipation of pregnancy, and vigorous pushing of the fetal head against the pelvic floor. Fear of having a bowel movement after delivery is a strong concern for many women. Stool softeners and mild cathartics are often helpful. For women with a third- or fourth-degree laceration, no enemas or suppositories should be used. Foods high in fiber, frequent ambulation, and an increase in fruits and fluids assist women in becoming self-regulated. Many women do better with attempting a bowel movement and dealing with hemorrhoidal discomfort in their own home rather than in the hospital.

Vulvar and Lower Extremity Varices

Vulvar and lower extremity varices are often noted prior to the delivery as the weight of the uterus and the fetus place pressure on vulvar and lower-extremity veins. Postpartum inspection of vulvar varices is warranted to ensure that their swelling decreases over time. Protection of large varices by means of perineal padding helps to limit trauma. Lower extremities are monitored for signs or symptoms of superficial or deep vein thrombo-phlebitis such as swelling, pain, calf heat or tenderness, and increased calf circumference.

Sleep Disturbances

Sleep disturbances during the immediate postpartum period may be associated with multiple factors, including the need to urinate, episiotomy discomfort, concern that someone be awake to hear the infant, feeding cycles, and other varied physical complaints. Enhancing the sleep efforts of most women during the postpartum period assists them in having less fatigue. Prolonged sleep disturbances may be an early symptom of postpartum depression.

Recommended Reading

Benedetti, T. J. Obstetric Hemorrhage. In S. G. Gabbe, J. R. Niebyl, and J. L. Simpson (eds.), *Obstetrics: Normal and Problem Pregnancies* (2nd ed.). New York: Churchill-Livingstone, 1991. Pp. 573–606.

The Puerperium. In F. G. Cunningham, P. C. MacDonald, N. F. Gant, K. J. Leveno, and L. C. Gilstrap, III (eds.), *Williams Obstetrics* (19th ed.). Norwalk: Appleton & Lange, 1993. Pp. 459–473.

Driscoll, J., and Walker, M. *Taking Care of Your New Baby.* Garden City Park, NY: Avery, 1989.

Klaus, M. H., and Kennell, J. H. *Parent-Infant Bonding* (2nd ed.). St. Louis: Mosby, 1982.

Lawrence, R. A. *Breastfeeding: A Guide for the Medical Profession* (4th ed.). St. Louis: Mosby, 1994.

Other Disorders of the Puerperium. In F. G. Cunningham, P. C. MacDonald, N. F. Gant, K. J. Leveno, and L. C. Gilstrap, III (eds.), *Williams Obstetrics* (19th ed.). Norwalk: Appleton & Lange, 1993. Pp. 643–650.

Stuenkel, C. A., and Burrow, G. N. Postpartum Thyroiditis. In R. V. Lee, et al. (eds.), *Current Obstetric Medicine* (Vol. 1). St. Louis: Mosby Year Book, 1991. Pp. 349–365.

Varney, H. *Nurse-Midwifery* (2nd ed.). Boston: Blackwell, 1987

21

Family Planning

Carol A. Wheeler

The field of family planning and contraception is one that has continued to expand, allowing more options as individuals engage in sexual relationships. For many, health concerns, such as prevention of sexually transmitted diseases, become equally or more important than contraceptive efficacy. Contraceptive choices may be influenced by concern about health risks of one method versus another. Issues such as cost, convenience, and peer group popularity may also influence a decision on method used. It is vitally important that the clinician provide complete and useful information to assist the patient in the decision-making process.

Perhaps one of the biggest problems with family planning methods is not what is used or why it is used but the fact that only roughly one-half of women engaging in intercourse for the first time use any form of contraception. Particularly prevalent among teenagers is the sense that "it won't happen to me." Teens have many misconceptions about their chances for fertility. Concerns over lack of spontaneity, guilt, identity problems, and the need to prove masculinity or femininity all interfere in making appropriate choices. Not only must the health care provider be aware of the technical aspects of each method, but he or she must be cognizant of the psychosocial aspects of contraceptive choices. The optimum method for a 15-year-old sexually active adolescent may not be the best choice for a 35-year-old married woman who smokes cigarettes. Individual counselling and choice are key issues.

Some interesting data collected by the Alan Guttmacher Institute help illustrate the magnitude of these issues. By their early twenties, 86 percent of women have had sex at least once and close to 80 percent are sexually active. Involuntary infertility is infrequent in women younger than 25 years of age (< 2%) for reasons such as low incidence of endometriosis and a high rate of regular ovulation. Because more than half of the pregnancies in the United States each year are unintended, the need for contraception is great. One in 10 women between 15 and 34 years of age are pregnant each year. Women spend on average at least 30 years of their lives in the reproductive years. Control over timing and frequency of pregnancy is critical to them and their partners. Women of the 1990s, many with careers, want to be able to make these choices.

Contraceptive Effectiveness

Any discussion of contraception must include an understanding of its efficacy in prevention of contraception. The two main distinctions are the *theoretical effectiveness* and the *use effectiveness*. The theoretical effectiveness is based on the "perfect" user who consistently uses the method in an optimal manner. The use effectiveness defines the ability of the method to prevent pregnancy when actually used and includes inconsistent or inappropriate use. A barrier method such as a diaphragm may have a much lower use effectiveness than theoretical effectiveness because of improper or infrequent use. Even an oral contraceptive that is prescribed without proper counselling about expected side effects may be used infrequently enough to become ineffective. Rhythm or periodic abstinence methods may have a high theoretical effectiveness but classically have very low use effectiveness due to difficult compliance or complexity.

One of the most commonly employed methods of comparing contraceptive efficacy is the Pearl method. The Pearl pregnancy rate is:

$$\frac{\text{No. of accidental pregnancies}}{\text{Total months of contraceptive use}} \times 12 = \text{No. of pregnancies per woman per year}$$

Subtracting the Pearl pregnancy rate from one gives the Pearl use effectiveness. Some problems exist with this method of evaluation since the longer a group of users is observed, the higher the use effectiveness will be since those who use the method improperly will become pregnant early.

Life-table analysis also has been used to evaluate contraceptive effectiveness. Life tables account for varying lengths of use by looking month by month at pregnancy rates and taking into account those who have stopped using a contraceptive method or become lost to follow-up. This method has the advantage that the use-effectiveness will not give different results if some women use the contraceptive for a long time or if some become pregnant after a short period of use. Life tables can involve complex calculations and may account for multiple effects on pregnancy risks. No matter what type of analysis is used, efficacy comparisons between contraceptive types should be made using the same type of analysis.

Contraceptive Safety

Issues regarding safety which are critical in the minds of patients and physicians, have recently attracted the attention of the federal government. Any method should be tested and evaluated in a large enough population to detect any significant risks. Unfortunately, it may be difficult to detect infrequent risks related to a method until it has been used by larger groups. On the other hand, an apparent risk in a small sample may not be statistically significant when applied to the whole population. These issues have particularly come into play when oral contraceptive use has been studied.

Studies of contraceptive use are particularly prone to bias (or distortion). A woman's recall of her contraceptive use may be influenced by a bad outcome or side effect. Appropriate control groups may not be employed and this will frequently bias results. Careful and critical analysis of all studies of contraceptive safety issues must be performed.

Unfortunately, because of the legal climate in the United States, incomplete or inappropriate data may lead to unjustified litigation. This climate has made informed consent a critical part of any contraceptive counselling. Patient package inserts have become frightening and unreadable. The task of the clinician to clarify and simplify this information is overwhelming. Constant communication with the patient and an informed support staff will help ensure that the patient is comfortable and knowledgeable regarding the contraceptive choice.

Methods of Contraception

Natural Methods

Natural family planning includes the rhythm method (calendar method), cervical mucus method, and lactational amenorrhea (breast-feeding). Also included are methods such as coitus interruptus (withdrawal), and post-coital douching.

Periodic abstinence is the only method approved by the Roman Catholic Church. This method has been available for centuries and does not involve the use of drugs or devices. The strict calendar method is best used in a woman with very regular cycles since it involves calculation of the fertile days and abstention for a period of time, often for as much as 1 to 2 weeks per month. The general rule is to subtract 18 days from the length of the shortest menstrual cycle and 11 days from the longest cycle length. This gives the cycle days between which the couple must abstain. For example, a woman with cycles ranging from 27 to 32 days would abstain from day 9 to day 21. Because of these long periods of abstinence, pregnancy rates reflect a use failure rate as high as 50 percent.

The calendar method is often combined with the temperature method, which involves daily temperature recording to detect the postovulatory

Human Reproduction: Growth and Development

temperature rise. Coitus then may be resumed 3 days after the temperature rise. The cervical mucus method involves self-testing for the classic cyclic changes in the mucus such as increased quantity and water content at midcycle. Spinnbarkeit, or the ability of the mucus to stretch in a manner similar to egg white, is also increased at midcycle. Coitus should be avoided at this time when cervical mucus is optimal for conception. Use effectiveness rates for such combination methods may be as high as 75 to 90 percent.

Breast-feeding as a method of contraception is widely practiced in third-world nations and has proponents of its use in the United States and Europe. Mothers who fully breast-feed and maintain frequent, intense feedings are less likely to ovulate. Women may experience lactational amenorrhea for as brief as 2 to 3 months or as long as 2 to 3 years. Three months postpartum, at least one-third of lactating women have resumed menses; by 9 months this proportion rises to two-thirds. If a woman is completely breast-feeding and has *no* return of bleeding, lactational amenorrhea can be used for contraception for 6 months with a 2 percent risk of pregnancy. After this time or if menstruation has resumed, lactation is unreliable as a sole method of contraception.

Postcoital douching with various substances is very ineffective since sperm are found in the cervical mucus within 90 seconds of ejaculation. Coitus interruptus involves withdrawing the penis prior to ejaculation and requires a highly motivated male partner. This is extremely difficult because often the preejaculatory fluid contains adequate sperm to effect a pregnancy. Use effectiveness rates may be in the range of 60 to 75 percent.

In summary, the natural methods are the safest and least expensive methods of contraception with virtually no physical side effects. Unfortunately, for the majority of patients they are very ineffective methods and do not provide a consistently reliable method of contraception.

Spermicide Methods

Spermicides, such as nonoxynol-9, are widely available without a prescription as foams, creams, jellies, suppositories, and in the contraceptive sponge. A variety of chemicals and carriers are involved in these products. They act both as functional barriers (blocking sperm entry into the cervix) and sperm immobilizers. A total of six spermicides are approved for use in the United States. These spermicides are menfegol, octoxynol-9, nonoxynol-9, dodecaethyleneglycol monolaurate, laureth 10S, and methoxypoly-oxyethyleneglycol 550 laurate. One study suggested teratogenic effects of spermicides, but larger, more recent studies have failed to show an association. In addition, most patients who conceive while using these preparations discontinue their use prior to embryogenesis. The biggest problems with these agents are vaginal irritation or allergies and inconsistency in their use. Failure rates with these methods vary from 1 to 30 percent.

One method of spermicide delivery that merits special attention is the contraceptive sponge (Fig. 21-1). The sponge, which is made of polyurethane foam impregnated with nonoxynol-9, is placed in the vagina up to 24 hours prior to intercourse. It is easy for the patient to use and does not require any fitting. It does have the possible risk of increased incidence of toxic shock syndrome, although this is not universally agreed on by investigators.

Condoms

Publicity and popularity of the use of condoms has risen dramatically in the late 1980s and 1990s with increased awareness of sexually transmitted diseases, particularly the human immunodeficiency virus. The 1991 Ortho Annual Birth Control Study showed an increase in the use of condoms from 9 percent in 1985 to 16 percent in 1991 in women ages 15 to 44 years. There also has been a change in who buys the condoms—now roughly half of all condoms are purchased by women.

Most condoms are made of latex rubber. An alternative, the "lambskin" condom, actually from the intestine of lambs, may be advantageous for the man who is allergic to rubber and may also offer greater sensitivity. Latex condoms, however, offer greater protection against sexually transmitted diseases and are preferable because of that protection. Condoms come with or without lubrication, and may be smooth or textured. They are

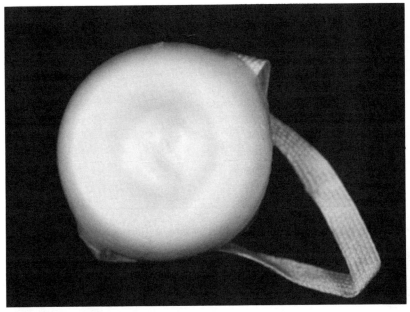

Fig. 21-1. Contraceptive sponge.

easily obtained and relatively inexpensive compared to other forms of contraception.

Failure rates vary depending on the consistency of condom use. Their use must be initiated immediately after erection since some of the preejaculatory fluid may contain viable sperm. In highly motivated populations, failure rates may be only 5 to 17 percent. In less committed users, failure rates may be as high as 15 to 20 percent.

The female condom was approved by the Food and Drug Administration in May, 1993. These protect against both pregnancy and sexually transmitted diseases. They consist of polyurethane sheaths with two flexible rings; the ring at the closed end fits over the cervix and the other ring covers the labia. This method offers women a new option for contraception, although its availability is currently limited. Pregnancy rates are expected to be approximately 15 percent although very limited data are available.

Diaphragm

The diaphragm is a circular, dome-shaped device made of latex rubber with a firm outer ring that is placed in the vagina and covers the cervix (Fig. 21-2). It is combined with spermicidal jelly or cream to act as both a physical and a chemical barrier to sperm. The device is fitted by a health care provider and inserted no more than 2 hours prior to intercourse by the user. If inserted more than 2 hours before intercourse, additional

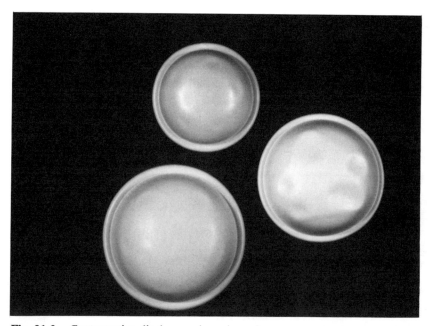

Fig. 21-2. Contraceptive diaphragms in various sizes.

spermicide must be used at the time of coitus. It should be left in place at least 6 hours after intercourse. Repeated acts of coitus require additional spermicide.

The major advantages to the diaphragm are its safety, relatively low cost, and moderate protection against sexually transmitted diseases. Disadvantages of the diaphragm include difficulty in fitting some women and displacement during intercourse, which may lead to method failure. Some patients may be allergic to the rubber or spermicide. An increase in vaginal infections and cystitis has been reported in some users. The diaphragm should not be left in place for more than 24 hours because of concern over possible linkage with toxic shock syndrome.

Diaphragms are available in several types and sizes ranging from 55 to 105 mm in diameter. Spermicide is placed inside the rim and the device is folded for vaginal placement. Patient placement should be checked by the health care provider since placement may be difficult. The diaphragm should be refitted after childbirth or after weight gain or loss of 20 lb.

Theoretical failure rates are as low as 2 to 3 percent, but use failure rates range from 2 to 20 percent. One of the biggest reasons for failure is simply irregular or erratic use because of inconvenience. It is more suited to the older woman in a stable relationship than to the teenager.

Cervical Cap

The use of the cervical cap was first described by a German gynecologist in 1838. Its popularity has varied since that time, with a fairly widespread use in Great Britain during the 1930s and 1940s. It was in limited use in the United States during that time. This device was approved by the Food and Drug Administration in May 1988 for use in the United States, and although its popularity is limited it is an important contraceptive option.

The cervical cap available in the United States (the Prentif cavity-rim cervical cap) is a flexible, rubber cuplike device fitted around the base of the cervix. The cap is smaller than a diaphragm (1.25 to 1.5 in. long) and available in four sizes (22–31 mm in internal rim diameter) (Fig. 21-3). In a manner similar to the diaphragm, spermicidal cream or jelly is placed inside the cap prior to insertion. Unlike the diaphragm, however, it may be left in place up to 48 hours and repeated intercourse does not require the use of additional spermicide.

The cap must be fitted by a health care provider trained specifically in its use. It is somewhat more difficult to fit and use than the traditional diaphragm. It may be less noticeable to the partner and may be used by some women who are unable to be fitted with the diaphragm. Its overall effectiveness is thought to be comparable to the diaphragm with a Pearl failure rate of 16.9 to 20 per 100 women-years. Theoretical effectiveness may approach 95 percent depending on consistency of use.

Some patients may not be candidates for the cervical cap. Women with an abnormally shaped or sized cervix may be difficult to fit. Those with

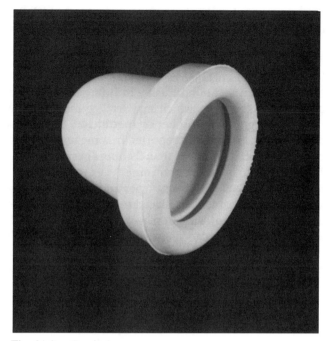

Fig. 21-3. Cervical cap.

active cervicitis, vaginitis, or an abnormal Pap smear should not use the cap. Although the method is generally safe, there are some minor side effects. Initial data from the National Institutes of Health trials showed that in the first 3 months of use 4 percent of users had Pap smear changes from class I to class III. Reanalysis of these data has shown that this risk is not significantly different from that seen in diaphragm users.

Other concerns with the cervical cap include possible toxic shock syndrome, but no cases have been reported. The cap should not be worn during menses because of this potential problem. Some women may experience small vaginal lacerations due to difficult insertion or allergic reactions to the rubber or spermicide. Patients also may notice odor or increased vaginal infections.

Intrauterine Device

Although it has fallen in and out of popularity over the last several decades, the intrauterine device (IUD) is one of the most effective forms of contraception. The IUD (Fig. 21-4) is a small loop or piece of plastic that is placed in the uterus. It may contain a form of progesterone or be covered with fine copper wire. The mechanisms of action for prevention of pregnancy are probably multiple. It is thought that the IUD evokes an inflammatory response in the endometrium and prevents implantation. It may also interfere with sperm or oocyte transport.

The IUD has a string that trails from the device to the vagina. The Dalkon shield, an IUD removed from the market, had an unacceptably high incidence of associated pelvic inflammatory disease (PID) believed to be related to a multifilament string. The two IUDs currently available in the United States are the copper T380A (ParaGard) and the Progestasert. The ParaGard may remain in place for 10 years; the Progestasert must be replaced annually. Both types have a monofilament tail.

Because of the PID risk, the IUD should be used only by a woman in a mutually monogamous relationship. Some physicians think that nulliparous women should not use an IUD because of concerns over long-term fertility as well as risk of expulsion due to small uterine size. Data from the Women's Health study, originally performed in 1983 by the Centers for Disease Control (CDC) to evaluate PID, were reanalyzed in 1988 and showed no significant increase in PID in women at low risk for sexually transmitted diseases.

Some patients are better suited to IUD use than others. It is an excellent option for the woman over age 35 who is unsure about sterilization and may have medical contraindications for the oral contraceptive. Women with a history of PID, ectopic pregnancy, or multiple sexual partners should avoid the IUD.

The most common side effects of IUD use are increased menstrual flow and dysmenorrhea. These effects may be less of a problem with the

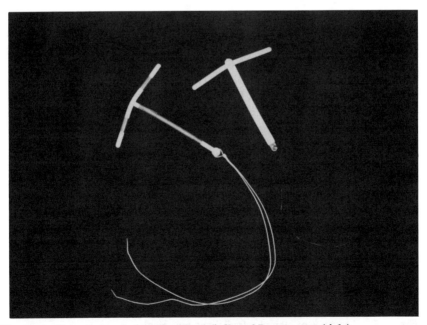

Fig. 21-4. Intrauterine devices: ParaGard (left) and Progestasert (right).

progesterone-containing IUD. Expulsion of the IUD may occur most frequently in the 3 months after insertion. The IUD is most often inserted during menses, and one complication occasionally related to insertion is perforation of the uterus.

The biggest advantage of the IUD is the high rate of compliance since it requires virtually no user involvement other than periodically checking for the string. Use-failure rates range from 1 to 3 percent. Discontinuation rates due to side effects may be as high as 30 to 40 percent at the end of 1 year, however. Although pregnancies with an IUD in place are rare, the risk of ectopic pregnancy is high should a pregnancy occur since the IUD is ineffective in preventing extrauterine pregnancies. Should an intrauterine pregnancy occur with an IUD in place, the IUD should be removed if the string is visible because of an unacceptably high risk of a septic abortion.

Steroid Contraception

Steroid Biochemistry

The development of steroid contraception began with the isolation of estradiol and progesterone in 1935. These orally inactive compounds were modified to produce the steroids currently used for contraception. The addition of an ethinyl group at the 17 position led to ethinyl estradiol, a very potent estrogen. The 3-methyl ether of ethinyl estradiol is mestranol, the other contraceptive estrogen. Mestranol is thought to be a weaker estrogen and is not used in the low-dose oral contraceptives (Fig. 21-5).

Orally active progestins are of two major types. Derivatives of 17 alpha-hydroxyprogesterone (a 21-carbon compound) are orally potent when formed from substitutions at the 17 and 6 carbon positions. These include medroxyprogesterone acetate and megestrol acetate, which are widely used in gynecologic practice (Fig. 21-6).

The second group of orally active progestins are derived from modi-fications of testosterone. Ethinyl substitution leads to the orally active ethisterone (Fig. 21-7). With removal of carbon 19, the compound changes from an androgen to primarily a progestin (norethindrone). Modifications

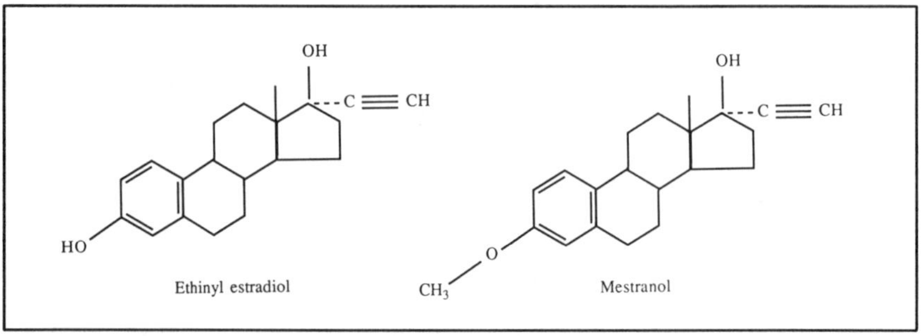

Fig. 21-5. Structures of ethinyl estradiol and mestranol.

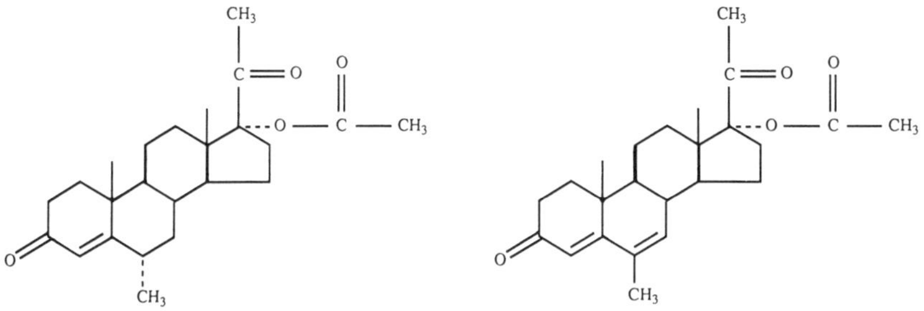

Medroxyprogesterone acetate (Provera)

Megestrol acetate

Fig. 21-6. Structures of medroxyprogesterone acetate and megestrol acetate.

of norethindrone include norethindrone acetate, norethynodrel, norgestrel, and ethynodiol diacetate, the other commonly used progestins (Fig. 21-8). Three other progestins are currently used in Europe (desogestrel, norgestimate, and gestodene) and are becoming available in the United States.

Oral Contraceptives

The most frequently used contraceptive method in the United States is the combination oral contraceptive. This highly efficacious form of contraception contains both a progestin and an estrogen component. The mechanism of action of this method is primarily by inhibition of ovulation at both the pituitary and hypothalamic centers. In general, the estrogen component suppresses follicle-stimulating hormone and the progestin suppresses luteinizing hormone. The estrogen component also stabilizes the endometrium to permit regular shedding. Overall, progestin effects are believed to predominate due to its relatively large dose in comparison to estrogen. These progestin effects include thickening of the cervical mucus, decidualization of the endometrium, and a decrease in tubal motility.

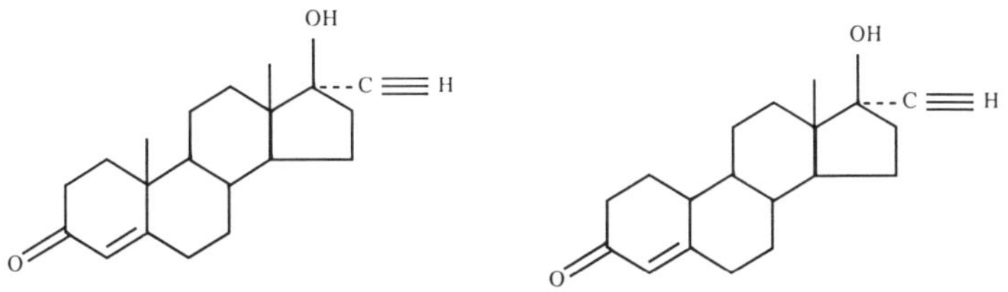

Ethisterone

Norethindrone

Fig. 21-7. Structures of ethisterone and norethindrone.

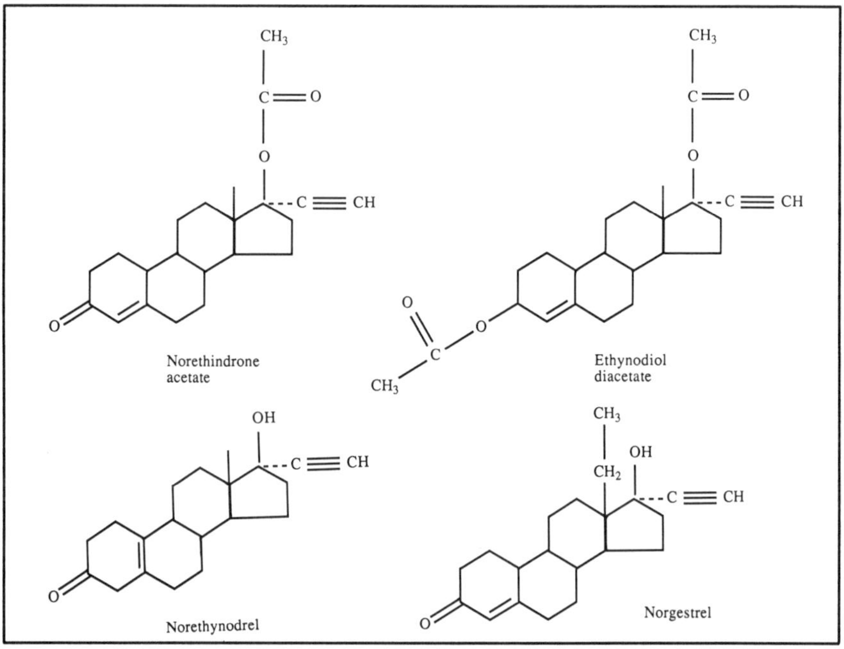

Fig. 21-8. Structures of norethindrone acetate, ethynodiol diacetate, norgestrel, and norethynodrel.

The typical oral contraceptive package contains 21 days of a drug containing both components (Fig. 21-9). Following these 21 days of treatment, there is a 7-day pill-free (or placebo) interval. Most patients experience a withdrawal bleed during this pill-free interval. The actual dose and combination of estrogen and progestin varies among manufacturers but most contain between 30 and 50 µg of estrogen. This amount is in contrast to the oral contraceptives of the 1960s, which contained as much as 150 µg of estrogen. In addition to a decreased estrogen dose, total progestin dose has decreased as well, often by "phasing" or varying the progestin during an individual cycle. Typically, a triphasic preparation varies the dose of progestin every 7 days to try to decrease breakthrough bleeding. The overall steroid dose has been minimized as much as possible in an attempt to limit minor and major side effects. This change is important to consider when looking at oral contraceptive risks since most data are based on older, higher dose formulations and may not apply to the pills used today.

The combined oral contraceptive has an extremely low failure rate in a compliant population. Taking into account the multiple sites of action, the theoretical failure rate should be approximately 0.1 percent. The actual failure rate is closer to 2 to 3 percent due to failure to take every pill. One disadvantage of the low-dose pills currently used is that missing only one or 2 pills may lead to ovulation and the possibility of conception.

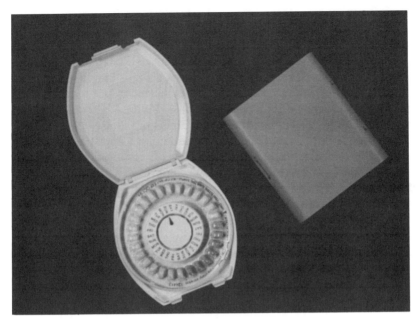

Fig. 21-9. Commercially available oral contraceptive packages.

In addition to contraceptive benefits, the oral contraceptive has many noncontraceptive advantages. Patients who take the pill experience more regular menses, less dysmenorrhea, and less menorrhagia. In addition, the likelihood of fibrocystic disease of the breast, PID, rheumatoid arthritis, ovarian cancer, and endometrial cancer is decreased by the pill.

Bothersome side effects sometimes noted by women who are taking oral contraceptives include nausea, breakthrough bleeding, and amenorrhea. Headaches, mood changes, and a decrease in libido are occasionally seen. Generally, however, oral contraceptives are well tolerated and can be used for extended periods of time without interruption. There is no evidence that a rest period off oral contraceptives is beneficial, and, in fact, often this can lead to an unintended pregnancy. Inadvertent use during early pregnancy is currently thought to have no significant impact on the incidence of congenital anomalies in the offspring. Combination oral contraceptives are usually avoided during lactation because of a negative impact on milk production.

Perhaps the most confusing area of oral contraception is the question of oral contraceptive risks. The biggest concern is a possible link between pill use and cardiovascular disease. The data are clear that there is a statistically significant increase in ischemic heart disease in smokers over the age of 35 who use the pill. The patient under age 35 and the nonsmoker over age 35 do not appear to have the same associated risk. For a more detailed discussion, the reader should consult the recommended reading list.

A second major concern in the area of oral contraception is a possible link with breast cancer. Many large-scale studies have attempted to quantify risks of breast cancer in subsets of oral contraceptive users. The largest United States study that evaluated the risk of breast cancer in oral contraceptive users was the Cancer and Steroid Hormone Study (CASH) (sponsored by the CDC). The CASH study showed a slight increase in breast cancer diagnosis in young current or former pill users but a decrease in diagnosis at an older age. The data from other studies are confusing but must be put into perspective with all the benefits of pill use.

The metabolic effects of the combined oral contraceptive are relatively minor and show some variation depending on the dose and types of estrogen and progestin used. Some formulations may alter the lipoprotein profile by increasing low-density lipoprotein and decreasing high-density lipoprotein, but most pills have no clinically significant impact on lipids. Impaired glucose tolerance was noted in patients who took the higher dose oral contraceptives in the past. The majority of patients do not have significant changes in carbohydrate metabolism of clinical relevance when taking the current pills.

Aside from gallbladder disease, which is clearly increased in pill users, and the cardiovascular risk in smokers older than 35 years, for most women the benefits of oral contraceptive use far outweigh the risks. The risk associated with unintended pregnancy and childbearing far exceed the pill risks at all ages.

Absolute contraindications for oral contraceptive use include: undiagnosed genital bleeding, suspected pregnancy, known or suspected breast cancer, smokers over the age of 35, markedly impaired liver function, and history of or active thrombophlebitis. Relative contraindications (where clinical judgment should be used) include: hypertension, migraine headaches, uterine fibroids, diabetes mellitus, gallbladder disease, and sickle-cell disease. Many of these patients require very effective methods of contraception and may be given oral contraceptives with careful monitoring.

Another form of oral contraception is the progestin-only pill, or minipill. This pill contains a low dose of a progestin (norethindrone or norgestrel) taken in a continuous fashion. Because this pill does not reliably inhibit ovulation, its effects are primarily at the level of the endometrium and cervical mucus. Failure rates for the progestin-only pill are 1 to 9 percent in the first year of use. Irregular bleeding and amenorrhea are frequent problems and commonly lead to discontinuation of the method. These pills have a place for the patient who cannot or should not take estrogen and are particularly useful for the lactating woman since they do not interfere with breast-feeding.

Long-acting Steroid Contraceptives

Two long-acting steroid contraceptives are currently available in the United States. These include an injection (depot medroxyprogesterone acetate, or Depo-Provera) and an implant (levonorgestrel, or Norplant). These are convenient to use and are administered by a health professional, which ensures compliance.

Depot medroxyprogesterone acetate (DMPA) has been used extensively worldwide but only recently was approved for use in this country due to earlier concerns regarding potential carcinogenicity. This concern was based on data showing an increase in breast cancer in beagle dogs treated with DMPA. It is now widely believed that the beagle is not a suitable model for contraceptive safety evaluation because of a peculiar sensitivity in the beagle dog's breast. This drug generally causes amenorrhea and is given every 3 months by intramuscular injection. Significant irregular bleeding may be a problem for many women and can lead to discontinuation. Failure rates of less than 0.5 percent are reported, and the high level of effectiveness is ascribed to inhibition of ovulation by the high dosage of progestin. Depot medroxyprogesterone acetate is an attractive form of contraception for the patient who has difficulty maintaining compliance with the other steroidal methods of contraception.

Norplant is a reversible long-acting subdermal implant containing the progestin levonorgestrel. Six 34 mm long Silastic capsules are placed beneath the skin in the upper arm to provide continuous contraception for 5 years. The progestin inhibits ovulation in most users and also causes thickened cervical mucus. The capsules are inserted by a trained health care provider while the woman is under local anesthesia and they require removal when contraception is no longer desired or after 5 years for replacement. Because compliance is not a problem (in contrast to oral contraceptives), use effectiveness is almost identical to theoretical effectiveness. The failure rate in the first year of use is 0.2 percent.

The most common side effects with the Norplant method are related to menstrual disturbances. The types of bleeding noted range from complete amenorrhea to frequent, irregular menses. The patient must be counselled regarding this bleeding in order to ensure continuation with the method. Other occasional minor side effects are headache, nausea, and dizziness, but these tend to improve over time. Metabolic effects are minimal and make this method a good choice for patients with medical problems who require long-term effective contraception.

Sterilization

Female
Sterilization is one of the most common contraceptive methods used in the United States. Among women ages 40 to 44, one study showed 68 percent chose sterilization as their method. Female sterilization involves interruption of the fallopian tube by removing a segment or blocking it. This method should always be considered permanent and should not be performed if the patient is unsure of her decision. Reversal of tubal ligation

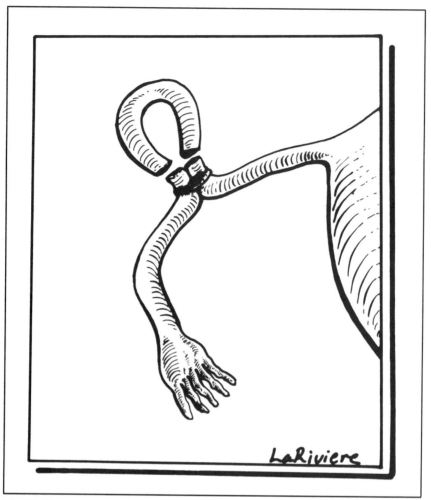

Fig. 21-10. Pomeroy technique of tubal ligation.

is feasible in some situations but should not be considered in the decision-making process surrounding tubal ligation.

There are no absolute contraindications to tubal ligation. In general, the procedure is performed either at the time of a delivery or as an interval procedure temporally removed from a pregnancy. Hysterectomy has been used as a sterilization technique, but should not be done simply for this indication. The approaches to tubal ligation are both vaginal and abdominal. Vaginal tubal ligations are not commonly performed but involve a culdotomy incision for tubal access. Infection rate is higher with the vaginal route than the abdominal route and the vaginal route may be more difficult technically.

Abdominal approaches to sterilization involve either a laparotomy or laparoscopy. For those patients who are undergoing a cesarean section, the procedure may be done at the time of the delivery by a number of different techniques. One of the most common, the Pomeroy technique, involves excision of a segment of the fallopian tube. A loop of the mid-portion of the fallopian tube is gently grasped and the base of the loop is ligated with absorbable suture. The loop is then excised. The ends of the tube ultimately separate after the suture has dissolved (Fig. 21-10). This same technique may be employed through a minilaparotomy incision immediately postpartum (when the uterus is high and the tubes are easily accessible) or as an interval procedure. Other surgical approaches are sometimes used but accomplish essentially the same thing.

Laparoscopic methods of sterilization became popular in the 1970s. These are outpatient surgical procedures that usually require general anesthesia. Tubal interruption is accomplished by the use of cautery, clips, or rings. Female sterilization failure rates are 0.5 percent during the first year and are often due to unrecognized pregnancies at the time of the procedure. Pregnancies that occur after a tubal ligation have a high likelihood of being ectopic, with ectopic rates ranging from 14 to 90 percent after the first year. Complications related to tubal sterilization are related to the procedure itself, with major surgical complications in less than 1 percent of cases. There are essentially no long-term complications or side effects, although some researchers have suggested the existence of a posttubal ligation syndrome consisting of abnormal menses and dysmenorrhea. Most investigators think this is probably not a real effect but relates to the discontinuation of oral contraceptives in many patients.

Male

Vasectomy, or occlusion of the vas deferens, is an outpatient surgical procedure performed while the patient is under local anesthesia (Fig. 21-11). It has less risk than female sterilization since vasectomy does not require peritoneal entry. The failure rate is similar to that of female sterilization provided adequate time with follow-up semen analysis performed to ensure its adequacy. Because it takes 74 days to produce sperm, part of which involves storage in the epididymis, 4 to 6 weeks and 10 to 12 ejaculations should occur prior to assessing the success of the procedure by semen analysis. One long-term sequela of vasectomy is the development of antisperm antibodies that can limit the success of vasectomy reversal. Another issue of potential concern was described in a study published in 1993 in the *Journal of the American Medical Association*; it suggested a possible link between vasectomy and the later development of prostate cancer. The relative risk in this study was small and more data should be collected to determine whether or not this is a true causal relationship. Ultimately, the decision regarding sterilization should be put into a risk-benefit perspective to ensure informed decision making, just as any other family-planning choice.

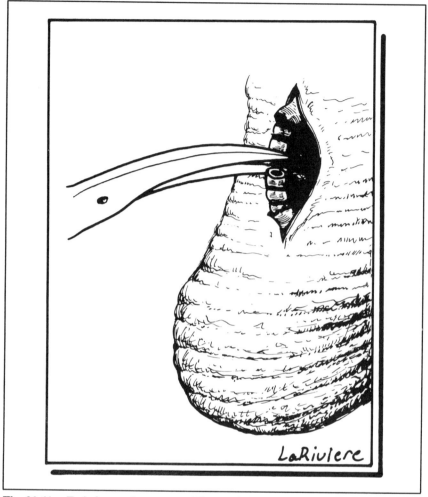

Fig. 21-11. Techniques of vasectomy. The vas deferens is sectioned between clips.

Recommended Reading

Corson, S. L., Derman, R. J., and Tyrer, L. B. *Fertility Control.* Boston: Little, Brown, 1985.

Harlap, S., Kost, K., and Forrest, G. O. T. *Preventing Pregnancy, Protecting Health: A New Look at Birth Control Choices in the United States.* The Alan Guttmacher Institute, New York, NY, 1991.

Lee, N. C., Rubin, G. L., and Boruck, R. The intrauterine device and pelvic inflammatory disease revisited: New results from the Women's Health Study. *Obstet. Gynecol.* 72:1, 1988.

Ortho Pharmaceutical Corporation. 1991 Ortho Annual Birth Control Study. Raritan, New Jersey, 1991.

Powell, M. G., et al. Contraception with the cervical cap: Effectiveness, safety, continuity of use, and user satisfaction. *Contraception* 33:215–232, 1986.

Speroff, L., and Darney, P. F. *A Clinical Guide for Contraception.* Baltimore: Williams & Wilkins, 1992.

Care of the Newborn

William Cashore

Following birth, the initiation of breathing, and the separation of the umbilical cord, the initial essential requirements of the newborn infant for transition to extrauterine life include oxygen, warmth, and nutrition.

The initiation of breathing and the transition of the circulation from fetal to neonatal pathways are described in Chap. 6. In the first few minutes and hours after delivery, the effectiveness of this cardiorespiratory adaptation is monitored by the physicians, midwives, or nurses attending the baby at delivery and in the nursery. As one indicator of the transition, an Apgar score is assigned at 1 and 5 minutes after birth, and also at 10 or 15 minutes after birth if the initial transition to normal breathing and circulation is slow or if the infant required resuscitation. After the initial examination of the infant and assignment of the Apgar score, vital signs (temperature, pulse, and respiration) are monitored regularly during the first few hours. Table 22-1 gives normal ranges for vital signs for the newborn.

To provide adequate care for the newborn who is depressed or distressed at birth, birth attendants should be suitably trained in neonatal resuscitation and the delivery area should be adequately equipped with humidified oxygen, suction equipment, inflatable bags, face masks, and laryngoscopes and endotracheal tubes of suitable size. Someone in the delivery area or readily available on call should be fully trained in neonatal cardiopulmonary resuscitation. Although the need for full cardiopulmonary resuscitation of newborn infants is relatively uncommon, a small number of infants may need suctioning, supplementary oxygen, or a brief period of assistance with initiating respiration even after an apparently normal pregnancy, labor, and delivery. If there was evidence of fetal distress before delivery, the infant is more likely to require assistance to initiate breathing and sustain adequate oxygenation.

Table 22-1. Normal vital signs in the newborn period

Heart rate	90–140/minute
Respirations	30–60/minute
Temperature	36.5–37.0°C (97.8–98.6°F)
Mean blood pressure*	40–55 mm Hg

*In many nurseries, this vital sign is not checked routinely.

If assisted ventilation or cardiopulmonary resuscitation are required for newborns, the rates of ventilation and chest compression are higher than for adults. Humidified oxygen should be administered at 40 to 60 breaths per minute, and chest compression should be administered at a rate of 100 to 120 per minute. During resuscitation, chest compression and ventilation should be synchronized at ratios of 3 : 1 or 2 : 1, with the usual rate being 120 chest compressions per minute and 60 breaths per minute during the resuscitation. As noted above, far more infants require brief periods of suctioning or respiratory assistance than require a full cardiopulmonary resuscitation.

Temperature Control

The basic concepts of thermal neutrality and heat production in newborn infants are reviewed in Chap. 6. The practical approach to temperature control in the newly born infant is the application of several simple measures to maintain a thermal-neutral environment just after delivery. To prevent cooling of the skin by evaporation of amniotic fluid at body temperature, the infant should be dried quickly with a warm towel. Except for surface cleaning of accumulated blood, meconium, and secretions, the baby should not be washed or bathed until the temperature is stable several hours after birth. In some hospitals, babies are placed in a radiant heater or warming crib immediately after delivery. A suitable and appealing alternative for most deliveries is to wrap the baby in a warm cotton blanket and hand the baby to the mother. Unless the room temperature is extremely cold, close contact between the mother and her newborn will usually suffice for temperature regulation.

After their initial examination and evaluation, babies should be dressed in a shirt and cap, wrapped in a light blanket, and placed in the mother's arms or in a bassinet with a flat, firm mattress. The cap is important because many newborns have little scalp hair, the area of skin exposed is considerable, and comparatively high rates of blood flow to the face and head early in postnatal life produce considerable heat loss from the head and upper body. Convective and radiant heat loss may be decreased by as much as 25 to 30 percent by the use of a stocking cap after birth.

Some hospitals admit babies to incubators for their initial observation and stabilization in the nursery, but other satisfactory alternatives are using a warm blanket to swaddle the baby in an open crib or keeping the mother and baby together with a single nurse performing the postnatal observations on both patients. By 4 to 6 hours of age, neonatal core temperature should be stable and is usually 0.5°C lower than that of an older child or adult. By that time, a lightly dressed term infant covered with a light blanket should be able to maintain stable temperature in an open crib in a normally heated room. Temperature instability after the first several hours should be further evaluated by the practitioner attending the infant in the nursery. Because infants are not efficient heat producers, the stresses of asphyxia, infection, etc., may produce hypothermia rather than fever, especially in preterm newborns.

Cold exposure is a significant metabolic stress during the period of neonatal adaptation. Hypothermia tends to perpetuate metabolic acidosis and impair the capacity of the infant to self-regulate the circulatory and respiratory changes that follow delivery. In addition, heat loss for any reason, whether metabolic, radiant, or convective, entails loss of calories and consumption of body energy stores. These caloric losses must be fed back to the baby in order to stabilize weight, so that babies in a temperature environment below their thermal-neutral zone gain weight poorly and need a larger caloric intake to sustain temperature, metabolism, and growth.

Feeding Normal Newborns

Human milk is the ideal nutrient for human babies. If labor and delivery are uneventful and the mother and baby are stable immediately afterwards, nursing can begin at any time. The intake in the first few days is mainly colostrum, and may be somewhat lower in breast-fed than formula-fed infants; however, the physiologic adaptation of most newborns means that their volume intake in the first 1 to 2 days postnatally may be as low as 50 to 60 ml/kg/day, or just enough to sustain urine output and water requirements. By the second to third day, the infant usually feeds more eagerly, and the lactating mother responds by increased milk production.

Frequency of nursing and the strength of the suckling impulse promote and sustain maternal milk production. Although hospital and home feeding schedules tend to be arranged in 4-hour cycles, some infants who are fed on demand nurse more frequently. The usual gastric emptying time for a term newborn is 2 to 3 hours, after which the baby begins to wake up and act hungry. Nursing 6 to 8 times a day is suitable for many newborns, but some may be nursed 8 to 10 times a day or more often, depending on the amount of time the baby and mother spend together, and the natural feeding schedule that evolves between the mother-baby pair. For the perinatal period and the first several months thereafter, breast milk is completely adequate nutritionally.

Formula-feeding is also widespread, either as a supplement to nursing or as a complete replacement for it. Although less ideal than breast milk, contemporary formulas are modified in their manufacture to resemble human milk much more closely than the cow's milk that was once the basis for formulas mixed at home. Prepared formulas are adequate in all essential nutrients and vitamins, and present-day formulas are also supplemented with sufficient iron to prevent the development of iron-deficiency anemia in the first year. Low-iron formula or cow's milk–based formula without added iron may be iron-deficient for rapidly growing infants in the second half of the first year, so iron supplements should be included in or given with the formula for all formula-fed babies.

A few infants with unusual metabolic diseases or unusual intolerances to human milk components may benefit from special formulas that are made to meet specific nutritional needs of infants with unusual metabolic or allergic problems (e.g., low-phenylalanine formula for children with phenylketonuria [PKU]).

The milk intake required to sustain growth is approximately 150 to 160 ml/kg/day, and provides 100 to 110 kcal/kg/day. Some vigorous infants take even higher volumes than those noted. In general, the persistalsis that feeding initiates results in a bowel movement after each feeding, so that mothers who nurse frequently may need to be prepared for more frequent diaper changes. The requirements of the newborn infant for water and various nutrients are listed in Table 22-2.

Prophylactic Medications and Metabolic Screening in the Newborn

At birth or during the nursery stay, several prophylactic medications are given and several screening tests are done. Some of these are required by state laws or health regulations, whereas others are part of standard pediatric practice in most nurseries.

Eye prophylaxis against *Neisseria gonorrhoeae* is required at birth in most states. This can be accomplished by instilling a 1 percent silver nitrate solution or 1 percent erythromycin ointment in both eyes. Silver nitrate is effective against all strains of gonorrhea, but may produce a more intense

Table 22-2. Nutrient requirements for newborn infants

Water	150–160 ml/kg/day
Calories	100–110 kcal/kg/day
Protein	2–3 g/kg/day
Carbohydrates	15–16 g/kg/day
Fat	3–4 g/kg/day

conjunctival reaction, with redness and swelling of the eyelids, than does erythromycin, which is equally effective against most strains of *N. gonorrhoeae*. Although it produces a less severe conjunctival reaction and is effective in most instances, erythromycin may be less effective when strains of penicillin-resistant gonorrhea are prevalent in the community. The effectiveness of erythromycin ointment in preventing postnatal chlamydial disease has not been proved. Since either topical agent is acceptable to ameliorate or prevent gonococcal eye disease, the choice of agent may be guided by parent or physician preference, institutional policies, or cost of the medication.

A number of state health departments, and many pediatric practices elsewhere, now recommend initiating hepatitis B immunization at birth. The rationale for this practice is that (1) most mother-to-baby transmission of hepatitis B is perinatal or postnatal; (2) up to 70 percent of newborns infected in the perinatal period become lifetime chronic carriers of the hepatitis B virus, with its attendant complications; and (3) immunization of infants in high-risk areas has been effective in reducing the chronic carrier state. Recombinant hepatitis B vaccine (2.5 mcg) given in the nursery should be followed by subsequent immunizations at 1 to 2 months and 6 to 12 months of age. This approach to early immunization should protect most infants and young children against early acquisition and chronic carriage of hepatitis B.

The administration of 1 mg of vitamin K at birth to prevent hemorrhagic disease of the newborn is also standard practice in most nurseries. Early administration of injectable vitamin K is highly effective in preventing this uncommon but potentially catastrophic complication, characterized by gastric, intracranial, or subcutaneous hemorrhages in otherwise well newborns during the first week. Because the synthesis of vitamin K depends on bacterial cofactors, breast-fed infants or those with delayed bowel colonization because they are not fed early are at somewhat more risk for this preventable disorder. Oral vitamin K is partially effective but not consistently absorbed, and is not available in most hospitals.

Filter-paper samples of blood (and sometimes urine) are obtained from all newborns before hospital discharge to screen for certain treatable metabolic diseases that are not easily detectable in the newborn period. Although the list of diseases screened for may vary somewhat, all state health departments have mandatory metabolic screening procedures for newborns. Uncommon metabolic diseases such as congenital hypothyroidism, PKU, galactosemia, and congenital adrenal hyperplasia are often not evident at birth. Their severe and sometimes life-threatening developmental consequences can be prevented or ameliorated by early recognition and treatment. Screening programs are designed not necessarily to establish the diagnosis of a rare disease on the basis of the screening tests, but to identify infants whose initial screening results indicate a need for further definitive testing and follow-up. Table 22-3 lists some common metabolic screening tests of newborns.

Table 22-3. Neonatal metabolic screening tests

Disorder	Consequences	Metabolic screening test
Hypothyroidism	Delayed growth and development	T_4, thyroid-stimulating hormone
Phenylketonuria	Severe retardation	Phenylalanine
Galactosemia	Acidosis, growth failure, severe infections	Galactose
Congenital adrenal hyperplasia	Virilization, salt-losing crises	17-hydroxy progesterone
Maple syrup urine disease	Acidosis, hypoglycemia	Leucine

Laboratory Studies of Newborn Infants

There is little need for "routine" laboratory studies in newborn infants. For example, routine blood counts, blood glucose, or bilirubin determinations at or shortly after birth do not identify or predict serious neonatal disorders with enough frequency to make such routine testing worthwhile. However, certain laboratory tests are appropriate in specific situations.

Infants of diabetic mothers should be followed by serial blood glucose determinations during their first several postnatal hours, or until they are fed and stable. As indicated in Chap. 6, some decline in blood sugar is an expected event during neonatal adaptation. Infants of diabetic mothers, however, have poorer self-regulation of plasma glucose levels than do most other term infants. Ideally, screening for hypoglycemia in these infants should employ a rapid and quantitative method for true glucose determination. Analytic methods for cribside determination of the actual plasma glucose level are under development, but not yet standard in all nurseries. The use of reagent strips is less reliable, because accurate determination of reagent-strip color changes is difficult in the normal and hypoglycemic ranges of neonatal plasma glucose values (e.g., 0–40 mg/dl). One useful strategy is to obtain a true glucose determination at 30 to 60 minutes of age in all newly admitted infants of diabetic mothers.

Depending on the stability of maternal glucose control, the condition of the infant, and the subsequent clinical course, abnormal values should be closely followed and promptly treated, and normal values should be followed with repeat glucose determinations as needed within the first 6 to 12 hours, especially in newborns who are not yet being fed. Although mild decreases in plasma glucose to low normal values are relatively common, sustained true hypoglycemia should be treated by administering adequate glucose (approximately 4–6 mg/kg/min, and occasionally more) by intravenous infusion. Profound or symptomatic hypoglycemia is potentially damaging to vital organs, including the central nervous system, and should be considered a medical emergency.

The infant's blood type should be determined in all infants of Rh-negative mothers, and in all infants with early jaundice (e.g., appearing on the first day), especially if the mother has blood group O. If the baby's major or minor (Rh) type is incompatible with the maternal type, a direct anti-globulin (Coombs') test should be performed, on a postnatal rather than a cord blood sample if active hemolysis is suspected.

Follow-up of a suspected hemolytic event also should include measurement of serum bilirubin (see below) and determination of red-cell morphology and indices if the hemolytic reaction is diagnosed by a positive antiglobulin test and appears severe enough to need treatment. Unless there is good reason to suspect hemolysis or infection in a newborn, routine performance of a complete blood count is not indicated. The range of normal hemoglobin, hematocrit, and white counts in newborns is generally above that of a normal adult, and the normal range is very wide in the first 12 hours after birth. Laboratories in hospitals with small obstetric services may not publish standard neonatal hematologic values, so that normal neonatal values for hemoglobin, hematocrit, white-cell count and differential may be identified as abnormal when laboratory reports use normal adult values. These factitious "abnormal" hematologic findings may create some confusion about diagnosis and follow-up in the nursery. In general, not enough information is gained from routine neonatal blood counts to make them appropriate. Hemoglobin and hematocrit may be performed if anemia or severe polycythemia is suspected; white counts and differential counts may be performed if there is good reason to suspect perinatal or neonatal infection. All such laboratory values identified as abnormal should be interpreted in their clinical context. When abnormal laboratory values are unexpectedly identified in babies who look normal, consultation with an experienced neonatal pediatrician or neonatologist may sometimes resolve the discrepancy without need for further extensive laboratory evaluation of the patient.

Serum bilirubin is the most common laboratory test performed in newborn infants, and jaundice is the most common neonatal condition requiring follow-up and treatment. Before birth, fetal bilirubin crosses the placenta to the maternal circulation and is metabolized by the mother. The bowel does not function as a route of bilirubin excretion, and hepatic conjugation and transport of bilirubin are somewhat suppressed. Postnatal maturation of the hepatic and enteric pathway for conjugation and excretion of bilirubin develops gradually during the first postnatal week. As a result, many newborns have mild elevations of serum unconjugated bilirubin, and some become visibly jaundiced. The milder form of this condition is called *physiologic jaundice of the newborn. Neonatal hyperbilirubinemia* represents a pattern of neonatal bilirubin accumulation and jaundice outside the expected normal range for mild jaundice, because serum bilirubin rises too early, too rapidly, or the elevation of serum bilirubin persists longer than expected. Most hyperbilirubinemia is physiologic, especially in breast-fed infants. In a few cases, however, the bilirubin remains elevated because of hemolysis, infection, or inhibition of bilirubin transport.

In general, jaundice evident at birth, jaundice appearing on the first day, or serum-indirect bilirubin exceeding 15 to 16 mg/dl at any time fall into the hyperbilirubinemic category. The jaundice itself related to these events is usually harmless, but two precautions must be observed. Early appearance or persistence of high bilirubin levels may be related to an underlying hematologic or hepatic disorder. Also, extremely high and uncontrolled bilirubin levels can produce a type of encephalopathy known as *kernicterus*, which in turn may eventuate in a subcortical type of choreo-athetoid cerebral palsy. This generally does not occur unless there is massive overproduction of bilirubin or a complete inability to excrete it, so that serum-indirect bilirubin levels persist in the range of 20 to 30 mg/dl or even higher. However, the incidence of moderate to moderately severe hyperbilirubinemia is high enough in newborn infants that determination of serum bilirubin is one of the most common laboratory tests performed in newborns.

Figure 22-1 shows the pathway for production, distribution, and excretion of bilirubin. Figure 22-2 shows the decision-making pathway that many clinicians follow if an infant appears inappropriately jaundiced. The first decision

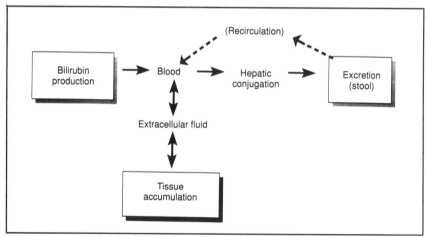

Fig. 22-1. Bilirubin production, tissue distribution, and excretion. The rate of recirculation of bilirubin from the bowel to the blood cannot be estimated clinically. Enterohepatic recirculation of bilirubin may be increased in unfed or breast-fed infants and may limit the expected physiologic decline in serum bilirubin or the anticipated response to phototherapy.

is whether the clinical jaundice, often first noticed by a physician or nurse who is examining the infant, warrants a bilirubin determination. Transcutaneous reflectance or color matching may assist in the initial estimate of the severity and extent of jaundice, which in general proceeds cephalad to caudad in the newborn. Once the serum bilirubin is found to be inappropriately elevated, additional testing is sometimes needed to determine whether a hemolytic process is occurring, especially one related to maternal-fetal blood group incompatibility. However, a complete blood count is not a necessary part of the initial evaluation of a newborn for jaundice, especially if there is no other clinical reason to suspect hemolysis or infection.

Following determination of the bilirubin level, or a series of bilirubin levels, further decisions may be necessary as to initiating phototherapy to control the serum bilirubin levels and facilitate excretion, or to perform an exchange transfusion if there is evidence of severe hemolysis or severe hyperbilirubinemia. Exchange transfusion, reserved for the most serious

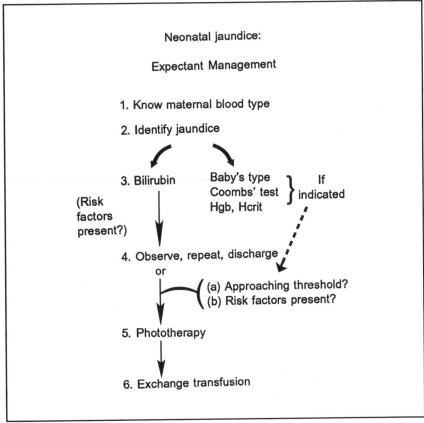

Fig. 22-2.   Clinical decision making in the management of neonatal jaundice.

cases, promptly lowers the serum bilirubin level to about half the pre-exchange value, and also eliminates the susceptible cells and the antibodies that may be causing a hemolytic reaction. Generally, however, phototherapy is sufficient for moderate to moderately severe cases of exaggerated hyperbilirubinemia in the range of 15 to 25 mg/dl. The clinical outcome of treated hyperbilirubinemia is generally very favorable, although kernicterus is occasionally reported in severe untreated cases.

Respiratory Distress

Mild degrees of nondistressed tachypnea are common in newborn infants, and may be related to cold stress or to pulmonary retention of amniotic fluid in the first few hours. Respiratory rates persisting above 60 per minute or any abnormalities of heart rate or respiration related to other possible causes, such as risk of maternal infection or presence of congenital anomalies, should be promptly evaluated. If respiratory distress or tachypnea persists beyond the transitional period, the infant should be examined by a pediatrician. In most cases, a chest x-ray film should be taken, and in many cases a white count, differential count, and cultures should be obtained as a screen for perinatal infection. Milder forms of transitional neonatal respiratory distress are usually self-limited, whereas those related to a significant disease process persist and tend to become more severe during the first few hours. The well-known advances in the management of neonatal respiratory disease that have contributed to increased survival, especially of low-birth-weight infants, need not be repeated here.

Before discharge of the newborn infant, a complete physical examination should be done, the mother should be counselled about well baby care, and arrangements should be made for home care and pediatric follow-up care. With earlier discharges (1–2 days) now becoming the norm, vigilance by the hospital staff and careful planning for discharge in the transition home are very important to the later well-being of newborn infants. Early discharges can be safely accomplished in most stable newborns if adequate follow-up is provided and if the mother is adequately instructed in well baby care and in potential danger signs that her infant is not doing well. Follow-up in many discharge programs includes a home visit, repetition of the metabolic screen after the first few days of feeding, and detailed written instructions given by the pediatrician or hospital staff to the mother at the time that the baby leaves the hospital. With these precautions, early discharge is safe for most patients.

Recommended Reading

Behrman, R. E. The Fetus and the Neonatal Infant. In R. E. Behrman (ed.), *Nelson's Textbook of Pediatrics* (14th ed.). Philadelphia: W. B. Saunders. Pp. 421–429.

Cashore, W. J. Hyperbilirubinemia. In J. J. Pomerance and C. J. Richardson (eds.), *Neonatology for the Clinician.* Norwalk: Appleton & Lange, 1993. Pp. 231–241.

Cochran, W. D. Management of the Normal Neonate. In F. A. Oski, et al. (eds.), *Principles and Practice of Pediatrics* (2nd ed.). Philadelphia: Lippincott, 1994. Pp. 302–308.

Levy, H. L. Screening of the Newborn. In H. W. Taeusch, R. A. Ballard, and M. E. Avery (eds.), *Schaffer and Avery's Diseases of the Newborn* (6th ed.). Philadelphia: Saunders, 1991. Pp. 111–119.

Medical Complications of Pregnancy

Karen Rosene-Montella

The management of the pregnant patient presents unique challenges to the physician. When studying the medical complications of pregnancy, both the physiology of normal pregnancy and the pathophysiology of specific disease states should be considered.

This chapter addresses specific disease states, and the framework in which the pregnant patient with a medical problem should be approached. For each disease category a specific set of questions should be asked:

1. What is "normal" for pregnancy?
2. What is the effect of the pregnancy on the disease?
3. What is the effect of the disease, its evaluation, and its treatment on the pregnancy and the fetus?
4. Should the pregnancy affect my decision making; i.e., should diagnostic or therapeutic intervention be delayed or modified because of the pregnancy?

Maternal Medical Diseases

Cardiovascular Disease
Significant maternal cardiovascular disease complicates 1 to 2 percent of all pregnancies. Although this incidence has not changed since the 1970s, the relative proportion of patients with rheumatic heart disease rather than

congenital heart disease has changed. This is due in part to the decreasing incidence of rheumatic fever, and in part to the increasing success of surgery for congenital heart disease. Since more women with congenital cardiac lesions are surviving into the childbearing years, with improved exercise function, a greater proportion of maternal cardiac disease cases will come from this group. In addition, there will continue to be an increase in coronary disease in pregnancy as the average age of childbearing rises simultaneous with an increase in the incidence of coronary artery disease in women.

Maternal cardiac physiology is altered as outlined in Chap. 10. Of particular importance when considering the diagnosis of cardiac disease are: (1) the 40 to 50 percent increase in blood volume; (2) the 30 to 50 percent increase in cardiac output; (3) the presence of a systolic murmur in 86 percent of normal pregnant women; (4) the decrease in systemic vascular resistance; and (5) the 300- to 500-ml autotransfusion from the uteroplacental circulation that occurs at the time of delivery. The impact of the pregnancy on the disease as well as the impact of the disease on fetal and maternal morbidity and mortality is dependent on the functional class, defined by the New York Heart Association classification (NYHA) (Table 23-1) and the underlying defect, including the degree to which cardiac output is fixed, and will be influenced by the development of other pregnancy-related complications.

Table 23-1.   New York Heart Association functional classification of cardiac disease*

Class I
  No functional limitation of activity
  No symptoms of cardiac decompensation with activity

Class II
  Mild amount of functional limitation
  Patients are asymptomatic at rest
  Ordinary physical activity results in symptoms

Class III
  Limitation of most physical activity
  Asymptomatic at rest
  Minimal physical activity results in symptoms

Class IV
  Severe limitation of physical activity
  Patients may be symptomatic at rest
  Any physical activity results in cardiac symptoms

*Adapted from New York Heart Association. *The Criteria Committee of the New York Heart Association Nomenclature and Criteria for Diagnosis of Diseases of the Heart and Great Vessels* (8th ed.). New York: New York Heart Association, 1979; with permission.

The risk of maternal mortality associated with specific cardiac lesions is outlined in Table 23-2. The NYHA functional class is an additional determinant as noted in Tables 23-1 and 23-2. Functional classes 3 and 4 are associated with a 25 to 50 percent maternal mortality rate. Pregnancy complications that can worsen the initially assigned risk include pregnancy-induced hypertension, hemorrhage, hypotension (related to blood loss or anesthesia), and infection. Counselling the pregnant patient with cardiac disease also should address the risk of heart disease in the offspring, which may be as high as 14 percent when the mother has cyanotic heart disease.

Specific Cardiac Lesions

Acquired Valvular Heart Disease   *Aortic stenosis* accounts for 10 percent of acquired valvular disease in pregnancy. Mild to moderate stenosis is well tolerated. Patients with severe disease (defined by a pressure gradient between the left ventricle and the aorta during systole of >100 mm Hg) have a 17 percent mortality rate according to one study. The major physiologic consideration is the fact that cardiac output is limited by the degree of stenosis. If preload is reduced by hypotension or hypovolemia, or significant bradycardia occurs, the resultant decrease in cardiac output can be life-threatening. Invasive cardiac monitoring and avoidance of conduction anesthesia are often employed to monitor and maximize filling pressures.

Table 23-2.   Risk of mortality associated with specific cardiac lesions*

Low risk of maternal mortality (less than 1%)
Septal defects
New York Heart Association (NYHA) classes I and II
Patient ductus arteriosus
Pulmonic/tricuspid lesions
Moderate risk of maternal mortality (5–15%)
NYHA classes III and IV mitral stenosis
Aortic stenosis
Marfan syndrome with normal aorta
Uncomplicated coarctation of the aorta
History of myocardial infarction
Tetralogy of Fallot
High risk of maternal mortality (25–50%)
Eisenmenger's syndrome
Pulmonary hypertension
Marfan syndrome with abnormal aortic root
Peripartal cardiomyopathy

*Adapted from S. L. Clark. Labor and delivery in the pregnant patient with structural cardiac disease. *Clin. Perinatol.* 13:697, 1986.

Antibiotic prophylaxis against subacute endocarditis (SBE) is indicated as well (Tables 23-3 and 23-4).

Aortic insufficiency accounts for approximately 2.5 percent of valvular lesions and is generally well tolerated.

Mitral stenosis (MS) is the most common acquired valvular lesion complicating pregnancy, and it accounts for 80 to 90 percent of such lesions. The hemodynamic defect is that of obstruction to left atrial outflow. The resultant elevation of left atrial and pulmonary vascular pressures and decreased cardiac output makes MS the most likely valve lesion to cause congestive heart failure and pulmonary edema during pregnancy. The specific pregnancy-related risks for pulmonary congestion include the demand for increased cardiac output and the increase in pulmonary blood volume, which reach a maximum in the early to mid–third trimester, and the increased heart rate, which decreases diastolic filling time. Increased left atrial volume and pressure predispose the patient to atrial arrhythmias and to the associated risk of thrombus formation. The pregnant patient with chronic atrial fibrillation is at further increased risk for formation of atrial thrombus because of the hypercoagulable state of pregnancy. The combination of an increased synthesis of clotting factors, decreased fibrinolysis, and the venous stasis caused by progesterone-induced smooth-muscle relaxation contribute to the hypercoagulability of pregnancy. In addition, if a clot does form in the left atrium, atrial fibrillation can trigger the breaking off of emboli that can enter the cerebral circulation and cause stroke. For this reason, the pregnant patient with chronic atrial fibrillation should be anticoagulated with heparin to avoid embolic complications.

Table 23-3.   Cardiac conditions

Endocarditis prophylaxis recommended
  Prosthetic heart valves
  Previous bacterial endocarditis, even in the absence of heart disease
  Most congenital cardiac malformations
  Rheumatic and other acquired valvular dysfunction, even after valvular surgery
  Hypertrophic cardiomyopathy
  Mitral valve prolapse with valvular regurgitation

Endocarditis prophylaxis not recommended
  Isolated secundum atrial septal defect
  Successful surgical repair of secundum atrial septal defect, ventrical septal defect, or patent ductus arteriosus
  Previous coronary artery bypass graft surgery
  Mitral valve prolapse without valvular regurgitation
  Physiologic, functional, or innocent heart murmurs
  Previous rheumatic fever without valvular dysfunction
  Cardiac pacemakers and implanted defibrillators

Table 23-4. American Heart Association recommended standard prophylactic
regimen for genitourinary tract surgery and instrumentation[a]

Drug	Dosing regimen[b]
	Standard regimen
Amoxicillin	3 g orally 1 hour before procedure; 1.5 g 8 hours after initial dose.
Ampicillin plus gentamicin	2 g ampicillin IM or IV plus gentamicin 1.5 mg/kg IM or IV given 30 minutes before procedure. May repeat 8 hours later.
	Amoxicillin/penicillin-allergic patients
Erythromycin or	Erythromycin ethylsuccinate, 800 mg, or erythromycin stearate, 1 g orally 2 hours before procedure, then half the dose 6 hours after initial dose.
Clindamycin	300 mg orally 1 hour before procedure and 150 mg 6 hours after initial dose.
Vancomycin plus gentamicin	1 g vancomycin IV given over 60 minutes plus 1.5 mg/kg gentamicin IM or IV, each given 60 minutes before procedure. Doses may be repeated once 8 to 12 hours later.

[a]Includes those with prosthetic heart valves and other high-risk patients.
[b]Initial pediatric doses are as follows: amoxicillin, 50 mg/kg; ampicillin, 50 mg/kg; gentamicin, 2 mg/kg; erythromycin ethylsuccinate or erythromycin stearate, 20 mg/kg; clindamycin, 10 mg/kg; vancomycin, 20 mg/kg; and gentamicin, 2 mg/kg. Follow-up doses should be one-half the initial dose. Total pediatric dose should not exceed total adult dose. The following weight ranges may also be used for the initial pediatric dose of amoxicillin: <15 kg, 750 mg; 15–30 kg, 1500 mg; and >30 kg, 3000 mg (full adult dose).

General management of the pregnant patient with mitral stenosis should include SBE prophylaxis, with fluid and activity restriction if left atrial or pulmonary pressures are elevated or congestive heart failure is present. Arrhythmias and pulmonary edema should be treated as they occur. If pulmonary congestion develops, treatment is directed towards limitation of activity, which will limit cardiac work and myocardial oxygen demand, and volume restriction. The use of diuretics to relieve volume overload and digoxin to improve myocardial contractility, its positive inotropic effect, may be indicated.

Mitral insufficiency accounts for approximately 6 percent of valvular lesions and is well tolerated. Even when it is secondary to mitral valve prolapse, which is generally benign, the presence of mitral regurgitation requires endocarditis prophylaxis. The turbulence in blood flow associated with valvular leakage or thickening of valve leaflets make the valve a potential nidus of infection in situations in which there may be bacteremia.

Congenital Valvular Heart Disease   Sixty percent of congenital lesions in pregnant women are characterized by left-to-right shunts in which some portion of blood flow is shunted directly from the left heart, the higher pressure system, to the right heart and then recirculated in the normal fashion. These lesions include ventricular and atrial septal defects (VSD, ASD) and patent ductus arteriosus (PDA). *Ventricular septal defect* in the absence of pulmonary hypertension, which could cause reversal of the shunt, is well tolerated. Most large defects will have been surgically closed during childhood. The only special considerations for uncomplicated VSD during pregnancy are the need for endocarditis prophylaxis, avoidance of hypotension significant enough to cause shunt reversal, and the recurrence risk in the offspring of 3 to 5 percent.

Isolated ASD requires no special care during pregnancy. Endocarditis prophylaxis is not needed for the uncomplicated common form of ASD since it has not been shown to increase the risk of heart infection in the presence of bacteremia. As with VSD, avoidance of hypotension and the inheritance risk of 3 percent are the only considerations unique to pregnancy.

Patent ductus arteriosus, if not associated with pulmonary hypertension, poses no increased risk during pregnancy. Subacute bacterial endocarditis prophylaxis is required during delivery.

The remaining 40 percent of congenital cardiac lesions are characterized by right-to-left shunts in which blood is shunted from the right heart directly to the left side of the heart without passing through the lungs or pulmonary circulation, so that blood that has not been properly oxygenated enters the systemic circulation directly. These lesions include tetralogy of Fallot, Eisenmenger's syndrome, and pulmonary hypertension. *Tetralogy of Fallot,* which is characterized by ventricular septal defect, obstruction to right ventricular outflow, an overriding aorta that straddles the VSD, and right ventricular hypertrophy, if corrected during childhood is well tolerated during pregnancy. Uncorrected tetralogy greatly increases maternal and fetal morbidity and mortality. The severity of the clinical presentation and its impact on pregnancy are determined by the extent of the obstruction to right ventricular outflow. When the obstruction is severe, pulmonary blood flow is markedly reduced and a large volume of desaturated systemic venous blood is shunted from right to left across the ventricular septal defect. The resultant hypoxemia causes increased red blood cell production and hematocrit elevations. Patients who have hematocrits greater than 60 percent, syncopal episodes, a PaO_2 less than 70 mm Hg, or significantly elevated right heart pressures have the worst prognosis. Venous return should be maintained to maximize filling pressures and cardiac output by avoiding hypotension and volume depletion, particularly during labor and delivery. This maintenance is imperative since an increase in blood flow across the right-to-left shunt can occur if filling pressures fall below a critical value. Antibiotic prophylaxis for endocarditis is indicated.

Eisenmenger's syndrome, characterized by a large right-to-left shunt through a VSD or patent ductus arteriosus, with its pulmonary hypertension and high pulmonary vascular resistance, carries a maternal mortality rate of 50 to 70 percent. Sudden death due to hypoxemia or hypotension from decreased cardiac output can occur at any time during pregnancy or typically postpartum, so many authorities recommend termination of pregnancy. The management, should a patient elect to continue her pregnancy, is that described below for pulmonary hypertension.

Significant *pulmonary hypertension,* of any cause, is a contraindication to pregnancy. The maternal mortality rate exceeds 50 percent, with a 40 to 50 percent perinatal mortality rate. The underlying hemodynamic defect in primary pulmonary hypertension is an increased resistance to pulmonary blood flow. Initially there is a marked elevation of pulmonary artery pressure with normal cardiac function. As the disease progresses, cardiac output falls and myocardial depression develops secondary to chronic right ventricular pressure overload. Since the pulmonary pressures and cardiac output are fixed and usually unresponsive to vasodilator therapy, any increase in cardiac work or blood volume is not well tolerated. Invasive hemodynamic monitoring to detect changes in pulmonary pressures, or a rise in pulmonary capillary wedge pressure, which heralds left ventricular failure, is often used during labor, delivery, and the early postpartum period. Maintenance of blood pressure and volume to maximize preload and diastolic filling are important. Regional anesthesia carries the risk of hypotension and further decrease in cardiac output, so intrathecal morphine, which causes little change in maternal hemodynamics, is a good anesthetic choice. Oxygen or drugs such as morphine, which may lower pulmonary pressures, should be considered in an attempt to lessen shunt flow if needed. Heparin and antibiotic prophylaxis against endocarditis are indicated as well.

Additional congenital lesions not characterized by shunt are *coarctation of the aorta* and *Marfan syndrome* with cardiac involvement. Isolated coarctation of the aorta, if surgically corrected prior to pregnancy, carries no increased maternal risk. Patients with uncorrected lesions are at risk for aortic dissection, bacterial endocarditis, cerebral hemorrhage, and other complications of long-term hypertension. These risks are all increased by pregnancy. There is a further increased risk of endocarditis when there is coexistence of a bicuspid aortic valve, a frequent association with aortic coarctation. Treatment should include control of hypertension, antibiotic prophylaxis, and avoidance of pushing during the second stage of labor (Valsalva maneuver), which can decrease cardiac output by decreasing venous return.

The cardiac manifestations of Marfan syndrome, which include mitral and aortic valve disease as well as aortic aneurysm, make it particularly dangerous in pregnancy if aortic involvement is present. There is an increased risk of aortic dissection and rupture, a decreased maternal life expectancy, and a 50 percent recurrence risk in the offspring. Should a patient with aortic dilatation choose to maintain a pregnancy, beta-adrenergic blockers should be used to minimize pressure on the wall of the aorta.

Prosthetic Heart Valves   Patients with prosthetic heart valves and normal cardiac function tolerate pregnancy well. Their major risk is that of valvular thrombosis, so anticoagulation with subcutaneous heparin, aimed at maintaining partial thromboplastin time at 1.5 to 2 times control, is indicated throughout pregnancy and postpartum. Further discussion of anticoagulation in pregnancy can be found in the section on thromboembolic disease. Subacute bacterial endocarditis prophylaxis is indicated for all patients with prosthetic heart valves at the time of delivery.

Cardiomyopathies   *Peripartum cardiomyopathy* is a disease of the cardiac muscle that is characterized by congestion and dilatation of the left ventricle, which occurs in late pregnancy or in the first 6 months postpartum. Unfortunately, most reports of this disease have failed to exclude other etiologies, such as viral, ischemic, or infiltrative cardiomyopathies. For this reason it is difficult to assess the risk of recurrence in future pregnancies. The only available data suggest that there is a 50 percent mortality rate and a 50 percent recurrence risk in subsequent pregnancies. Therefore, unless an underlying cause has been found, patients with this condition should be advised against further pregnancies. Additional known risk factors include multiple gestation, pregnancy-induced hypertension, multiparity, and black race.

The defect in *idiopathic hypertrophic subaortic stenosis,* which is inherited as an autosomal-dominant trait, is a dynamic obstruction at the left ventricular outflow tract such that the severity of obstruction is dependent on the width of the outflow tract during systole. Any situation that decreases venous return and thus ventricular volume increases obstruction in the outflow tract. Similarly, exercise and drugs that enhance myocardial contractility can decrease ventricular size and increase the obstruction. For this reason it is important to avoid hypovolemia, hypotension, the Valsalva maneuver, supine position, and epidural anesthesia. Patients also have an increased risk of sudden death; this risk is decreased by the use of beta-adrenergic blockers in symptomatic patients with documented ventricular arrhythmias.

Coronary Artery Disease   Risk factors for coronary disease should be sought in the intake history. Most coronary artery disease (CAD) in pregnant women is first diagnosed during the pregnancy since this is a time of increased myocardial oxygen demand during which regular health care is obtained. In addition to the traditional risk factors such as hypertension, smoking, and elevated cholesterol, glucose intolerance is a significant risk factor for women. Management of CAD during pregnancy does not differ from management in the nonpregnant state. Maternal myocardial infarction during the 3 months prior to delivery, or at delivery, has a 25 to 50 percent mortality rate.

Arrhythmias Treatment of cardiac arrhythmias during pregnancy involves careful consideration of the effect of the arrhythmia and its treatment on the fetus. Arrhythmias should be treated before they can cause prolonged maternal hypotension, hypoxia, or ischemia in order to maintain placental perfusion and fetal oxygenation, with drugs believed to be safe to the fetus. Appropriate dosages and levels of drugs must be attained in the face of the pregnancy-related 40 to 50 percent increase in the glomerular filtration rate, blood volume, and renal blood flow. Fetal heart rate monitoring during the initial administration of cardiac drugs may be helpful.

Paroxysmal supraventricular tachycardia, which occurs in the presence of functional differences in conduction and refractoriness in the atrioventricular (AV) node or an AV nodal bypass tract, is the most common arrhythmia during pregnancy. Digoxin and beta-adrenergic blockers, which slow conduction velocity through the AV node, have been used safely in all trimesters of pregnancy. A discussion of specific ß blockers can be found in the section on hypertension. Procainamide and quinidine, type I antiarrhythmics that slow atrial and ventricular conduction velocities and reduce refractoriness in the His-Purkinje system, also have been used without adverse fetal effects. The calcium channel blockers that decrease conduction velocity and increase refractoriness, nifedipine and verapamil, are not teratogenic but have been suggested in animal models as a cause of fetal acidosis and sudden fetal demise, possibly secondary to decreased placental perfusion. Low- to moderate-voltage direct current cardioversion has been used without adverse effects. Disopyramide, an anticholinergic agent, has been associated with hypertonic uterine activity and so should not be used. Flecainide and mexiletine, which decrease conduction velocity at fast heart rates, have both been used safely against *ventricular arrhythmias* in pregnancy, but have not been well studied. Amiodarone prolongs action potential duration by an increase in refractoriness of all cardiac tissue. Although it is effective against atrial and ventricular tachyarrhythmias, it should be used only as a last resort because of the large quantities of iodine in it that can cause fetal and maternal hypothyroidism. Lidocaine and bretylium, the ventricular antiarrhythmics of choice in the nonpregnant stage, have been associated with neonatal respiratory depression and neurobehavioral changes but may be used in emergencies with close fetal and maternal monitoring.

Thromboembolic Disease
Pulmonary embolism (PE) is now the major nonobstetric cause of maternal mortality in developed nations. The incidence of thromboembolic disease is 0.2 percent of all pregnancies without predisposing risk factors,

rising to 0.4 to 1.0 percent postpartum. Patients with a prior history of a documented thromboembolic event, independent of the circumstances surrounding the event, have a 12 to 20 percent recurrence risk during pregnancy. According to retrospective data, the incidence of thromboembolic disease in pregnancies associated with deficiencies in the fibrinolytic proteins C or S is 50 percent, and as high as 70 percent in the presence of antithrombin III deficiency. Lupus anticoagulant is an additional risk factor for thrombosis but the exact incidence is less clearly defined because of confounding factors.

Since pulmonary embolization occurs in 30 to 50 percent of cases of untreated proximal deep vein thrombosis (DVT), and if untreated carries a maternal mortality rate of 20 to 30 percent, the importance of early diagnosis and treatment is enormous. Heparin prophylaxis should be considered in high-risk patients with prior thromboembolic disease. Full-dose therapeutic heparin may be necessary in the presence of deficiencies of the fibrinolytic system. Antiphospholipid (APL) antibodies including the lupus anticoagulant (so named because it prolongs phospholipid-dependent clotting reactions) are a group of antibodies of the IgG or IgM class that bind to phospholipid in platelets and endothelial cells, promoting both venous and arterial thrombosis. Antiphospholipid antibody–associated placental thrombosis and infarction may result in intrauterine fetal death or growth retardation. In pregnancies complicated by APL antibodies and a history suggestive of prior placental thrombosis, the use of low-dose aspirin in conjunction with steroids to suppress antibody production or heparin to prevent thrombosis has resulted in live-born term infants in 70 percent of cases.

Additional risk factors for thromboembolic disease include bed rest, cesarean section (increases incidence ninefold), age >35 years, multiparity, trauma, obesity, and disorders associated with increased blood viscosity.

What is it about pregnancy that predisposes a young, healthy population to thromboembolic disease? The combined hormonal effects of an increase in clotting factors and a decrease in fibrinolysis create a hypercoagulable state that begins early in gestation and lasts for approximately 6 weeks postpartum. There is increased vein distensibility and a 50 percent decrease in venous flow velocity in the lower extremities by the third trimester, which creates marked venous stasis as well.

The clinical diagnosis of DVT, or PE, with its 20 to 30 percent mortality rate, is inaccurate much of the time, so it is important to utilize effective diagnostic procedures. A standard technetium (Tc 99) mm perfusion and ventilation lung scan to diagnose PE exposes the fetus to 0.2 rad of radiation, well below the Nuclear Regulatory Commission recommendation to stay below a total pregnancy exposure of 5 rad. The more promptly and frequently the mother voids, the lower the fetal dose of radiation will be since the majority of exposure occurs while the technetium mm is in the maternal bladder. If DVT is suspected, ultrasonography with Doppler should be done first since this test avoids any radiation exposure. Combined with Doppler flow or impedance plethysmography, ultrasound is now thought to be as accurate as contrast venography in the diagnosis of DVT. If a venogram is necessary, the radiation exposure to the fetus will be aproximately 0.25 rad. Similarly, pulmonary angiography, which may be necessary in the face of a nondiagnostic lung scan, exposes the fetus to a maximum dose of 0.25 rad.

Heparin therapy is the treatment of choice in documented proximal DVT or PE in pregnancy. It is administered intravenously for 7 to 10 days, and then by subcutaneous injection that can be done at home. Despite the ease of administration of oral warfarin, this drug freely crosses the placental barrier and is contraindicated in all trimesters of pregnancy. Warfarin embryopathy, characterized by nasal hypoplasia and epiphyseal stippling, occurs with first-trimester exposure only. Central nervous system defects and fetal hemorrhage, however, can occur following warfarin exposure in any trimester.

Recommendations for administration of heparin are summarized in Table 23-5. Heparin does not cross the placenta, is not excreted in breast milk,

Table 23-5. Heparin administration in pregnancy*

Condition	Recommendation
Previous venous thrombosis or pulmonary embolism in prior pregnancy	Heparin ≥5000 units every 12 hours until mid–third trimester and then increase to 7500–10,000 units twice a day.
Venous thrombosis or pulmonary embolism during current pregnancy	Heparin in full IV doses for 7–10 days, followed by every 12-hour subcutaneous injections to prolong 6-hour postinjection activated partial thromboplastin time (aPTT) to 1.5 times control until delivery. Warfarin can then be used postpartum.
Patient who requires long-term anticoagulation is planning pregnancy	Either heparin every 12 hours subcutaneously to prolong 6-hour postinjection aPTT to 1.5 times control, or frequent pregnancy tests and substitute heparin (as above) for warfarin when pregnancy is achieved.
Mechanical prosthetic heart valves	Heparin every 12 hours subcutaneously to prolong 6-hour postinjection aPTT to 1.5 to 3 times control.

*Modified from 1992 American College of Chest Physicians (ACCP), Consensus Conference Recommendations. (Chest Suppl.). 102:4, 1992.

and has not been associated with an increase in adverse fetal outcomes when comorbid conditions are controlled for. Maternal adverse effects include osteoporosis with exposures of >15,000 units per day for 6 months or longer, thrombocytopenia, and bleeding complications. Because of the dose-related risk of oseoporosis with heparin, warfarin should be used postpartum. Two studies have failed to demonstrate neonatal anticoagulant effects when nursing mothers take warfarin, so this drug may be used safely during breast-feeding.

Septic pelvic thrombophlebitis, ovarian vein thrombosis, and central retinal vein thrombosis are additional thrombotic events that can occur during pregnancy and postpartum. Amniotic fluid embolism may occur intrapartum or peripartum when membranes are ruptured and amniotic fluid accidently enters the central venous circulation. The presence of amniotic fluid in the pulmonary circulation can cause acute severe adult respiratory distress syndrome as a result of both pulmonary microvascular thrombosis and parenchymal damage from amniotic particulate matter in the lungs. Patients who survive the initial hypoxic event then may suffer from disseminated intravascular coagulation (DIC), again as a result of the potent thromboplastic properties of the amniotic fluid that has entered the systemic circulation.

Hypertensive Disorders

The hypertensive disorders of pregnancy can be classified by the following diagnostic criteria:

Hypertension   Diastolic BP ≥ 90 mm Hg or systolic BP ≥ 140 mm Hg or diastolic BP increase from prepregnancy or first-trimester BP by 15 mm Hg or systolic by 30 mm Hg on two occasions at least 6 hours apart, or diastolic BP > 110 or mean arterial pressure >105 mm Hg on one occasion

Preeclampsia   Hypertension after 20 weeks' gestation with proteinuria >300 mg in 24 hours or >100 mg/dl in a random specimen

Chronic hypertension   Hypertension present prior to 20 weeks' gestation or persisting > 42 days postpartum

Eclampsia   Seizures in the presence of preeclampsia

Superimposed preeclampsia   Preeclampsia in a pregnancy with preexisting chronic hypertension

Preeclampsia complicates approximately 7 percent of all pregnancies, and two-thirds of these cases occur in primigravidas. Additional maternal risk factors for pregnancy-related hypertension include family history of preeclampsia in the patient's mother or sister, chronic hypertension, renal disorder, diabetes, APL antibody syndrome, and advanced maternal age. Fetal predisposing factors include twin gestation, molar pregnancy, fetal hydrops, or triploidy. Preeclampsia is thought to be a vasospastic disorder that may result from an imbalance between thromboxane and prostacyclin in the placental and systemic circulation. In its classic form, preeclampsia consists of edema, hypertension, hyperreflexia, and proteinuria. The diagnosis of preeclampsia is often difficult to make since the presentation is extremely variable. Tables 23-6 and 23-7 summarize the signs, symptoms, and laboratory findings, any of which can be the presenting manifestation of preeclampsia. It is a multisystem disorder that in its most severe form can cause cerebral hemorrhage; liver rupture from an expanding subcapsular hematoma or edema; malignant hypertension; renal failure with glomerulo-endotheliosis at biopsy; or disseminated intravascular coagulation. The only known definitive treatment is delivery, although any of the manifestations may occur postpartum as well. Control of blood pressure is discussed in the following section on chronic hypertension. Seizure prophylaxis with intravenous magnesium sulfate is the standard in most North American centers. Phenytoin has been demonstrated to be equally effective in at least one prospective study.

Chronic hypertension during pregnancy has been shown to increase both maternal and fetal morbidity and mortality. Potential maternal complications include abruptio placentae and intracranial bleeding. Increased fetal morbidity including intrauterine growth retardation and higher fetal

Table 23-6.   Signs and symptoms of preeclampsia and eclampsia

Cerebral
  Headache
  Dizziness
  Tinnitus
  Drowsiness
  Change in respiratory rate
  Fever

Visual
  Diplopia
  Scotomata
  Blurred vision
  Amaurosis

Gastrointestinal
  Nausea
  Vomiting
  Epigastric pain
  Hematemesis

Renal
  Oliguria
  Anuria
  Hematuria
  Hemoglobinuria

Table 23-7. Laboratory findings in preeclampsia

Most frequent findings
   Urine protein ≥ 300 mg/24 hours
   Serum creatinine ≥ 0.8 ng/dl
   Hemoconcentration with increased hematocrit
   Uric acid > 4.5 mg/dl
   Decreased platelet count
   Elevation of serum transaminase

Other findings
   Other evidence of disseminated intravascular coagulation including ↑partial
      thromboplastin time, ↓ fibrinogen
   Decreased antithrombin III
   Decreased urinary calcium excretion

and perinatal mortality rates have been documented if the mean arterial pressure exceeds 90 mm Hg during the second trimester. There is an increased incidence of preeclampsia, the superimposition of which doubles the perinatal mortality risk. Although treatment of hypertension alone has not been shown to prevent the onset of preeclampsia, the use of 80 mg per day of aspirin to lower the thromboxane to prostacyclin ratio, thus theoretically decreasing vasoconstriction, has been associated with a significantly lower incidence of preeclampsia in patients with chronic hypertension in some studies. Dietary calcium supplementation is also under investigation as a means of decreasing the risk of preeclampsia.

The choice of antihypertensive agents is limited by the efficacy of a given drug and its safety for the fetus. As a result of early studies of propranolol, β blocker, suggested an association with neonatal respiratory depression and intrauterine growth retardation; thus, for a long time β blockers were initially avoided as antihypertensive therapy in pregnancy. There are now extensive prospective data comparing the selective B_1 agents including atenolol and metoprolol with the most frequently used agents, hydralazine, a direct vasodilator, and methyldopa, a centrally acting drug. Equivalent or improved blood pressure control, maternal volume expansion, fetal growth, placental weight, and patient compliance have all been demonstrated in the β blocker–treated mothers. The safety and efficacy of labetalol, which combines beta-adrenergic blockade with alpha blockage, has been demonstrated as well. Labetalol's vasodilatory effect, lack of bradycardia, and its rapid action both orally and intravenously make it an ideal drug in this setting. Methyldopa therapy initiated between 16 and 20 weeks' gestation has been associated with decreased head circumference in one study, but has not been shown to cause developmental delay in the offspring of treated mothers.

The calcium channel blockers, nifedipine and verapamil, are efficacious but have been associated with decreased placental perfusion and fetal acidosis in animal models. In addition, the hypotensive effect of nifedipine is markedly potentiated by magnesium sulfate. The angiotensin-converting enzyme (ACE) inhibitors, captopril, enalapril, and lisinopril, are theoretically ideal drugs in a condition known to increase sensitivity to angiotensin. Unfortunately, there are numerous case reports of fetal oliguria, oligohydramnios, fetal and neonatal renal failure, and fetal demise during exposure to ACE inhibitors in pregnancy so they are contraindicated in this setting.

Hypertensive emergencies, during which intravenous therapy is required, pose additional problems. The most frequently used drugs in the non-pregnant patient, diazoxide and nitroprusside, both have deleterious side effects in pregnancy. Diazoxide may cause marked neonatal hyperglycemia, particularly in premature infants, and nitroprusside has been associated with fetal thiocyanate toxicity. Hydralazine, the most commonly used drug during severe hypertension in pregnancy, is a direct vasodilator and is theoretically a good choice in the presence of increased systemic vascular resistance. However, the 20- to 30-minute onset of action and the flushing, headache, and reflex tachycardia limit its usefulness. Labetalol, also a vasodilator, has the advantage of a rapid onset of action without reflex tachycardia, and like hydralazine, can be administered as multiple boluses or as a continuous infusion. In the presence of high cardiac output, a pure, rapidly acting β blocker such as esmolol may be a better choice.

Dermatology

Skin changes that occur in normal pregnancy include hyperpigmentation, telangiectasia similar to spider angiomata, palmar erythema, skin tags, and striae. *Telogen effluvium* is the name given to the alopecia that can occur postpartum. Dermatologic conditions unique to pregnancy are summarized in Table 23-8. The effect of pregnancy on underlying skin disorders is variable. The major precaution with respect to dermatologic drug use is that isotretinoin is a potent teratogen that is contraindicated during pregnancy and should be avoided unless effective contraception is being used.

Endocrine Disorders

Thyroid Disease

The interpretation of thyroid function studies during pregnancy necessitates an understanding of the alterations that accompany normal pregnancy. The major change is the doubling in the level of thyroid-binding globulin (TBG), the protein to which the thyroid hormone thyroxine (T_4) is bound, by 8 to 10 weeks' gestation. This doubling results in an increase in total T_4 and decrease in the thyroid hormone–binding ratio (THBR), the new term for T_3 resin uptake. The THBR is an indirect estimate of free T_4 that is obtained by adding labeled T_3 to patients' serum and measuring how much of it remains free for binding to a matrix. The amount that remains available for binding is less in pregnancy since there is an increase in TBG. For this reason it is necessary to use a free T_4 value or free thyroxine index to assess true thyroid function during pregnancy. Thyroid-

Table 23-8. Rashes of pregnancy*

	Estimated percent of all pregnancies	Lesion morphology	Most common location	Important laboratory features	Usual trimester of onset	Increased fetal mortality
Pruritus gravidarum	15	Pruritus, no rash	Anywhere	Sometimes increased liver function test results	3	No
Prurigo gestationis (Besnier)	2	Excoriated papules	Trunk, extremities	None	2 or 3	No
Papular dermatitis (Spangler)	0.03	Papules	Trunk, extremities	Decreased estrogen, increased human chorionic gonadotropin	1, 2, or 3	Yes (?)
Polymorphic eruption of pregnancy (pruritic urticarial papules and plaque of pregnancy)	0.5	Papules, plaques, uticaria	Abdomen, thighs	None	3	No
Herpes gestationis (pemphigoid gestationis)	0.01	Papules, vesicules	Anywhere, biopsy	Direct immuno-fluorescence	2	Yes (?)
Impetigo herpetiformis	Very rare	Pustules	Intertriginous, trunk	Biopsy	1, 2, or 3	Yes
Autoimmune progesterone dermatitis	Only 1 reported case	Acneiform	Buttocks, extremities	Progesterone	1	Yes (?)

*Adapted from R. K. Creasy, and R. Resnick. *Maternal Fetal Medicine: Principles and Practice.* Philadelphia: Saunders, 1989.

stimulating hormone (TSH) produced by the pituitary gland is regulated by a feedback mechanism, increasing in response to low levels of thyroxine and decreasing in the presence of excess thyroxine. Since this feedback mechanism functions unchanged during pregnancy, an elevated TSH can be used to confirm the presence of primary hypothyroidism in pregnancy. With currently available sensitive immunoradiometric TSH assays, it has been found that TSH levels are lowered early in pregnancy, gradually rising to prepregnancy levels at term. For this reason the presence of low TSH during pregnancy cannot be used to confirm the diagnosis of hyperthyroidism.

Hyperthyroidism occurs in approximately 0.2 percent of pregnancies, and is most often caused by Graves' disease (autoimmune), followed in frequency by an autonomously functioning thyroid nodule and thyroiditis. Because of the intrinsic thyrotrophic activity of human chorionic gonadotropin, the incidence of hyperthyroidism in the presence of hydatiform mole or choriocarcinoma is quite high. The diagnosis of hyperthyroidism should be suspected clinically when there is tachycardia and poor weight gain, but it may also present as nausea and vomiting. A diagnosis may be confirmed by the presence of an elevated T_4 index. The effect of thyrotoxicosis on pregnancy is an increased risk of spontaneous abortion, prematurity, intrauterine growth retardation, and maternal thyroid storm. There is a 1 to 2 percent incidence of neonatal thyrotoxicosis in the presence of maternal Graves' disease. This incidence is independent of maternal thyroid function since it is caused by maternal thyroid-stimulating immune globulin (TSIG), an IgG that freely crosses the placenta and can stimulate fetal and neonatal thyroid activity.

Treatment with iodine-containing substances during pregnancy should be avoided, since the fetal thyroid gland, which is visible by 5 to 6 weeks, is able to synthesize hormone and trap iodine, an excess of which can cause goiter, by 8 to 10 weeks. Radioactive iodine freely crosses the placenta and is contraindicated in pregnancy, particularly after 10 weeks, since it can cause total ablation of the fetal thyroid gland as well as the adjacent parathyroids. The treatment of choice for hyperthyroidism during pregnancy is propylthiouracil (PTU), which blocks formation of thyroxine as well as peripheral conversion of T_4 to T_3. The goal of treatment is to maintain the free T_4 index at the upper limits of normal, and maintain maternal weight gain, while keeping the maternal dose of PTU, which crosses the placenta, as low as possible in an attempt to avoid fetal hypothyroidism.

Hypothyroidism has a major effect on fertility since it is associated with a greater than 50 percent anovulation rate and a very high incidence of first-trimester spontaneous abortions. Once pregnancy is achieved, however, the largest series reports 90 percent live births, 5 percent spontaneous abortions, 5 percent perinatal deaths, and no increase in congenital anomalies in a group of untreated hypothyroid patients. Transient neonatal hypothyroidism can occur in the presence of the maternal antibody associated with autoimmune thyroiditis, a blocking IgG that inhibits binding of TSH to its receptor.

Treatment of hypothyroidism is with L-thyroxine, in a dose adequate to maintain a normal maternal TSH level. Since thyroxine does not cross the placenta in appreciable amounts, and the fetal thyroid functions autonomously, fetal effects of thyroid replacement are not a concern. Recent data suggest that the need for thyroxine increases during pregnancy as reflected by a gradual increase in TSH levels.

Postpartum thyroid disorders occur following 5 to 10 percent of all pregnancies and carry an approximately 80 percent recurrence risk in subsequent pregnancies. Autoimmune or lymphocytic thyroiditis is the most frequent disorder. It is characterized by the presence of microsomal thyroid antibodies, lymphocytic infiltration of the gland, and a low radioactive iodine uptake during thyroid scanning. As destruction of the gland occurs, excess thyroid hormone pours out. The resultant transient hyperthyroidism has a peak incidence at 2 months postpartum, can occur at 2 to 12 months, and is usually followed by transient hypothyroidism, the occurrence of which peaks at 4 to 6 months postpartum. Graves' disease can recur postpartum as well, usually by 2 to 3 months. Sheehan's syndrome, postpartum pituitary necrosis, should be suspected if hypothyroidism follows postpartum hemorrhage with hypotension. It is usually heralded by a failure to lactate.

Parathyroid Disorders   Hyperparathyroidism, which can cause significant maternal hypercalcemia, occurs rarely in pregnancy but has significant maternal and fetal effects. In the presence of untreated hyperparathyroidism and the resultant hypercalcemia there is a 40 to 50 percent incidence of maternal kidney stones and a 50 percent overall fetal loss secondary to spontaneous abortion, fetal demise, and preterm delivery. Additional maternal complications include pancreatitis, hyperemesis, muscle weakness, and psychiatric disorders. Neonatal hypocalcemic tetany is frequently seen since maternal hypercalcemia of any etiology can cause suppression of the fetal parathyroid, which functions autonomously by 10 to 12 weeks' gestation.

Neonatal calcium and vitamin D toxicity can occur if the mother being treated for hypoparathyroidism is breast-feeding, since therapy includes calcium and vitamin D replacement.

Since fetal calcium levels are dependent on maternal levels, maternal hypocalcemia due to poor intake, excessive loss, or hypoparathyroidism will result in fetal hypocalcemia as well. Transient neonatal hyperparathyroidism as a result of maternal-fetal hypocalcemia with secondary elevation in fetal and neonatal parathyroid hormone levels has been reported.

Pituitary and Adrenal Disorders   The most common pituitary abnormality in women of childbearing age is a prolactin-secreting adenoma. Microadenomas have little impact on pregnancy and, despite earlier reports of growth during pregnancy, appear not to be affected by the pregnancy. Macroadenomas, however, are associated with a complication rate during pregnancy that approaches 20 percent, primarily in the form of headache and visual disturbance. The differential diagnosis of hyperprolactinemia is summarized in Table 23-9. Bromocriptine, a dopamine agonist used in the treatment of hyperprolactinemia, is not known to be teratogenic and has not been associated with increased fetal loss. Sheehan's syndrome, post-partum pituitary necrosis, occurs following prolonged hypotension or bleeding and is more frequent if there is already an underlying pituitary lesion. Diabetes insipidus, a vasopressin deficiency resulting from a disorder of the posterior pituitary, occurs rarely during pregnancy. Diabetes insipidus can be treated safely with nasal administration of arginine vasopressin at any time during gestation and during breast-feeding.

The adrenal disorders of overproduction, including pheochromocytoma, Cushing's syndrome, and primary hyperaldosteronism, occur infrequently in pregnancy. The importance of their recognition is usually related to the differential diagnosis of hypertensive disorders since the treatment differs greatly in the presence of an underlying adrenal abnormality. Undiagnosed

Table 23-9. Differential diagnosis of hyperprolactinemia*

Physiologic
  Pregnancy and lactation
  Sleep
  Stress
  Exercise
  Coitus
  Nipple stimulation

Hypothalamic lesions
  Infiltrative disease, e.g., sarcoidosis
  Tumors

Pituitary lesions
  Prolactin-secreting adenomas
  Nonprolactin-secreting tumors adjacent to prolactin-secreting cells
  Empty sella syndrome

Medications
  Psychotropic agents: phenothiazines, tricyclic antidepressants, opiate alkaloids
  Antiemetics and antihistamines: metoclopramide, cimetidine
  Antihypertensives: reserpine, methyldopa
  Hormones: estrogens, thyrotropin-releasing hormone

Other endocrine disorders
  Hypothyroidism

*Adapted from R. S. Abrams: Medical problems in pregnancy. *Med. Clin. North Am.* 3:3, 1989. Appleton & Case.

pheochromocytoma, which is characterized by extraordinarily high levels of adrenalin or noradrenalin, is associated with a high mortality rate during labor and delivery. Primary hyperaldosteronism may improve during pregnancy secondary to the blocking effect of progesterone on aldosterone, and so often is not apparent until severe hypertension occurs postpartum. Addison's disease, or adrenal insufficiency that presents as weakness, diarrhea, or orthostatic hypotension, is also rare during pregnancy.

Diabetes Mellitus

Diabetes in pregnancy is the perfect model from which to understand the potential impact of maternal metabolism on the fetus. The essential defect in diabetes is an absence or decrease in insulin production by the pancreas or a diminished response to insulin at the receptor site. Regardless of the etiology, the hyperglycemia that results may affect the developing fetus. Glucose freely crosses the placenta so maternal hyperglycemia results in fetal hyperglycemia and an increase in fetal insulin production. High levels of glycosolated hemoglobin, an indirect measure of chronic maternal hyperglycemia, during organogenesis are associated with an increase in the incidence of congenital anomalies. When hyperglycemia is present later in gestation, fetal macrosomia, neonatal hypoglycemia, hypocalcemia, hyperbilirubinemia, and infant respiratory distress syndrome can result.

Gestational diabetes, carbohydrate intolerance that occurs during pregnancy, is considered when random administration of a 50-g oral glucose load at 24 to 28 weeks' gestation results in a 1-hour plasma glucose of >130 mg/dl, and is confirmed when two or more abnormal values on a 3-hour glucose tolerance test are met or exceeded. Type I and type II diabetes refer to preexisting diabetes that is either insulin-dependent (type I) or noninsulin-dependent (type II) in the nonpregnant state. Either type may be treated with insulin but only type I requires insulin to avoid ketoacidisis. Independent of the classification, hyperglycemia, defined as fasting plasma glucose above 105 mg/dl or 2-hour postprandial plasma glucose greater than 120 mg/dl, is associated with increased perinatal morbidity and mortality.

It is controversial whether maternal complications of diabetes such as nephropathy, retinopathy, and neuropathy are permanently affected by, and have an effect on the outcome of pregnancy. A marked increase in proteinuria in patients with diabetic nephropathy is normally seen by the third trimester as a result of the physiologic increase in the glomerular filtration rate. Deterioration in renal function and worsening of hypertension occur in about one-third of cases. However, long-term prognosis, i.e., the appearance of end-stage renal disease, may not be influenced by pregnancy. The perinatal risks of maternal preexisting diabetes with nephropathy include an increase in the incidence of intrauterine growth retardation, stillbirths, and the neonatal mortality rate, which are further increased by the presence of hypertension and or creatinine ≥ 1.5 mg/dl.

The effect of pregnancy on diabetic retinopathy is not clearly known and requires further study since it is a disease that progresses over time even in the absence of pregnancy. Of the diabetic neuropathies, the most important for pregnancy is diabetic gastroparesis, which should be considered in the evaluation of any gastrointestinal complaint in the pregnant women with diabetes. Diabetic atherosclerotic vascular disease, presenting as coronary artery disease, increases maternal morbidity and mortality to an unknown degree.

In conclusion, the initial evaluation of any pregnant patient with pre-existing diabetes may require a careful ophthalmologic, cardiac, and neurologic examination, tests of renal function, and an electrocardiogram.

Gastrointestinal Disorders

The diagnosis of gastrointestinal disease during pregnancy may be obscured by numerous physiologic and anatomic changes that can occur during normal gestation. The progesterone effect of smooth-muscle relaxation causes: (1) decreased lower esophageal sphincter pressure, which increases symptomatic gastroesophageal reflux; (2) gallbladder relaxation and stasis with increased stone formation (an effect enhanced by the estrogen effect on bile lithogenecity) and an increased likelihood of pancreatitis; and (3) delayed gastric emptying and decreased bowel motility, increasing the risk of gastric content aspiration and constipation. The gravid uterus displaces abdominal organs, making abdominal palpation more difficult, and the diagnosis of an acute abdomen, e.g., appendicitis, confusing. The nausea and vomiting that occur during normal pregnancy must be differentiated from that occurring secondary to intrinsic gastrointestinal disease or obstruction. In addition, there are liver diseases unique to pregnancy that will be considered below.

Peptic ulcer disease and esophagitis occur during pregnancy and should be treated similarly to the nonpregnant state. Antacids and the type 2 histaminic receptor blockers, which block production of gastric acid, as well as sucralfate have been used safely in all trimesters of pregnancy. If abdominal pain or bleeding persist despite treatment, endoscopy is the diagnostic procedure of choice. Mallory-Weiss tear, a traumatic laceration in the lower esophagus, can occur in the presence of hyperemesis gravidarum and should be considered in the differential diagnosis of hematemesis.

Hepatobiliary diseases are the most common gastrointestinal disorders during pregnancy. Cholelithiasis and cholecystitis, for which ultrasound is the diagnostic procedure of choice, and pancreatitis are all treated as in the nonpregnant state. Viral hepatitis, the most frequent cause of jaundice in pregnancy, should always be excluded as a cause of liver function abnormalities. Perinatal transmission of hepatitis B can occur at delivery and during breastfeeding, so infants born to mothers who carry hepatitis B surface antigen should receive hepatitis B immune globulin and vaccine at birth. Hepatitis C may also be associated with significant perinatal transmission.

Intrahepatic cholestasis of pregnancy, acute fatty liver, and preeclampsia are all causes of liver dysfunction unique to pregnancy that occur most frequently late in gestation and postpartum. The differential diagnostic features of these third-trimester disorders are outlined in Table 23-10. Hyperemesis gravidarum, which occurs most frequently during the first trimester, should also be considered since it can alter liver function tests as well. Intrahepatic cholestasis accounts for approximately 20 percent of cases of jaundice during pregnancy. It presents most often as pruritis in conjunction with elevated alkaline phosphatase and bile acids. Intrahepatic cholestasis of pregnancy is a cause of postpartum hemorrhage presumably due to inadequate synthesis of vitamin K–dependent clotting factors by the liver. There is an increased incidence of fetal mortality and morbidity due to premature labor and decreased birth weight. Acute fatty liver of pregnancy, characterized by fatty infiltration of the liver associated with liver failure, a coagulopathy, and often renal failure, is a disease of unknown etiology that occurs in late pregnancy. Improvement may follow delivery but the maternal mortality rate remains high. Severe preeclampsia can be associated with abnormalities in liver function due primarily to ischemia, edema, subcapsular hematoma, and rarely, spontaneous rupture of the liver.

Inflammatory bowel disease occurs in about 1 to 2 percent of pregnancies. There is an increased infertility rate in patients with Crohn's disease, but not in patients with ulcerative colitis. The disease activity is generally not effected by pregnancy, but active disease accompanied by malabsorption, weight loss, and the potential for infection and perforation may have a major effect on the pregnancy and on perinatal outcome. Fetal death and intrauterine growth retardation have both been reported in this setting, as well as delayed wound healing, maternal incisional infections, and breakdown of episiotomy. Of those patients who initially are diagnosed during pregnancy, 50 percent require surgery during gestation. There is a 25 to 40 percent relapse rate postpartum independent of disease activity during pregnancy. In addition, there is a small increase in the spontaneous abortion rate in women with inflammatory bowel disease. Treatment is similar to that in the nonpregnant state, and includes bowel rest, corticosteroids, and sulfasalazine.

Hematologic Disorders

Disorders of coagulation, bleeding and platelet disorders, and the anemias represent important diagnostic and therapeutic challenges during pregnancy.

As outlined in Chap. 10 and the section on thromboembolic disease, normal pregnancy is a hypercoagulable state, due to increases in many of the clotting factors, decreased fibrinolysis, and venous stasis. A superimposed coagulation disorder, either acquired, such as lupus anticoagulant, or congenital, such as a deficiency of antithrombin III, protein C, or protein S, can have a significant impact during pregnancy. The presence of

Table 23-10. Characteristic features of various liver dysfunctions

Liver dysfunction	Onset (trimester)	Symptoms	Aspartate transferase (u/liter)	Bilirubin (mg/dl)	Alkaline phosphatase	Coagulopathy	Serology
AFLP	Third (typically >36 weeks)	Nausea, vomiting, malaise	<1000	<10	Moderate increase	+	
ICP	Early third, late second	Pruritis with or without jaundice	<300	<5	Seven- to 10-fold increase	± Increased prothrombin time	
Preeclampsia and eclampsia	Third (usually)	Headache, RUQ; pain, malaise, edema	<300	<2	Slight increase	±	
HELLP syndrome	Third (85%), second (15%)	RUQ pain, malaise, nausea	>70 (third trimester), <1000 (second trimester)	2–5	Slight increase	± Disseminated intravascular coagulation, decreased platelets	
Infarct	Third	RUQ pain, fever	>3000	2–10	Slight increase	Decreased platelets, increased platelets	
Viral hepatitis	Any trimester (third most often)	Fever, malaise, nausea, jaundice	>1000	>5	Moderate–marked increase	± (Severe case)	Often +

Key: RUQ = right upper quadrant; AFLP = acute fatty liver of pregnancy; HELLP = hemolysis, elevated liver enzymes, and low platelets; ICP = intrahepatic cholestasis of pregnancy.

the APL antibodies, antiphosphatidyl serine and anticardiolipin, and the lupus anticoagulant have each been associated with placental thrombosis and infarction, recurrent miscarriage, intrauterine growth retardation, and fetal demise. Maternal thromboembolic disease complicates 50 percent or more of pregnancies in which there are deficiencies in antithrombin III, protein C or protein S, necessitating a prophylactic heparin regimen that prolongs partial thromboplastin time in these cases.

Bleeding and platelet disorders that complicate pregnancy include congenital disorders such as hemophilia and von Willebrand's disease, which may require factor transfusions, and acquired disorders such as immune thrombocytopenia and disseminated intravascular coagulation. A careful history seeking prior family or patient bleeding complications should be obtained so that treatment to avoid serious, unexpected hemorrhage due to congenital coagulopathies can be instituted. Disseminated intravascular coagulation (DIC) should be suspected when bleeding occurs in association with abruptio placentae, amniotic fluid embolism, sepsis, and fetal demise. Bleeding in association with preeclampsia or acute fatty liver of pregnancy may be secondary to thrombocytopenia, decreased liver synthesis of clotting factors, or to DIC. The hemolytic uremic syndrome may occur peripartum as well. When the diagnosis of autoimmune or alloimmune thrombocytopenia is made in pregnancy, an additional consideration is the potential risk of thrombocytopenia to the fetus since IgG antiplatelet antibodies that cross the placenta may be present. The diagnosis of maternal IgG-mediated fetal thrombocytopenia has become more accurate due to the use of percutaneous umbilical blood sampling close to term.

The most common anemias during pregnancy are iron and folate deficiencies, related to the increased fetal demands, both of which are treated with oral replacement therapy.

The maternal effects of the hemoglobinopathies, exemplified by sickle cell anemia, include increased risks for urinary tract infection, cholelithiasis, and both pulmonary and systemic vaso-occlusive events related to clumping of sickled red blood cells with resultant thrombosis. Fetal effects include a greater likelihood of intrauterine growth retardation, fetal demise, and premature birth. Since hemoglobin is the oxygen carrier responsible for delivery of oxygen to both fetal and maternal tissues, its availability is of vital importance. The level of hemoglobin at which there are adverse fetal or maternal effects is controversial. Many experts recommend transfusion to maintain hematocrit above 25 percent or exchange transfusion to maintain hemoglobin A levels of 25 percent or greater.

Infectious Disease

The diagnosis and treatment of infections during pregnancy challenge the physician to consider both the impact of the pregnancy-related changes in the maternal immune system and the impact of the disease and its treatment on the fetus. Although there is no known change in humoral immunity during pregnancy, there appears to be a significant decrease in cell-mediated immunity. This decrease results in increased severity and occasional dissemination of viral illnesses such as varicella, and the occurrence of infections such as listeriosis that are usually seen only in immunocompromised hosts. Other potential etiologic agents of infection include a wide range of bacterial (streptococci, E. coli, staphylococci, enterococci, listeria, and various anaerobes) and viral (human immunodeficiency virus [HIV], rubella, herpes, cytomegalovirus [CMV], parvovirus) organisms as well as chlamydia, mycoplasma, treponemes, and toxoplasmosis. These agents can be responsible for pneumonia, chorioamnionitis, pyelonephritis, meningitis, endometritis, and mastitis during pregnancy or postpartum. This can result in sepsis, preterm labor, rupture of membranes, intrauterine growth retardation, fetal demise, or congenital anomalies. A thorough catalogue of these agents is beyond the scope of this textbook.

The infections with significant perinatal implications for which there is the most information available include group B streptococcus and Chlamydia trachomatis and the TORCH infections (toxoplasmosis, rubella, CMV, and herpes simplex viruses). Group B beta-hemolytic streptococcus is one of the most common causes of neonatal sepsis in the United States and has a high mortality rate, particularly in the premature neonate. As many as 20 percent of pregnant women may be colonized with group B streptococcus at some time during gestation and treatment does not necessarily eradicate a carrier state. For this reason attempts at prevention of neonatal infection have been aimed at detection of mothers and neonates at particularly high risk of infection. Most authors now recommend culturing all patients with preterm labor, premature rupture of membranes, or a prior maternal or neonatal history of group B streptococcus colonization or infection. Treatment can be withheld pending culture results only if delivery can be delayed. If delivery is imminent, treatment with ampicillin is initiated since maternal treatment in labor has been shown to decrease the risk of neonatal infection. Chlamydia infection, which is present in 2 to 30 percent of pregnant women, has a high transmission rate from mother to infant during delivery. If transmission occurs it can result in neonatal conjunctivitis or pneumonia. The effects of chlamydia infection on the pregnancy are less clearly defined but are thought by some investigators to be associated with preterm labor, premature rupture of membranes, and postpartum endometritis.

Toxoplasmosis, caused by the protozoan *Toxoplasma gondii*, is usually acquired by ingestion of cysts as a result of eating undercooked meat of an infected animal or of exposure to infected cat feces. The danger from this infection, which presents as mild malaise and lymphadenopathy, is to the fetus rather than to the mother. Toxoplasmosis may lead to spontaneous abortion, stillbirth, or congenital infection that may be characterized by chorioretinitis and varying degrees of mental retardation. The risk of fetal infection increases with gestation but the severity of the infection decreases as pregnancy progresses.

Rubella was the first virus that was demonstrated to have teratogenic potential. The degree of teratogenicity is not related to the severity of maternal infection, which may be mild or asymptomatic, but rather to the time in gestation that infection occurs. If maternal infection occurs during the first 10 weeks of gestation, approximately 90 percent of infants will be affected; this number falls to 20 percent after about 17 weeks' gestation. The clinical manifestations of congenital rubella syndromes vary with the timing of maternal infection. Prior to 8 weeks, cardiac defects and cataracts predominate; after 8 weeks, deafness and other neurologic deficits are more common. Transmission and neonatal infection may occur perinatally as well, during delivery or breast-feeding.

Cytomegalovirus is the most common congenital infection, with an incidence of 0.2 to 2.2 percent of live births. Congenital infection may occur following primary or recurrent infection and may vary from mild asymptomatic infection to significant CNS defects, chorioretinitis, and hepatosplenomegaly. Although the risk of congenital infection is as high as 40 to 50 percent of infected mothers, only about 5 percent of infected infants have severe CMV disease.

Herpes simplex virus infection early in pregnancy may result in spontaneous abortion but has not been clearly associated with congenital malformation. Neonatal herpes, due to genital transmission at the time of delivery, may result in life-threatening generalized neonatal infection. Untreated localized neonatal infection may progress to disseminated disease, CNS, or eye involvement in the majority of cases. Treatment should be aimed at detection of maternal disease and prevention of perinatal transmission by avoidance of vaginal delivery in mothers with active lesions.

Human parvovirus, the etiologic agent in fifth disease, is now a known cause of nonimmune hydrops. The hydrops may be secondary to fetal myocarditis with heart failure or anemia due to bone marrow involvement.

The two newest infectious diseases caused by agents known to cross the placenta include HIV and Lyme disease. Women who are seropositive for HIV are at risk to develop opportunistic infections if they carry a pregnancy to term. This risk may be due to the disease itself or a result of the progressive decline in helper T-cell number and overall cell-mediated immunity during gestation. Transplacental transmission of the virus occurs in 20 to 65 percent of cases, and results in a significant neonatal infection rate. Most neonates are at least transiently HIV-positive due to passive transfer of maternal antibody. Human immunodeficiency virus positivity is a risk factor for maternal pneumonia as well as for intrauterine growth retardation, prematurity, and low birth weight. Treatment with zidovudine may decrease the risk of development of the infectious complications in the mother and is now known to decrease the placental or perinatal transmission of the virus to the fetus if used antepartum, intrapartum and then given to the neonate. Transmission to neonates occurs in 25 percent of breast-fed infants who were HIV-negative at birth.

Lyme disease, caused by the spirochete *Borrelia burgdorferi,* is now the most common vector-borne infection in the United States, and is transmitted by the *Ixodes* tick. Lyme disease during pregnancy is associated with an increased risk of spontaneous abortion, premature labor, and intrauterine growth retardation. Large epidemiologic studies in the United States and Europe have failed to find an association between congenital anomalies and antibody to *B. burgdorfi* in cord blood. Autopsy cultures of fetal tissues, however, have demonstrated growth of *B. burgdorfi* in the liver, spleen, kidney, and heart in neonates of infected mothers, from presumed placental transmission of the spirochete. Fetal heart failure related to myocardial inflammation has been reported as well. However, considering the widespread prevalence of infection in endemic areas and the rarity of adverse fetal outcomes, transplacental infection is unusual and fetal disease is rarely severe.

When antibiotic use is necessary during pregnancy, the extent to which the drug crosses the placenta, the potential fetal toxicity, and pregnancy-induced modification in pharmacokinetics must be considered. The importance of sputum, blood, urine, endometrial, and cervical cultures, which may help to avoid inappropriate or unnecessary antimicrobial coverage, must be emphasized. The normal maternal physiologic changes that affect pharmacokinetics include a greater volume of distribution, reduced plasma protein, increased renal clearance, increased hapatic metabolism, and more erratic gastrointestinal absorption. Decreased dosing intervals, increased doses, and closer monitoring of levels may be needed to achieve adequate drug levels in pregnancy. Safety categories of specific antibiotics are outlined in Table 23-11.

Renal Disease

The normal physiologic changes in pregnancy that should be considered in the assessment of renal disease include a 50 percent increase in the glomerular filtration rate (GFR), renal blood flow, and plasma volume. Decreased tubular reabsorption of urate, glucose, and most amino acids, as well as the increased GFR, result in the increased excretion of uric acid, glucose, and protein and a decreased plasma osmolality. Anatomically, the kidneys increase in size and there is dilatation of the pelves, calyces, and ureters, resulting in the so-called hydronephrosis of pregnancy, which is more prominent on the right.

Renal disease in pregnancy can be categorized as unrelated to pregnancy or specifically associated with, or unique to pregnancy (Table 23-12). Pregnancy-unrelated renal diseases include acute and chronic renal failure, nephrotic syndrome, glomerulonephritis, and pyelonephritis. Preeclampsia, HELLP (hemolysis, elevated liver enzymes, low platelets) syndrome, acute fatty liver, and idiopathic postpartum renal failure or hemolytic uremic syndrome are all pregnancy-associated illnesses of which renal failure or intrinsic renal disease are a major part.

Table 23-11. Antibacterial agents in pregnancy

Agent	Placental passage	Excretion in breast milk	Comments	FDA rating
Penicillins				
Penicillin G	Readily crosses placenta to produce fetal serum levels of up to 100% maternal levels	Trace levels only	Safe for use in pregnancy	B
Ampicillin, amoxicillin	As for penicillin G	Low or trace levels only	Safe for use in pregnancy	B
Amoxicillin clavulanate	As for penicillin G	Low or trace levels only	Limited experience but no evidence of fetal toxicity	
Carbenicillin	Not known	Not known	Limited experience suggests no evidence of fetal toxicity	B
Flucloxacillin	Low, probably due to high degree of protein	Trace levels only	No evidence of fetal toxicity	Not used in the United States
Nafcillin	As for flucloxacillin	Trace levels only	No evidence of fetal toxicity	B
Cephalosporins				
Cephalothin	Low degree of transfer only	Low or trace levels only	No evidence of fetal toxicity	B
Cephalexin	Moderately, especially in late pregnancy	Trace levels only	Safe for use in pregnancy	B
Cefuroxime	Moderate, fetal serum levels 20–30% of maternal levels	Trace levels only	No evidence of fetal toxicity	B

Ceftazidime	Not known	Trace levels only	No evidence of fetal toxicity, but experience is limited	
Imipenem	Not known	Not known	No experience with its use in pregnancy; evidence of fetal toxicity in animal studies using high doses	
Aminoglycosides				
Gentamicin	Moderately; fetal serum levels of up to 40% of maternal levels are achieved	Not known	Fetal ototoxicity may occur but degree of risk to fetus is unknown	C
Tobramycin	As for gentamicin	Not known	As for gentamicin	D
Netilmicin	Not known	Not known	As for gentamicin	C
Amikacin	As for gentamicin	Not known	As for gentamicin	C
Other antibacterials				
Chloramphenicol	Readily; fetal serum levels up to 100% of maternal levels	High levels achieved, up to 50% of serum levels	Circulatory collapse ("gray baby syndrome") may occur if given in late pregnancy or labor; the drug should be avoided except for life-threatening infections.	C

(Continued)

419

Table 23-11. *(Continued)*

Agent	Placental passage	Excretion in breast milk	Comments	FDA rating
Other antibacterials *(Cont.)*				
Ciprofloxacin	Not known	Not known	Arthropathy has been demonstrated in young animals and use of this agent is not recommended in pregnancy.	
Clindamycin	Moderately	Low to moderate levels (10–20% of serum levels)	No evidence of fetal toxicity	B
Erythromycin	Crosses placenta to a low and variable extent	High, up to 100% of serum levels	Erythromycin estolate is contraindicated due to potential for reversible hepatotoxicity in mother; erythromycin does not cause fetal toxicity.	B
Fusidic acid	Not known	Not known	Limited clinical experience in pregnancy has not shown evidence of fetal toxicity.	
Metronidazoale	Readily crosses placenta	High levels achieved, approaching serum levels	No evidence of fetal toxicity, but it is mutagenic and carcinogenic in animals in high doses; short-course, high-dosage regimens should not be used.	B

Drug	Crosses placenta	Breast milk	Comments	Category
Nalidixic acid	Yes, but only to a small extent	Low levels are achieved	Although there is no evidence of fetal toxicity, use of nalidixic acid is not recommended in pregnancy.	B
Nitrofurantoin	Readily; fetal serum levels up to 100% of maternal levels	Low levels are achieved	Many years of clinical experience have shown nitrofurantoin to be safe for use in pregnancy.	B
Spectinomycin	Not known	Not known	There is no evidence of fetal toxicity	B
Tetracycline	Readily, fetal serum levels up to 100% of maternal levels	Moderate to high levels are found in breast milk, but bioavailability is low due to chelation with calcium.	All tetracyclines are contraindicated in pregnancy due to fetal toxicity (teeth discoloration and inhibition of bone growth) and maternal toxicity (acute fatty liver and renal failure). In nursing mothers, absorption from breast milk is minimal but use of these agents is not recommended.	D

(Continued)

Table 23-11. *(Continued)*

Agent	Placental passage	Excretion in breast milk	Comments	FDA rating
Other antibacterials *(Cont.)*				
Trimethoprim	Readily; fetal serum levels up to 100% of maternal levels	High, levels up to 100% of serum levels	Teratogenic in animals due to mode of action (folate antagonism); not recommended in pregnancy, especially in first trimester	C
			May precipitate megaloblastic anemia in pregnant women, which may be prevented by administration of folinic acid	
Sulfamethoxazole	Readily crosses the placenta	Low levels only	May cause kernicterus if given to mother in late pregnancy; not recommended in pregnancy	B (Rated D at term)
Vancomycin	Not known	Not known	Experience is very limited; drug should be used only when there is an absolute indication for it	C

Table 23-12. Causes of acute renal failure in pregnancy

I. Prerenal
  A. Unrelated to pregnancy
    1. Volume depletion
      vomiting, diarrhea, diuretics, bleeding
    2. Decreased extracellular fluid
      congestive heart failure, cirrhosis, nephrotic syndrome
    3. Decreased cardiac output
    4. Hypotension
  B. Associated with pregnancy
    1. Hyperemesis gravidarum
    2. Uterine hemorrhage
    3. Septic abortion

II. Postrenal
  A. Unrelated to pregnancy
    1. Bladder outlet obstruction
    2. Bilateral ureteral obstruction
  B. Associated with pregnancy
    1. Uterine compression of ureters
      multiple gestations, polyhydramnios
    2. Nephrolithiasis

III. Intrinsic renal disease
  A. Unrelated to pregnancy
    1. Acute glomerulonephritis
    2. Acute interstitial nephritis
    3. Intratubular obstruction
    4. Acute tubular necrosis
  B. Associated with pregnancy
    1. Acute tubular necrosis
    2. Pyelonephritis
    3. Bilateral renal cortical necrosis
    4. Preeclampsia
    5. HELLP syndrome
    6. Acute fatty liver
    7. Idiopathic postpartum renal failure

The renal changes present in preeclampsia and its variant HELLP syndrome are a result of the primary underlying vasospastic disorder. A decrease in GFR and renal plasma flow is seen as a result of local and generalized vasoconstriction. In addition, glomerular endotheliosis, the glomerular intracapillary cell swelling that is the characteristic lesion of preeclampsia, is seen. This combination of reduced intravascular volume and an ischemic renal lesion may result in oliguria, edema, and in severe cases, acute tubular or cortical necrosis.

Acute fatty liver is a disease of unknown etiology that is characterized by jaundice, severe hepatic dysfunction, and often DIC in the late third trimester or postpartum. The hepatic lesion is that of microvesicular fat deposition in hepatocytes. The association of acute renal failure with acute fatty liver was previously thought to be as high as 60 percent, but appears to be much less in more recent reviews. The kidney lesion is that of fatty vacuolization and minimal tubular structural damage. The cause of the renal failure is unknown but is thought to be related to hemodynamic factors and to DIC.

Idiopathic postpartum renal failure occurs from days to weeks after delivery and presents as rapidly progressive anuric or oliguric renal failure accompanied by microangiopathic hemolytic anemia or a consumptive coagulopathy. The pathophysiology is similar to that of thrombotic thrombocytopenic purpura, with arteriolar fibrin and platelet deposition; however, the etiology remains obscure. The prognosis continues to be poor with the majority of patients requiring long-term dialysis.

Renal failure can best be assessed by categorizing it into prerenal, postrenal, or intrinsic renal disease as in the nonpregnant state. Prerenal azotemia occurs with volume depletion secondary to diarrhea, vomiting as seen in hyperemesis gravidarum, uterine hemorrhage, ingestion of diuretics, and with edema-forming states such as cirrhosis, nephrosis, and congestive heart failure. Postrenal or obstructive causes include polyhydramnios or multiple gestation with obstruction by the gravid uterus, nephrolithiasis, and hydronephrosis. Intrinsic renal disorders include glomerulonephritis, interstitial nephritis secondary to drugs, renal cortical necrosis, and acute tubular necrosis.

Asymptomatic bacteruria is an important predictor of pyelonephritis in pregnancy, presumably because of the urostasis that is mediated by progesterone. If untreated during pregnancy, asymptomatic bacteruria will progress to pyelonephritis 20 to 40 percent of the time, and so should be treated for a minimum of 7 days. Despite treatment, the recurrence risk is approximately 20 percent so a test of cure culture is indicated. Pyelonephritis, 80 percent of which occurs in patients with previous asymptomatic bacteruria, requires high-dose intravenous antibiotics. It is an important cause of both preterm labor and adult respiratory distress syndrome in pregnancy and has a high recurrence rate. For this reason suppressive therapy is indicated for the duration of pregnancy in patients who have had recurrent urinary tract infection or a single documented episode of pyelonephritis.

The major determinants of perinatal outcome in the presence of renal disease are levels of hypertension and serum creatinine. In the presence of a creatinine of ≥1.5 mg/dl there is a significant increase in the likelihood of intrauterine growth retardation, prematurity, and maternal morbidity. Proteinuria, especially from diabetic nephropathy, increases markedly during pregnancy and can be as great as 8 to 10 g per 24 hours by term. This progressive increase in protein excretion parallels the progressive increase in glomerular filtration rate that accompanies normal pregnancy and does not necessarily reflect a worsening of renal disease. The consequent lowering of serum albumin and oncotic pressure can cause severe malnutrition and edema in the pregnant woman.

Neurologic Disorders

The major neurologic disorders encountered in pregnancy include epilepsy, cerebrovascular aneurysms, and arteriovenous malformations (AVM), and the neuromuscular disorders myesthenia gravis and multiple sclerosis.

Seizure disorders complicate 0.3 to 0.6 percent of all pregnancies. The effect of pregnancy on seizure frequency is variable, with 50 percent of patients reporting no change, 40 percent experiencing increased seizures, and about 10 percent reporting a decrease in seizure activity. The more severe the seizure disorder prior to pregnancy, the more likely is the patient to experience an exacerbation. It is generally accepted that the hyperventilation effect of progesterone lowers the seizure threshold but there appears to be no increase in the likelihood of status epilepticus during pregnancy. The occurrence of status epilepticus is associated with a high rate of fetal demise related to fetal hypoxemia and acidosis. Both maternal and neonatal hemorrhage can occur in patients taking hydantoin or phenobarbital due to a drug-induced decreased liver synthesis of vitamin K–dependent clotting factors.

The choice of anticonvulsant drugs is controversial. Congenital anomalies occur in the offspring of pregnant patients who are taking anticonvulsants with 2 to 3 times the frequency seen in the general population. The most commonly found anomalies include cleft lip, cleft palate, and cardiac malformations. The fetal hydantoin syndrome, characterized by distal phalangeal hypoplasia and possibly craniofacial and limb reduction defects, occurs in the offspring of patients who are taking phenytoin but also other anticonvulsants. There is a clear association between valproic acid and neural tube defects, so careful screening is needed. Trimethadione has been associated with cardiac and limb reduction defects, mental retardation, and craniofacial abnormalities in many exposed fetuses, and so should be avoided.

The major concern in patients with cerebrovascular disease is the effect that the Valsalva maneuver and increased intracranial pressure during the second stage of labor may have on the risk of an intracranial hemorrhage. The two major lesions of concern are congenital arteriovenous malformations and aneurysms, which occur in areas of congenitally weakened arterial walls. Since central venous pressure and thus the risk of bleeding is increased by pushing, most authors recommend cesarean section in the presence of a known AVM since the pressure in the venous portion of the AVM will increase with the Valsalva maneuver. Vaginal delivery is allowed in patients with a cerebral arterial aneurysm that has not bled, since the risk of rupture, while present, is not known to increase during labor and delivery, probably because there is no increase in arterial pressure with the Valsalva maneuver unless there has been a recent bleed.

Myesthenia gravis, an autoimmune neuromuscular disorder, is characterized by rapid fatigue of skeletal muscle and antibodies to acetylcholine receptors (anti-AChR), which creates a relative deficiency of acetylcholine protein at the postsynaptic site. The course of myesthenia generally is not affected by pregnancy but, as with multiple sclerosis, there is a high rate of exacerbation postpartum. Since many myesthenia gravis patients have circulating anti-AChR, an IgG class antibody, there is a neonatal myesthenia syndrome that occurs in 10 to 20 percent of offspring. Fatigue, particularly of maternal respiratory muscles, is a risk during labor and delivery.

Pulmonary Disease

An understanding of the normal physiologic changes in the respiratory system during pregnancy is essential to the interpretation of diagnostic tests of pulmonary function during gestation. The 40 percent increase in tidal volume, and thus minute ventilation, is manifested by an increase in arterial PO_2 to 106 to 108 mm Hg in the first trimester and 101 to 104 mm Hg by term, decreased arterial PCO_2 to below 30 mm Hg, and a compensatory fall in serum bicarbonate levels to 19 to 20 mEq/liter to maintain a normal pH. Normal arterial oxygen levels are based on measurement while the patient is in the left lateral supine or sitting positions.

Asthma complicates 0.4 to 1.3 percent of all pregnancies. In both retrospective and prospective analyses it appears that one-third of patients worsen, one-third improve, and one-third experience no change in their asthma during pregnancy. Severity of asthma and exacerbation during prior pregnancy both are predictive of worsening asthma during gestation. An improvement in disease is often seen at 36 to 40 weeks. Retrospective data suggest increased labor complications, prematurity, intrauterine growth retardation, and perinatal mortality in patients with asthma. However, at least one prospective study has failed to demonstrate an increase in fetal or maternal morbidity. Treatment of asthma is the same as in the nonpregnant state since lack of safety has not been demonstrated with the use of methylxanthines, inhaled beta agonists, cromolyn sodium, or corticosteroids during pregnancy.

Pneumonia in pregnancy is one of the leading causes of nonobstetric maternal mortality and a significant cause of preterm labor. Etiologic agents are thought to be similar to those in the nonpregnant population but have not been well studied. A recent review found HIV positivity and maternal drug use to be the major risk factors for pneumonia during pregnancy.

Tuberculosis, which was at one time unusual during pregnancy, is currently seen in immigrant populations, HIV-infected populations, and other parts of the world. There are no known deleterious effects of pregnancy on the course of the disease. There has been documented fetal infection believed to be acquired either transplacentally or through swallowing of infected amniotic fluid. Antituberculous drugs during pregnancy have been well studied. The use of ethambutol, which can be associated with optic neuritis in the adult, appears to be safe, with no optic tract abnormalities found in fetuses to date. Isoniazid does not appear to have adverse fetal effects but can cause maternal peripheral neuropathy related to pyridoxine deficiency, and some authors express concern about the maternal risk of hepatitis that increases with age as well. Eighth nerve damage has been found in 15 percent of neonates exposed to streptomycin in utero, and an association between rifampin and limb reduction defects has been suggested by case reports. Prophylactic regimens to treat purified protein derivative (PPD) conversions without evidence of active disease are generally delayed until postpartum.

Rheumatologic Disorders

Nowhere in obstetric medicine, except perhaps in diabetes, is the impact of maternal disease on the fetus more evident than in the autoimmune rheumatologic disorders. Maternal autoantibodies may be responsible for placental thrombosis, intrauterine growth retardation, congenital heart block, and fetal demise.

The presence of any of the APL antibodies, such as lupus anticoagulant, anticardiolipin, or antiphosphatidyl serine antibodies, correlates with the occurrence of placental thromboses and infarction, which lead to an increased risk of intrauterine growth retardation, intrauterine fetal demise, and preeclampsia. Although this class of antibodies is more prevalent in patients with systemic lupus erythematosis (SLE), they also may be found in the general population in the absence of known autoimmune disease. If an APL antibody is found in a patient who has experienced prior second-trimester fetal loss, the use of 80 mg of aspirin plus 40 to 60 mg of prednisone or subcutaneous heparin is thought by some authors to improve perinatal outcome. Randomized trials to establish an efficacious regimen are ongoing. Maternal anti-Rho antibody, SSA, is a known cause of fetal heart block and is present in 90 percent of mothers whose infants are affected.

The two major rheumatologic disorders seen during pregnancy are SLE and rheumatoid arthritis. The effect of pregnancy on SLE is variable, with the most recent studies showing no increase in the likelihood of exacerbation during pregnancy in patients without active disease at the time of conception. In patients with nephritis in remission, pregnancy does not alter the long-term renal prognosis. However, in patients with active glomerular inflammation, hypertension, or serum creatinine ≥ 1.5 mg/dl, there is a significant increase in maternal morbidity in the form of severe hypertension, proteinuria, and progressive renal impairment. There are reports of maternal deaths secondary to pulmonary hemorrhage and lupus pneumonitis in the postpartum period.

Because of the pregnancy-related increase in GFR and renal blood flow there is often a marked increase in proteinuria seen in patients with lupus nephritis independent of disease activity. It is extremely difficult to differentiate an exacerbation of SLE from preeclampsia. In patients in whom preeclampsia is suspected the major differential diagnostic features that favor lupus nephritis include extrarenal manifestations of SLE, hematuria, or red cell casts. The risk of heightened disease activity in patients with SLE is increased in the postpartum period. The fetal and neonatal effects of SLE include the antibody effects referred to previously as well as an overall increase in fetal loss and prematurity.

Rheumatoid arthritis is the only autoimmune disease that clearly improves during pregnancy and has no adverse effect on pregnancy outcome. However, 90 percent of patients who experience a remission during gestation relapse or flare within 6 months postpartum. The major therapeutic consideration involves the potential toxicity of gold and penicillamine. Gold has been shown to be teratogenic in animals and penicillamine, which freely crosses the placenta, has been associated with fetal connective tissue disease.

The medical problems in pregnancy discussed in this chapter represent challenging, exciting, underexplored areas of obstetrics and internal medicine. The student is encouraged to pursue them further and in more detail by reviewing the recommended reading list that follows.

Recommended Reading

Barron, W. M., and Lindheimer, M. D. *Medical Disorders During Pregnancy.* St. Louis: Mosby Year Book, 1991.

Berkowitz, R. L., Coustan, D. R., and Mochizuki, T. K. *Handbook for Prescribing Medications During Pregnancy* (2nd ed.). Boston: Little, Brown, 1986.

Briggs, G. C., Freeman, R. K., and Yaffe, S. J. *Drugs in Pregnancy and Lactation* (4th ed.). Baltimore: Williams & Wilkins, 1994.

Brody, S., and Weland, K. *Endocrine Disorders in Pregnancy.* Norwalk: Appleton & Lange, 1989.

Burrow, G., and Ferris, T. *Medical Complications During Pregnancy* (4th ed.). Philadelphia: Saunders, 1994.

Clark, S., et al. *Critical Care Obstetrics* (2nd ed.). Boston: Blackwell, 1991, updated edition.

Creasy, R., and Resnick, R. *Maternal Fetal Medicine: Principles and Practice* (3rd ed.). Philadelphia: Saunders, 1994.

de Swiet, M. *Medical Disorders in Obstetric Practice.* Boston: Blackwell, 1989.

Donaldson, J. D. Major Problems in Neurology. In *Neurology of Pregnancy* (2nd ed.). Vol. 19. Philadelphia: Saunders, 1989.

Elkayan, U., and Gleicher, N. *Cardiac Problems in Pregnancy* (2nd ed.). Alan R. Liss, 1990.

Gilstrap, L., and Faro, S. *Infections in Pregnancy*. Alan R. Liss, 1990.

Lee, R. V., Barron, W. M., Cotton, D. B., and Coustan, D. R. *Current Obstetric Medicine* (volume 1). St. Louis: Mosby Year Book, 1991.

Lee, R. V., Barron, W. M., Cotton, D. B., and Coustan, D. R. *Current Obstetric Medicine* (volume 2). St. Louis: Mosby Year Book, 1993.

Reece, E. A., and Coustan, D. *Diabetes Mellitus in Pregnancy: Principles and Practice*. New York: Churchill-Livingston, 1988.

24

Obstetric Complications

Donald R. Coustan

Pregnancy and birth are clearly normal, physiologic processes that occur universally, yet there is a widespread public perception that the medical profession treats pregnant women as "diseased," and birth as if it were pathologic. This chapter describes various complications that may supervene in an apparently normal pregnancy. It is important, however, to bear in mind that the vast majority of pregnancies proceed without mishap. The task of the obstetric caregiver is to allow normal events to occur with a minimum of intervention, yet to remain alert to the possibility of problems and be prepared to help the patient deal with them and deliver a healthy baby with minimal maternal risk.

Multiple Gestations

Definition and Incidence
When the conceptus splits into two (or more) complete embryos, a random event that occurs in approximately 1 in 250 pregnancies throughout the world, *monozygotic* twins result. By definition, such twins share gender, physical appearance, and their entire genome. When an ovary releases more than one ovum during a given cycle, and the multiple ova are fertilized, *dizygotic* twins or *trizygotic* triplets, etc., result. Genetically, such multizygotic fetuses are siblings who were conceived during the same reproductive cycle, but have no more in common than other brothers or sisters. Dizygotic twins do not appear to occur in a totally random fashion, as they are found much more frequently in some populations (Nigeria: 1 in 20 pregnancies) than in others (Japan: 1 in 250 pregnancies). In the United

States the incidence is approximately 1 in 80 pregnancies. Risk factors for dizygotic twinning, in addition to geography, include multiparity, advancing maternal age, and family history. These are risk factors for multiple ovulation.

Twinning is probably much more common than the above figures indicate, if twin pregnancies that are present early in pregnancy but not later are counted. This "vanishing twin" phenomenon represents very early spontaneous abortion of one embryo or fetus, with the other continuing as a singleton pregnancy. The aborted embryo or fetus is reabsorbed or may persist as a fetus papyraceous. The patient may not be aware of the event unless an early ultrasound is performed.

Causes and Risk Factors

Multiple pregnancies have been viewed by the public as a unique event, and various cultures have attached all sorts of special significance to twins and triplets. In recent years the advent of assisted reproductive technology has rendered multiple pregnancies more common. The use of the ovulation-inducing agent clomiphene citrate has been associated with a 5 to 10 percent likelihood of twins. When exogenous gonadotropic hormones are administered to induce ovulation, multiple pregnancies occur 10 to 20 percent of the time, depending on the protocol and dosage utilized. In vitro fertilization (IVF) programs report multiple pregnancy rates of 20 percent to as high as 50 percent, depending on the number of embryos put back into the uterus after "test tube conception" has occurred. Furthermore, the likelihood of higher-order multiple gestations, such as quadruplets, quintuplets, and above, is considerably increased with IVF. There is also some evidence to suggest that IVF embryos are more likely to undergo cleavage to form monozygotic twins.

Placentation

Although it is possible to determine whether twins are monozygotic or dizygotic by analyzing the DNA of each child, such testing is expensive and time-consuming. For this reason, twin pregnancies are often classified according to the relationship between their placentas (see Fig. 4-11). The placentas of dizygotic twins must, by definition, have two complete sets of membranous attachments, and are called *dichorionic-diamnionic.* Almost one-third of monozygotic twins also have dichorionic-diamnionic placentas, which occur if the splitting into two embryos occurs during the first 3 days after conception. However, if division occurs on days 4 through 8, a *monochorionic-diamnionic* placenta will result. This situation is most apparent at the membrane interface between the two amnionic sacs, which will contain the two amnionic layers (one from each embryo), but no chorion.

Approximately two-thirds of monozygotic twins have monochorionic-diamnionic placentas. The most unusual arrangement, occurring in approximately 10 percent of monozygotic twins, is the *monochorionic-mono-*

amnionic placenta. Here fission has occurred after the eighth day after fertilization, and both twins are contained within a single sac. Monoamnionic twins are at greatest risk for adverse outcomes, presumably due to the possibility of one twin becoming entangled in the umbilical cord of the other. If the embryo attempts to split after the twelfth day, the division is incomplete and *conjoined twins* result. This extremely rare phenomenon, which occurs once in approximately 600 twin births, is often incompatible with independent existence. Its presence generally attracts considerable attention in the lay press.

Diagnosis

Prior to the widespread availability of ultrasound technology, approximately 50 percent of twin pregnancies were undiagnosed prior to labor and delivery. Currently most twins are diagnosed during the first half of pregnancy, and it is rare for the diagnosis to be delayed until delivery. The most common clinical clue to the presence of multifetal gestation is a uterus that is growing faster than would be expected. The diagnosis is difficult without ultrasonography equipment. Auscultating fetal heart beats with a Doppler stethoscope at two different abdominal locations does not unequivocally prove the existence of more than one fetus, since heart sounds may be heard over the fetal chest, back, or placenta. If two different examiners simultaneously hear fetal heart tones at different abdominal sites, and the rates differ by 10 bpm or more, twins are extremely likely.

Sequelae

A number of adverse outcomes are more common with multifetal gestations. Congenital anomalies appear to occur at a rate about twice that in singletons. The twin-to-twin transfusion syndrome, seen only in twins with monochorionic placentas, is associated with unbalanced blood flow when the two twins share a placental vascular field. The "donor" twin is anemic and growth retarded, while the recipient twin is plethoric and often hydropic. Recently this phenomenon has come to be known as *"stuck twin" syndrome*; this term refers to the donor twin who has severe oligohydramnios, and on ultrasound appears to be "stuck in a corner" of the placenta. There is a high stillbirth and neonatal mortality rate in such situations, and many investigators believe that the problem goes beyond simply uneven blood exchange between the two fetuses. The "stuck" twin with oligohydramnios may be further disadvantaged because of the elevated surrounding pressure secondary to hydramnios in the sac of the sibling. This condition may decrease placental perfusion of the smaller twin and lead to worsening of its cardiovascular status. The use of serial amniocentesis to reduce the intrauterine pressure is currently being explored as a treatment option in such cases.

Another situation in which twins may manifest dissimilar birth weights arises when one twin has intrauterine growth retardation and the other does not. It appears that placental exchange is deficient in one but not the other twin, as though one twin captured most of the total functional placental mass. Although the smaller twin may have oligohydramnios on the basis of diminished renal plasma flow from hypovolemia, the larger twin is not plethoric and does not have hydramnios, and no unbalanced sharing of the circulation occurs. This phenomenon can occur with dizygotic as well as monozygotic twins.

Premature labor and birth are especially common with multiple gestations. The average duration of pregnancy is inversely related to the number of fetuses present. As many as 50 percent of twins are reported to deliver prior to 37 completed weeks. As assisted reproductive technology has become popular, multiple gestations contribute to an increasing proportion of low-birth-weight and very-low-birth-weight neonates, as well as perinatal mortality and morbidity. The cause of prematurity with multifetal pregnancies is not clear. Overdistention of the uterus is often proposed as a factor.

Measures used to decrease the likelihood of preterm birth include patient education to enable early recognition of preterm labor, decreased maternal activity, and home uterine monitoring to detect premature contractions; the latter modality is still considered experimental by many authorities. Routine hospitalization beginning in the middle of the second trimester has been tried but has not proved effective. When higher-order multiple pregnancies, such as quadruplets or quintuplets, occur, reduction procedures may be offered. One or more of the embryos is killed, often by intracardiac injection of a caustic substance such as potassium chloride. The remains of the dead fetus become compressed by the living fetuses, and a *fetus papyraceous* may result. The reduction procedure lowers the risk of prematurity by creating singleton or twin pregnancies.

When one of twin fetuses dies in utero, and remains in place while its sibling grows and develops, there is a theoretical possibility that maternal disseminated intravascular coagulation (DIC) will develop due to the retained dead twin. Although this situation has been reported, it is rare and takes many weeks to develop. There are case reports of successful heparin treatment of the mother. When one of a pair of monozygotic twins dies in utero, it is possible for its sibling to have sublethal damage to several organs. Central nervous system lesions, renal damage, and peripheral embolic lesions have all been reported. This situation, while fascinating, is rare (see Chap. 5).

Delivery

At the time of the onset of labor, twins may both present as vertex, or one or both may be breech or transverse lie. When the first twin presents as breech and the second as vertex, the potential exists for *interlocking* twins. In this situation the body of the first twin delivers, but the head of the second twin descends into the maternal pelvis below the head of the first twin. This positioning prevents the head of the first twin from delivering, and the twins are said to be interlocking. This catastrophe may be prevented by an assistant maintaining pressure to hold the second twin out of the maternal pelvis while the first twin is delivering, but is most often averted by cesarean section delivery.

Isoimmunization

Pathophysiology and Genetics—Rh (D)

Maternal antibodies that are directed against a blood-group antigen present on fetal erythrocytes may cross the placenta and cause fetal hemolysis. The incidence of this serious problem has been reduced significantly by the development of methods of passive maternal immunization against the most common antigen, Rh (D). Maternal antibodies cross the placenta if they are G-class immunoglobulins. Approximately 15 percent of the white population is negative for the Rh (D) factor; they usually are called "Rh-negative," and are potentially capable of producing antibodies against this factor if exposed to it. If spouses are selected randomly with respect to blood group, the chance of an Rh (D)–negative female marrying an Rh (D)–positive male is approximately 85 percent. The D antigen is dominant whereas d (the absence of D, also called "Rh-negative") is recessive; 45 percent of Rh (D)–positive individuals are homozygous for D, whereas 55 percent are heterozygous. The Rh (D)–negative mother is homozygous for d, and so her fetus must receive a d allele from her. The homozygous Rh (D)–positive father will contribute a D allele to every fetus. Such a fetus, who has received a D allele from the father and a d allele from the mother, will be Dd, heterozygous Rh (D)–positive. If the father is heterozygous for D the odds that a given fetus will be Dd, or dd (Rh [D]–negative) are each 50 percent.

The Rh (D)–negative mother who has never been exposed to the D antigen does not make antibodies against this antigen, and her first pregnancy with an Rh (D)–positive fetus is unaffected. However, there are a number of opportunities for Rh (D)–positive erythrocytes from the fetus to enter the maternal circulation during and after pregnancy. Although fetal and maternal circulations are separate, with three interposed fetal tissue layers (trophoblast, connective tissue, and capillary endothelium) in the placenta, microscopic breaks in the integrity of this barrier may occur. Transplacental hemorrhage has been found by detecting fetal erythrocytes in the maternal circulation in slightly less than 5 percent of first-trimester pregnancies, 10 percent of second-trimester pregnancies, and 45 percent of third-trimester pregnancies. It may also occur after spontaneous or therapeutic abortion, or ectopic pregnancy.

When the mother's immune system encounters the D antigen on Rh (D)–positive erythrocytes, it may respond by making antibodies directed against the D antigen. Such an immune response does not always occur, and factors involved include the volume of red cells in the maternal circulation and the innate ability of the maternal immune system to respond. In addition, ABO blood-group incompatibility between the mother and the fetus protect against isoimmunization, presumably by destroying fetal red cells before they can be taken up and processed by the maternal immune system.

Once the mother has mounted an immune response against the Rh (D) factor, and the nature of the antibodies has shifted from the initial IgM to IgC, the antibodies then may cross the placenta and attach to fetal Rh (D)–positive erythrocytes. Erythrocytes coated with antibodies will agglutinate in the laboratory when incubated with "Coombs' serum," which contains anti-human globulin. Thus, the blood of a D-positive neonate whose mother is immunized against the D antigen will display a positive "direct Coombs' " test. The "indirect Coombs' " test is used to detect the presence of anti-D antibodies in the maternal blood. Rh (D)–positive cells are added to maternal serum. If there are antibodies against the Rh (D) factor, they will coat the cells, which will then agglutinate when Coombs' serum (anti-human globulin) is added.

The indirect Coombs' test can be used to detect antibodies against other blood groups than Rh (D) so long as the blood group of interest is present on the cells that are used. The amount of antibody in the maternal serum can be estimated by using serial dilutions of maternal serum ("titering"), and expressing the level by the weakest dilution in which the indirect Coombs' test is still positive. For example, a 1:8 titer signifies a relatively low level of antibody, whereas a 1:512 titer is quite high. Threshold values differ among various laboratories, but a maternal indirect Coombs' titer of 1:32 is usually regarded as placing the fetus at significant risk.

Other methods of measuring maternal antibodies exist, and significant values differ depending on the method. When the antibody measurement is performed in a medium containing albumin, the "albumin titer" is usually slightly lower than the indirect Coombs' titer mentioned above. Maternal antibody titers may change as pregnancy progresses, probably reflecting the effects of challenges to the mother's immune system by small transplacental hemorrhages.

Sequelae

When significant amounts of anti-D antibody cross the placenta and coat fetal erythrocytes, a number of adverse consequences may result. Antibody-coated erythrocytes are destroyed in the fetal spleen, and anemia may result. The anemia causes fetal erythropoietin production that stimulates the marrow to produce red cells. If the marrow cannot respond adequately or the process occurs before 32 to 34 weeks of gestation, excessive erythropoiesis occurs in extramedullary sites, particularly the liver and spleen. In extreme cases, when fetal red cell production cannot keep up with destruction, a condition called *hydrops fetalis* results. The fetus develops edema and anasarca and may die in utero. The cause may be obstruction of the portal vascular system by erythropoietic tissue and interference with hepatic cell function.

Alternatively, hydrops may be due to severe anemia and forward heart failure. Increased portal pressure combined with low albumin production lead to edema and ascites, and placental edema may interfere with respiratory and nutritional exchange. If hydrops does not develop, or is not fatal in utero, problems may still befall the Rh (D)–positive neonate of an Rh-negative sensitized mother. As erythrocytes are destroyed in the spleen, the breakdown products of hemoglobin, primarily bilirubin, can be toxic to the central nervous system. The adult is normally able to conjugate bilirubin to a water-soluble product, bilirubin diglucuronide (also called "direct bilirubin") and then dispose of it. The fetus and neonate lack adequate amounts of the responsible enzyme glucuronyl transferase, and so cannot conjugate the bilirubin. During fetal life the "indirect" or unconjugated bilirubin can be removed and conjugated by the mother, and poses little threat. However, after birth, if hemolysis continues due to the continued presence of maternal anti-D antibodies, this indirect bilirubin may accumulate in the newborn and cause jaundice and possibly *kernicterus*, a condition of the central nervous system in which the bilirubin enters the lipid membranes of neurons, leading to neuronal destruction. The pathophysiology and treatment of isoimmunization in the neonate is discussed in Chaps. 5, 6, and 22.

Management
The use of amniotic fluid analysis to predict the severity of the fetal effects of isoimmunization became possible in the 1960s. A sample of fluid, obtained by amniocentesis, is placed in a spectrophotometer and the optical density at 450 nm is determined. The amount by which this optical density differs from a standard is called the Δ *OD 450*, and is proportional to the amount of heme pigment in the fluid. Graphs are available to correlate the Δ OD 450 at a particular gestational age with the likelihood of death in utero. If the risk is high, early delivery may be undertaken.

When the pregnancy is not far enough advanced to have a high likelihood of survival if delivered, another option is intrauterine transfusion. This procedure was first accomplished by infusing Rh (D)–negative red cells into the fetal peritoneal cavity, where they can be absorbed intact into the fetal circulation, and more recently by direct transfusion into the umbilical vein under ultrasound guidance. Details of these procedures, which are carried out in highly specialized tertiary perinatal centers, are beyond the scope of this textbook.

Prevention
Rh isoimmunization and its sequelae are becoming far less prevalent due to the development of a preventive approach to this problem. If the Rh-

negative mother is passively immunized with Rh (D) antibodies before or shortly after fetal erythrocytes enter her circulation, a primary immune response can be prevented. It is now standard practice to administer an injection of Rh immune globulin, purified after being obtained from the blood of individuals with high titers of Rh (D) antibodies, to an Rh (D)–negative unsensitized mother within 48 to 72 hours after the delivery of an Rh (D)–positive fetus. Such an approach has been highly successful in preventing maternal isoimmunization, which formerly occurred after approximately 10 percent of at-risk deliveries. The usual dose of 300 µg of immunoglobulin is effective in neutralizing approximately 30 ml of Rh (D)–positive blood, or 15 ml of Rh (D)–positive erythrocytes. Prophylaxis may fail when more than that volume of fetal red cells has entered the maternal circulation.

It is customary to perform a *Kleihauer Betke* test (see Chap. 9, Fig. 9-10) on maternal blood after delivery in order to ascertain whether there was a large fetal-maternal transfusion. In this test, a thin smear of maternal blood is exposed to an acid medium that denatures adult erythrocytes. Fetal erythrocytes stain more brightly than the denatured adult "ghost" erythrocytes, and the proportion of fetal to maternal cells can be used to estimate the volume of fetal blood that entered the mother's circulation.

If more than 15 ml of fetal erythrocytes are detected, additional doses of Rh immune globulin are administered. In addition to giving Rh immune globulin after delivery, it is now usual practice to administer a dose at 28 weeks' gestation to Rh-negative mothers, in order to protect the 1 or 2 percent who may become sensitized as a result of a third-trimester transplacental hemorrhage. Rh immune globulin is also given to unsensitized Rh (D)–negative mothers at the time of amniocentesis, chorionic villus sampling, trauma, abortion, bleeding during pregnancy, or in the case of mismatched transfusion of Rh (D)–positive cells at any time.

Other Antigens

As Rh (D) isoimmunization has become less common, other blood group antigens have assumed greater relative importance as causes of incompatibility between mother and fetus. Theoretically, any antigen that is present on fetal cells but not maternal cells may sensitize the mother after transplacental hemorrhage, and the resulting IgG antibodies may produce hemolysis in the fetus. In fact, differing antigen systems show differing proclivities for causing adverse fetal outcomes. Maternal-fetal incompatibility in the ABO system may cause jaundice, but is not known to cause fetal hydrops. The Lewis antigens are not present on fetal red cells, and maternal antibodies against them do not cause hemolysis. In the Rh system, antibodies directed against c and E may cause severe hemolytic disease, whereas those against C and e generally cause only moderate disease. The Kell system antigens, K and k, can be associated with severe disease, as can one of the Duffy antigens, Fyª. A list of all such antigens can be found in the recommended reading at the end of the chapter. The sequelae and management of mothers with antibodies directed against these "irregular antigens" are similar to those for Rh (D), except that there is no prophylactic immune globulin to prevent maternal sensitization.

Third-trimester Bleeding

Vaginal bleeding during the third trimester occurs in approximately 4 percent of pregnancies. In many cases no cause is identified and the bleeding is ascribed to early labor ("bloody show"), whereas in some there is a vaginal or cervical lesion responsible for the bleeding. Rarely the blood is fetal in origin, coming from a *vasa previa* in which a fetal vessel courses aberrantly through the membranes and is torn as the cervix dilates or as the membranes rupture across it. The causes of third-trimester bleeding that are of most concern, however, are *placenta previa* and *abruptio placentae*.

Placenta Previa

Definition and Classification

Classically, it is taught that bleeding from placenta previa presents without pain, whereas bleeding from abruptio placentae is accompanied by abdominal pain and uterine contractions. Like all "rules of thumb," the above does not always hold true. For example, patients may not bleed from placenta previa prior to labor, and during labor the bleeding is not painless.

Placenta previa occurs when the placenta implants over the cervical os, an abnormal location (Fig. 24-1). Prior to the availability of ultrasonography, placenta previa was classified as total, partial, or marginal, based on digital examination of the cervix. Because such digital examinations may precipitate life-threatening hemorrhage when the cervix has begun to dilate, they are not performed prior to the time when delivery is planned. Modern ultrasonography, including the use of vaginal ultrasound probes, allows a much more precise characterization of placental implantation. Placental insertion may be described as *complete placenta previa*, in which the placenta is more or less centrally located over the cervix, or as *low lying placenta*, in which the placenta is in the lower uterine segment and its edge overrides the cervix. Although placenta previa is diagnosed in the second trimester in upwards of 5 percent of patients, it is present in the third trimester in only 0.5 to 0.9 percent. This apparent "migration" probably does not represent true movement of the placenta. As the cervix unfolds to become the lower uterine segment in preparation for labor, there may appear to be upward movement of the placental implantation site. It is also possible that the portion of the placenta nearest the cervix has a poor blood supply and undergoes atrophy.

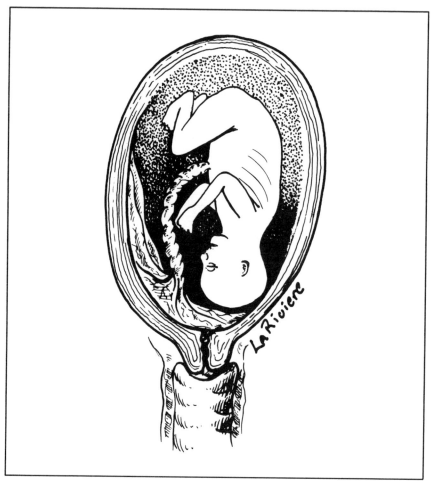

Fig. 24-1. Placenta previa in the third trimester. The placental edge extends to cover the uterine wall on both sides of cervix. This placenta is unlikely to "migrate."

Risk Factors

Risk factors for placenta previa include previous cesarean section, multiparity, and advanced maternal age. When there is a previous cesarean section there is a significant likelihood that the placenta will invade the underlying scar; this condition is called *placenta accreta*. This complication is associated with dangerous bleeding at parturition, whether by cesarean section or vaginally, and maternal death occasionally occurs. Removal of the uterus is generally the only effective treatment for placenta accreta.

Sequelae

The consequences of total placenta previa, in which the entire cervix is covered by the placenta, are quite serious. As the cervix effaces and dilates, the attachment of the placenta to the uterine wall inevitably becomes dislodged, and profuse hemorrhage is highly likely. Maternal death may result if rapid action is not taken. Furthermore, the placenta occupies the lower uterine segment, so that delivery is obstructed. The fetus is much more likely to present as breech or transverse lie because the head is prevented from assuming its usual place in the lower pole of the uterus.

Management

Management of placenta previa depends on the clinical circumstances and gestational age at diagnosis. For example, a patient whose placenta previa is diagnosed when she undergoes ultrasound examination to assess fetal growth at 22 weeks' gestation, and who has not experienced bleeding, probably requires no special management other than a repeat ultrasound in the third trimester. The chances are approximately 90 percent that placenta previa will no longer be present at the time of labor. The patient who presents with painless vaginal bleeding at 30 weeks' gestation, and on ultrasound examination has a complete placenta previa, is hospitalized and put at bed rest. Vaginal examinations are avoided, and attempts are made to delay delivery. Ultrasound examinations are repeated every few weeks to ascertain whether placental "migration" has occurred. Severe hemorrhage may require immediate cesarean section. Otherwise, planned cesarean section is performed once fetal lung maturity is present.

Abruptio Placentae

Definition and Pathophysiology

Abruptio placentae is defined as bleeding from the premature separation of a normally implanted placenta. It is also possible for an abnormally implanted placenta, such as placenta previa, to separate prematurely, and so combinations of abruptio and previa may be encountered. Clinically apparent abruptio is approximately twice as common as placenta previa. Although abruptions appear to be acute events, their development is not always sudden. The association of intrauterine growth retardation with abruption suggests an ongoing process, as does the recurrence risk in subsequent pregnancies, which is reported to be between 5 and 15 percent.

Abruptio is believed to begin with bleeding into the decidua, between the placenta and uterine wall (Fig. 24-2). The original source of bleeding may be fetal, but most often is maternal. The blood then accumulates beneath the placenta. If it does not find its way to the cervical os and out the vagina it is called *concealed hemorrhage*. If the bleeding stops there may be no adverse sequelae, or there may be compression of the placenta by the clot, leading to a scarred or depressed area visible at delivery. If a substantial proportion of the placental surface area is compromised by a single large blood collection or multiple smaller ones, maternal-fetal exchange may be compromised, leading to intrauterine growth retardation or

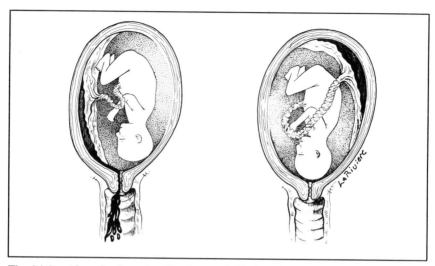

Fig. 24-2. Abruptio placentae. The "concealed" abruptio (left) has retroplacental hemorrhage but no clinically evident vaginal bleeding. The abruptio placentae (right) has resulted in overt hemorrhage.

hypoxia. More commonly the collection of blood reaches the edge of the placenta, makes its way between the membranes and uterine wall, and ultimately exits through the cervix, leading to externally visible bleeding. Abruptio placentae is often, but not always, accompanied by pain because the blood collecting between the placenta and uterus probably insinuates itself into the myometrium between muscle fibers. In addition, retroplacental blood stimulates uterine contractions.

Risk Factors
Reported risk factors for abruptio placentae include the history of abruption in a previous pregnancy, high parity, maternal hypertension, cigarette smoking, and occasionally uterine trauma. In recent years maternal cocaine use has been strongly associated with abruptio placentae.

Sequelae
Adverse sequelae of abruptio placentae include fetal hypoxia proportional to the degree of placental surface that has sheared off, and maternal hemorrhagic shock proportional to the blood loss. Clinically significant DIC occurs in approximately 10 percent of cases of abruptio, particularly in those severe enough to cause fetal demise. The mechanism for DIC in such cases is believed to be the release of thromboplastin from the injured placenta into the general circulation.

Diagnosis and Management

The clinical findings of vaginal bleeding, uterine tenderness, and contractions should suggest the diagnosis of abruption, but all these elements are not invariably present. When abruptio placentae is suspected, ultrasonography may identify retroplacental or retromembranous blood collection in less than half of cases, and cannot be used to rule out the condition. The presence of acute, clinically significant abruption is an indication for delivery of the pregnancy. Artificial rupture of the amniotic membranes should be performed to hasten labor. If the patient is in active labor, progress is often rapid and vaginal delivery can be anticipated. In fact, hypertonic uterine contractions, without the usual resting period in between, are commonly seen.

Fetal hypoxia may supervene, and the fetal heart rate tracing may become worrisome. Before performing a cesarean section to improve the fetal outcome, it is critical to ascertain that the mother is capable of clotting her blood, lest a fetal death be converted into combined maternal and fetal mortality. This capability can be ascertained at the bedside by drawing a nonanticoagulated tube of maternal blood and observing it for clot formation. If a clot fails to form within 8 minutes there is a high likelihood of a severe coagulopathy. It is also important to ascertain that the mother is hemodynamically stable and that blood replacement is available before performing surgery.

When abruption is diagnosed it is useful to measure clotting parameters. The presence of fibrin degradation products is one of the earliest events in the DIC associated with abruption. The serum fibrinogen level is a useful assessment in such patients. Normally somewhat elevated during pregnancy, fibrinogen levels below 100 mg/dl support the need for replacement, usually by fresh-frozen plasma. Platelet counts, prothrombin time, and partial thromboplastin times are usually abnormal only after fibrinogen has begun to fall.

Occasionally abruption is suspected but the diagnosis is not straightforward, and the pregnancy is at an early stage such that immediate delivery would put the neonate at significant risk from prematurity. Under such circumstances, assuming normal coagulation studies and no evidence of acute or chronic fetal compromise, and in the absence of labor, many clinicians allow the pregnancy to continue under close observation. Factors that were present to cause the initial abruption are presumably still present, so recurrence of the condition during the same pregnancy is to be anticipated.

Premature Rupture of the Membranes

Definition

Premature rupture of the membranes (PROM) is defined as the rupture of the amniotic membranes prior to the onset of labor. *Preterm PROM* (PPROM) is the premature rupture of membranes prior to 37 completed weeks of pregnancy. *Prolonged PROM* is usually defined as rupture of membranes lasting more than 24 hours before delivery. Preterm PROM is one of the more common causes of preterm labor and birth.

Etiology

The etiology of PROM is unclear. In most patients who are left alone (i.e., membranes are not artificially ruptured) the membranes rupture spontaneously during labor, usually as full dilation is approached. Increased intrauterine pressure may be invoked as the mechanical cause of rupture, which usually occurs over the cervical os where there is the least support of the integrity of the membranes; this is presumably not the case when membranes rupture prior to labor. Some studies have suggested that there are specific areas of "weakness," demonstrated histologically, over the cervix. This weakness may be due to decreased nutritional support because of the absence of a local blood supply in this area. Such findings do not explain why some patients experience PPROM and others do not. Some investigators have shown decreased elasticity in membranes that have ruptured prematurely, and others have demonstrated decreased collagen content. Such studies are not all consistent with each other, so consensus has not been reached.

Evidence exists for increased proteolytic activity in the amniotic fluid of individuals who experience PPROM. One possible source of proteases could be microbial invasion of the amniotic cavity. Cytokines, which may stimulate proteolytic activity, have been identified in the amniotic fluid of individuals with PPROM and infection.

A number of other studies support an infectious etiology in some cases of PPROM. Placentas from patients with PPROM frequently have bacterial invasion of the interface between fetal chorion and maternal decidua, and maternal and neonatal infection are common with PPROM.

Sequelae

Premature rupture of the membranes occurs at term in about 10 percent of pregnancies, whereas PPROM affects 2 to 3 percent. When membranes rupture at term, labor ensues within 24 hours in upwards of 80 percent of women. However, the earlier in pregnancy PPROM occurs, the longer is the average *latent period* (interval between rupture of membranes and onset of labor). When PPROM occurs prior to 26 weeks, approximately 70 percent of patients go into labor within a week, but 20 percent remain undelivered for a month or more. The mechanism by which PROM initiates labor appears to be a combination of factors. Injury to the membranes and decidua may bring about the release of arachidonic acid, a precursor in prostaglandin synthesis. Ruptured membranes provide a means of entry for vaginal microorganisms, so that microbial invasion may be a result as well as a cause of PROM. Cytokine bacterial products may stimulate prostaglandin production, thus increasing the likelihood of labor when PPROM is accompanied by infection. Although infection is clearly a concern with PPROM, the primary cause of perinatal mortality and morbidity is prematurity.

In addition to infection and preterm delivery, other sequelae of PPROM may include prolapse of the umbilical cord, compression of the umbilical cord due to lack of protection by ample amniotic fluid, and the *Potter's sequence*, or oligohydramnios sequence. This cluster of deformations, described in Chap. 8, may occur when PROM occurs before approximately 26 weeks' gestation, and includes pulmonary hypoplasia that is usually incompatible with life, abnormal facies, compression defects of the extremities, and amnion nodosum. It is similar to the effects of fetal renal agenesis. Not all babies born after very early PPROM suffer these problems, and prediction is not always possible.

Diagnosis

The diagnosis of PROM is relatively certain when three findings are present on examination with a sterile speculum: (1) a pool of fluid in the posterior vaginal fornix; (2) a relatively alkaline pH (>7.0) in the vaginal pool, as evidenced by a deep blue color when the fluid is placed on nitrazine paper; and (3) a "ferning" pattern (Fig. 24-3) when a thin smear of the fluid is allowed to air-dry on a slide and examined under a microscope. Sometimes there is no vaginal pool in a patient who gives a history of losing fluid from the vagina, so that the diagnosis is in doubt. In such cases, ultrasound examination may disclose decreased amounts of amniotic fluid *(oligohydramnios)*, which support the possibility of PROM. If uncertainty is still present, and it is thought that making a diagnosis is important, an amniocentesis may be performed and a dye such as indigo carmine can be instilled. Inspection of a sterile tampon placed in the vagina for an hour or so should then reveal a characteristic blue dye when PROM is present.

Management

The management of PROM at term is controversial, with some authors advocating immediate induction of labor to avoid infection, others suggesting a limited observation period of 12 to 24 hours prior to induction, and still others advocating observation until spontaneous labor supervenes. Investigations of this issue have yielded conflicting results, with some showing a higher cesarean section rate following immediate induction of labor, and others showing no difference. Although infection rates are higher the longer the latent period at term, it is difficult to determine whether the most important risk factor is duration of the latent period, or more likely the number of vaginal examinations performed during the latent period. Therefore most clinicians avoid digital vaginal examinations in such patients prior to the onset of labor. An initial sterile speculum examination to document PROM and observe the cervix is appropriate, since patients

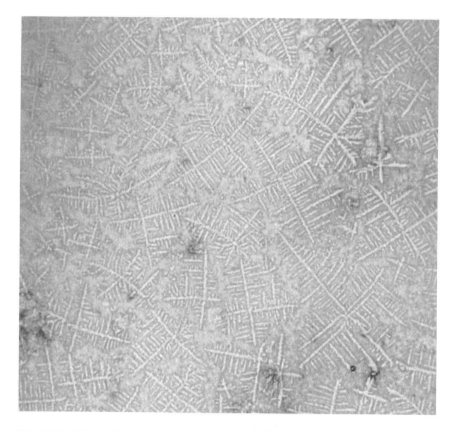

Fig. 24-3. Photomicrograph (original ×40) of positive "fern" test confirming the presence of amniotic fluid. Note the delicate fern-like arborizing pattern. (Courtesy of Drs. Calvin Oyer and Lynn Norton.)

with a "ripe" cervix will probably go into labor readily, either spontaneously or with oxytocin stimulation, whereas those with long closed cervices are most likely to benefit from a period of observation during which "ripening" may occur.

Patients with PPROM are usually managed conservatively by observation and bed rest. Since prematurity is more likely to be a problem than infection, labor is not induced unless there is an indication to do so (such as infection), or there is evidence of lung maturity when amniotic fluid is tested. Prophylactic antibiotics are often prescribed when PPROM occurs, because, unlike the situation of preterm labor with intact membranes, treatment has been shown to decrease maternal febrile morbidity and prolong pregnancy. The use of tocolytic agents when preterm labor starts is controversial, since available data suggest that tocolysis is unlikely to add more than 24 hours to the pregnancy, presumably because labor is often a sign of infection. Corticosteroid treatment to enhance fetal lung maturity is controversial in the face of PPROM, with the added risk of infection, but meta-analyses of published studies suggest that a benefit may be obtained at little risk.

Group B Streptococcus in Premature Rupture of the Membranes
One of the bacteria often implicated in infections associated with PROM is the group B ß-hemolytic streptococcus. This microorganism is of particular concern because it is the leading single organism causing life-threatening neonatal infections in the United States, and it infects approximately 1 in 1000 newborns. Upwards of 15 percent of women, depending on the population studied, are colonized with group B streptococcus during pregnancy. The organism may be transmitted from mother to infant during labor and delivery, with about half the cases of clinical neonatal infection being "early onset," evident during the first week of life. Early-onset infection with group B streptococcus has a high case mortality rate (approximately 15 percent). In addition to PROM, other risk factors for group B streptococcus sepsis in the neonate include prematurity, prolonged ruptured membranes, maternal fever in labor, and the history of a previous affected child. Some authorities recommend obtaining vaginal cultures to look for colonization in all pregnant women at the beginning of the third trimester. Women who screen positive are treated with antibiotics during labor if they have any of the above risk factors. Because of the expense associated with screening, and the possibility that women who are positive at 28 weeks' gestation will become negative before birth, and vice versa, other authorities have taken the approach of treating all women with risk factors when they are in labor, without having previously obtained cultures. Treatment with penicillin or ampicillin during labor appears to be highly effective in preventing neonatal infection.

Preterm Birth

Definition
Most babies are born at term, i.e., approximately 280 days from the commencement of the last menstrual period, assuming that ovulation and fertilization occur on about the fourteenth day of that cycle. When delivery occurs prior to 37 completed weeks, or less than 259 days from the commencement of the last menstrual period, it is considered *preterm*. Nearly 10 percent of births in the United States are preterm. Because gestational age may be difficult to determine with accuracy, many studies and pronouncements in the past have used the more conveniently measured *low birth weight* (<2500 g) interchangeably with prematurity. This practice is inappropriate. Because low birth weight (LBW) corresponds to an average gestational age approximately 2 weeks lower than the definition of prematurity, only approximately 6 percent of babies are LBW. Furthermore, a significant

proportion of LBW babies are not premature, but rather are "small for dates" at term. The term *very low birth weight* (VLBW) is used to describe babies weighing less than 1500 g at birth.

When *perinatal mortality rates* (stillbirths plus neonatal deaths in the first 28 days after birth, per 1000 births) are ranked, the United States usually compares poorly with many less affluent nations. Such comparisons are often used, in a political fashion, to castigate American medicine, and it is worth exploring the reasons for our relatively high perinatal mortality rate (approximately 10 per 1000). One reason for the difference is that in the United States various state regulations require the counting of stillbirths and live births beginning at 20 weeks, or at a birth weight of 350 g (compatible with approximately 20 weeks). Many other countries do not count neonatal deaths or stillbirths until 28 weeks' gestational age has been attained. Recent efforts to standardize these definitions still leave the United States trailing many other countries, and the primary reasons appear to be prematurity and LBW. At a given birth weight, a child born in the United States has a greater chance to survive the first 28 days of life than would a child anywhere else in the world. Presumably this is due to the presence of high-technology medical care for such infants. However, American children are more likely to be born prematurely or at LBW than are children in many other countries. Most authorities attribute this high rate of prematurity and LBW to socioeconomic factors, particularly the presence of pockets of poverty with malnutrition and limited access to medical care.

Sequelae

The leading cause of neonatal death among normally formed children is the cluster of sequelae of prematurity, including respiratory distress syndrome, intracranial hemorrhage, and necrotizing enterocolitis. Various studies suggest that the chance of survival for at least 28 days among babies born at 23 weeks or less is <2 percent, while at 24 weeks roughly 10 percent can be expected to live. By 26 weeks, in modern neonatal units, at least half of babies will survive, and by 28 weeks the figure approaches 80 percent (Table 24-1). In addition to their markedly increased death rate, premature babies, especially those of VLBW, are prone to chronic conditions such as cerebral palsy and bronchopulmonary dysplasia. Prematurity is a major public health problem in the United States, but its causes and prevention are imperfectly understood at present.

Etiology and Risk Factors

Preterm birth is usually, but not always, associated with preterm labor. Exceptions include medically indicated prematurity, when the obstetrician decides that maternal or fetal jeopardy require that labor be induced or cesarean delivery be performed prior to term. When spontaneous labor occurs prematurely, most often no specific cause can be assigned. Known maternal risk factors for preterm labor include nonwhite race, low socio-

Table 24-1. Survival rates by gestational age

Gestational age (weeks)	Survival rate (%)
22	0
24	10
26	55
28	77
30	91
32	96
34	99
36	99

Adapted from Copper, et al. A multicenter study of preterm birth weight and gestational age-specific neonatal mortality. *Am. J. Obstet. Gynecol.* 168:78–84, 1993.

economic status, low prepregnancy weight, and age below 18 or above 40 years. A history of previous preterm birth is the strongest single risk factor, with recurrence rates in the range of 20 percent or more. Lack of prenatal care is another extremely strong risk factor. Maternal cocaine use has been associated with preterm labor, as has cigarette smoking. High levels of maternal exercise and exertion have not been clearly linked to premature labor, nor has sexual intercourse. Nevertheless, individuals at particularly high risk for preterm birth are traditionally cautioned to avoid such activities.

A condition called *cervical incompetence* has been described in which the cervix opens painlessly prior to term and delivery ensues. This problem often can be successfully treated with a suture, called *cerclage,* to reinforce the cervix. Premature labor and birth occur with increased frequency when uterine abnormalities such as submucous leiomyomata are present, or when there is a congenital bicornuate or unicornuate uterus. Premature rupture of the amniotic membranes is one of the leading causes of preterm birth, and was discussed in the previous section of this chapter.

Pathophysiology

The physiology of labor is discussed in Chap. 17. Preterm labor is generally believed to occur by means of the same basic physiology as term labor, but at an inappropriate time. The pathophysiology of preterm labor is poorly understood. At least 15 percent of patients with preterm labor and intact membranes have positive amniotic fluid cultures, even in the absence of clinical signs of infection. The proportion of infections may be higher, since some organisms are particularly difficult to grow in culture. Cytokines, such as interleukin-6, have been identified in amniotic fluid of infected patients, and it is possible that they are involved in the initiation of contractions, perhaps by increasing the production of prostaglandins from precursors in the decidua and membranes. Oncofetal fibronectin, which is present in the extracellular matrix between the decidua and chorion, may be increased in the cervicovaginal secretions of patients destined to deliver prematurely compared with controls. This increase appears to support the concept that disruption of the chorion-decidua interface may be a precursor of preterm birth. Some investigators believe that measurement of fetal fibronectin will become a clinically useful way to detect individuals at risk for preterm birth.

Management

A number of different medical regimens have been developed in an attempt to arrest preterm labor, and the specifics of these *tocolytic* drugs are discussed in Chap. 17. Although virtually all of these drugs (betamimetics, magnesium sulfate, prostaglandin inhibitors, and calcium channel blockers) appear to be effective in stopping labor for the short term, evidence for a reduction in perinatal mortality or morbidity is tenuous. It is difficult to study such agents because the diagnosis of labor is generally retrospective, i.e., there must be significant cervical change in addition to uterine contractions. Clinicians are hesitant to wait for cervical change to occur when the patient appears to be laboring prematurely, lest the cervix advance to a point at which tocolysis is less likely to be effective. Many patients treated for premature labor are not truly in labor, and would not progress to premature delivery even if untreated. Since most tocolytic agents may cause significant maternal side effects, information regarding their efficacy and the appropriate conditions for their use is much needed.

Prevention

Many schemes for prevention of preterm birth have been studied; none appears to be clearly superior. A protocol of risk scoring and intensive counselling of both patients and health care providers, in order to recognize preterm labor at the earliest possible time, has been apparently effective in a middle-class population (compared to historical controls), but is ineffective among patients in lower socioeconomic groups. One possible explanation for this difference is the finding that preterm labor with intact membranes is a more common precursor to preterm birth in affluent populations, whereas preterm premature rupture of membranes is more likely in lower socioeconomic groups. Another problem is that currently available risk-scoring systems identify fewer than 50 percent of patients who ultimately deliver prematurely.

Some studies have suggested that uterine activity (i.e., contractions per unit time) increases prior to the onset of preterm labor, while the patient is often unaware of the contractions. This concept has led to the development of home uterine activity monitors that record uterine contractions on a daily or more frequent basis. The records are then transmitted by phone modem to a central office, where they are interpreted and the responsible physician is notified when worrisome changes occur. Such systems are extremely expensive, and it is not yet clear whether any benefit comes from the technology or from the fact that the patients talk, by phone, to a health care provider each day.

Randomized trials of antibiotic prophylaxis in patients with preterm labor and intact membranes have not consistently demonstrated efficacy in delaying delivery, although some studies have been promising. Adjunctive maternal therapy with corticosteroids decreases the likelihood of respiratory distress syndrome in infants born prior to 34-weeks' gestation. Glucocorticoids that cross the placenta (dexamethasone or betamethasone) are administered at least 24 hours prior to delivery. Maternal hyperglycemia and fluid overload are side effects that may ensue. The administration of artificial surfactant therapy to premature neonates in order to prevent or treat respiratory distress syndrome has greatly improved the prognosis in recent years.

One of the most important determinants of outcome in premature infants is delivery into a facility with a neonatal intensive care unit. The more premature the delivery, the more critical is the need for this technology. Numerous studies have demonstrated that it is much better to transfer the mother to such a facility with her fetus in utero than to await delivery and transport the neonate.

Prolonged Pregnancy

Definition and Incidence

Although approximately 90 percent of pregnancies have delivered by 42 weeks (294 days) after the first day of the last menstrual period (40 weeks after conception), some 10 percent do not and are considered to be *prolonged*, or *postdates*, pregnancies. Studies in the early 1960s demonstrated an approximate doubling of the perinatal mortality rate when pregnancy went beyond 42 weeks, with further increases if the woman was still pregnant at 43 weeks. Advances in fetal evaluation since the 1960s have markedly lowered the perinatal mortality rates associated with prolonged pregnancy, but significant morbidity continues to be a problem (Fig. 24-4).

Various studies report differing incidences of prolonged pregnancy. The primary reason for the discrepancies is the method used in establishing gestational dating. When last menstrual period alone is used, rates are approximately double those reported when accurate early ultrasound dating or basal body temperature charting is employed. In fact, some studies in which early ultrasound dating was combined with menstrual dating found that less than 3 percent of pregnancies were truly prolonged beyond 42 weeks. This finding strongly suggests that many patients with apparent prolonged pregnancy are actually misdated, and strengthens the case for establishing accurate dates as early in gestation as possible. When an obstetrician is confronted with a patient who appears to be 2 weeks "late," it is generally not possible to retrospectively confirm her gestational dates.

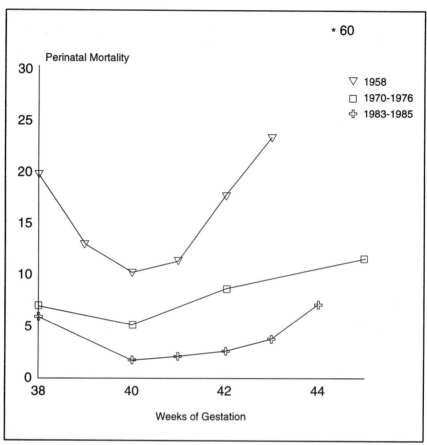

Fig. 24-4. Comparison of perinatal mortality rates with gestational age. Note the lowering of overall perinatal mortality rates, and the apparent blunting of the effects of prolonged pregnancy. (With permission from R. K. Freeman and D. C. Lagrew, Jr. Prolonged Pregnancy. In S. G. Gabbe, J. R. Niebyl, & J. L. Simpson [eds.]. *Obstetrics: Normal and Problem Pregnancies* [2nd ed.]. New York: Churchill-Livingstone, 1991. P. 947.)

Etiology

The causes of prolonged pregnancy are generally unknown. However, there are some "experiments of nature" that may be illuminating. In the pregnant sheep there is a rise in estrogen and a fall in progesterone, followed by a large increase in cortisol, just prior to the onset of labor. Labor can be induced in the sheep by the administration of cortisol. Although precisely similar events do not occur in the human, pregnancies with an anencephalic fetus, who has no anterior pituitary and thus cannot stimulate cortisol production from the adrenals, have a tendency to deliver at gestational ages widely varying around the normal term, either early or late. Placental sulfatase deficiency, an unusual sex-linked hereditary condition that includes ichthyosis, and in which very little estrogen is produced by the fetoplacental unit, is associated with delayed "ripening" of the cervix and prolonged pregnancy. In most cases of prolonged pregnancy none of the above conditions is apparent and the cause is unknown. It might be anticipated that gestational length, like most biologic variables, is distributed around a mean, and that approximately 2 percent of individuals are bound to be two or more standard deviations above the mean.

Sequelae

There are many consequences of prolonged pregnancy. Much attention has focused on the *postmature* pregnancy, the features of which are usually attributed to placental dysfunction. In fact, many authors term this the *dysmaturity syndrome*, in recognition of the fact that it can occur at earlier gestational ages as well. Affected fetuses tend to have wasting as evidenced by loss of subcutaneous fat, wrinkled skin, long nails, peeling skin, and meconium staining. They are often described as "wizened" and "hyperalert." Amniotic fluid is decreased, and neonatal hypoglycemia is common. Chronic hypoxia in utero may be the cause of neonatal polycythemia. Decreased fat stores may lead to poor thermal regulation in the neonatal period. These are probably the fetuses who were responsible for the increased stillbirth rate among postdates pregnancies in the 1960s and 1970s. This rate has now diminished markedly with the advent of modern methods of fetal evaluation.

Although the postmaturity syndrome has received much attention, it has been found in only 10 to 20 percent of pregnancies that continue beyond 42 weeks. A more common problem is fetal macrosomia, as the placenta may continue to support fetal nutrition beyond the due date. The large fetus is more likely to encounter difficulties such as the need for operative vaginal or abdominal delivery, or shoulder dystocia. Another problem occurring with greater frequency in the prolonged pregnancy is the presence of meconium in the amniotic fluid. Although once considered to be almost exclusively the result of fetal compromise, meconium passage is now viewed as a frequently normal fetal function and not necessarily evidence of hypoxia. However, its presence can be associated with neonatal complications known as the *meconium aspiration syndrome.* Meconium entering the lungs, either during prenatal gasping or with the first breath after birth, may cause significant pulmonary complications that can be fatal. The oligohydramnios that often accompanies prolonged pregnancy adds to the problem because the meconium that has been passed by the fetus in utero is not diluted by amniotic fluid, and remains viscous.

Management

The clinical management of prolonged pregnancy varies depending on the assessment of the cervix. When the cervix is "ripe," i.e., favorable for induction of labor, most clinicians stimulate labor at 41 to 42 weeks. All too frequently the cervix is unfavorable. Induction of labor under such circumstances is more likely to be unsuccessful, leading to cesarean section delivery. Furthermore, many patients with apparent prolonged pregnancy and unfavorable cervices are misdated, as described above. Available options include the use of prostaglandin vaginal or cervical gel to induce cervical ripening or observation with intensive monitoring of the fetal condition, awaiting spontaneous labor or cervical change. Specific methods of fetal assessment are described in Chap. 16.

Recommended Reading

Multiple Gestations
Adams, D. M., and Chervenak, F. A. Multifetal Pregnancies: Epidemiology, Clinical Characteristics, and Management. In E. A. Reece, et al. (eds.), *Medicine of the Fetus and Mother.* Philadelphia: Lippincott, 1992. Pp. 266–284.
Mulifetal Pregnancy. In F. G. Cunningham, P. C. MacDonald, N. F. Gant, K. J. Leveno, and L. C. Gilstrap III (eds.), *Williams Obstetrics* (19th ed.). Norwalk: Appleton & Lange, 1993. Pp. 891–918.

Isoimmunization
American College of Obstetricians and Gynecologists. Prevention of D isoimmunization. *ACOG Technical Bulletin* No. 147, October, 1990.
Bowman, J. M. Maternal Alloimmunization and Fetal Hemolytic Disease. In E. A. Reece, et al. (eds.), *Medicine of the Fetus and Mother.* Philadelphia: Lippincott, 1992. Pp. 1152–1182.

Third-Trimester Bleeding
Green, J. R. Placenta Previa and Abruptio Placentae. In R. K. Creasy and R. Resnik (eds.), *Maternal-Fetal Medicine* (3rd ed.). Philadelphia: Saunders, 1994. Pp. 602–619.
Nimrod, C. A. Third Trimester Bleeding. In E. A. Reece, et al. (eds.), *Medicine of the Fetus and Mother.* Philadelphia: Lippincott, 1992. Pp. 1363–1369.

Premature Rupture of the Membranes
American College of Obstetricians and Gynecologists. Group B streptococcal infections in pregnancy. *ACOG Technical Bulletin* No. 170, July, 1992.
Main, D. M., and Main, E. K. Preterm Birth. In S. G. Gabbe, J. R. Niebyl, and J. L. Simpson (eds.), *Obstetrics: Normal and Problem Pregnancies* (2nd ed.). New York: Churchill-Livingstone, 1991. Pp. 829–880.
Romero, R., Ghidini, A., and Bahado-Singh, R. Premature Rupture of the Membranes. In E. A. Reece, et al. (eds.), *Medicine of the Fetus and Mother.* Philadelphia: Lippincott, 1992. Pp. 1430–1468.

Preterm Birth

Creasy, R. K. Preterm Labor and Delivery. In R. K. Creasy and R. Resnik (eds.), *Medicine* (3rd ed.). Philadelphia: Saunders, 1994. Pp. 494–520.

Horton, J. A. (ed.). *The Women's Health Data Book.* Washington: Jacobs Institute of Women's Health, 1992.

Main, D. M., and Main, E. K. Preterm Birth. In S. G. Gabbe, J. R. Niebyl, and J. L. Simpson (eds.), *Obstetrics: Normal and Problem Pregnancies* (2nd ed.). New York: Churchill-Livingstone, 1991. Pp. 829–880.

Prolonged Pregnancy

Freeman, R. K., and Lagrew, D. C., Jr. Prolonged Pregnancy. In S. G. Gabbe, J. R. Niebyl, and J. L. Simpson (eds.), *Obstetrics: Normal and Problem Pregnancies* (2nd ed.). New York: Churchill-Livingstone, 1991. Pp. 945–956.

Resnik, R. Post-term Pregnancy. In R. K. Creasy and R. Resnik (eds.), *Maternal-Fetal Medicine* (3rd ed.). Philadelphia: Saunders, 1994. Pp. 521–526.

Shaw, K., and Paul, R. Postterm Pregnancy. In E. A. Reece, et al. (eds.), *Medicine of the Fetus and Mother.* Philadelphia: Lippincott, 1992. Pp. 1469–1481.

Index